EILEEN E. MORRISON, MPH, EdD, CHES

Professor, Health Administration
Texas State University
San Marcos, Texas

Ethics in HEALTH
ADMINISTRATION

A Practical Approach
for Decision Makers

Second Edition

JONES AND BARTLETT PUBLISHERS
Sudbury, Massachusetts

LONDON   SINGAPORE

World Headquarters

Jones and Bartlett Publishers
40 Tall Pine Drive
Sudbury, MA 01776
978-443-5000
info@jbpub.com
www.jbpub.com

Jones and Bartlett Publishers
Canada
6339 Ormindale Way
Mississauga, Ontario L5V 1J2
Canada

Jones and Bartlett Publishers
International
Barb House, Barb Mews
London W6 7PA
United Kingdom

Jones and Bartlett's books and products are available through most bookstores and online booksellers. To contact Jones and Bartlett Publishers directly, call 800-832-0034, fax 978-443-8000, or visit our website, www.jbpub.com.

Substantial discounts on bulk quantities of Jones and Bartlett's publications are available to corporations, professional associations, and other qualified organizations. For details and specific discount information, contact the special sales department at Jones and Bartlett via the above contact information or send an email to specialsales@jbpub.com.

This publication is designed to provide accurate and authoritative information in regard to the Subject Matter covered. It is sold with the understanding that the publisher is not engaged in rendering legal, accounting, or other professional service. If legal advice or other expert assistance is required, the service of a competent professional person should be sought.

Production Credits
Publisher: Michael Brown
Associate Editor: Maro Gartside
Editorial Assistant: Catie Heverling
Editorial Assistant Teresa Reilly
Senior Production Editor: Tracey Chapman
Senior Marketing Manager: Sophie Fleck
Manufacturing and Inventory Control Supervisor: Amy Bacus
Composition: DSCS/Absolute Service, Inc.
Cover Design: Kristin E. Parker
Cover Image: © Les Cunliffe/Dreamstime.com
Text Image: © photos.com
Printing and Binding: Malloy, Inc.
Cover Printing: Malloy, Inc.

Library of Congress Cataloging-in-Publication Data
Morrison, Eileen E.
  Ethics in health administration : a practical approach for decision makers /
Eileen E. Morrison. — 2nd ed.
    p. ; cm.
  Includes bibliographical references and index.
  ISBN-13: 978-0-7637-7327-4 (pbk. : alk. paper)
  ISBN-10: 0-7637-7327-1 (pbk. : alk. paper)
  1. Health services administration—Moral and ethical aspects. 2. Health services administrators—Professional ethics. 3. Medical care—Decision making—Moral and ethical aspects. 4. Medical ethics. I. Title.
  [DNLM: 1. Health Services Administration—ethics. 2. Decision Making—ethics. 3. Ethics, Medical. W 50 M878e 2009]
  RA394.M67 2009
  174.2—dc22

                                                                      2009015770

6048

Printed in the United States of America
13 12 11 10 09   10 9 8 7 6 5 4 3 2 1

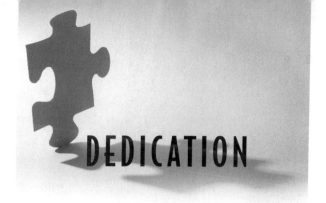

DEDICATION

This edition is dedicated to Grant, Kate, and
Emery Aidan, who always believe in me.

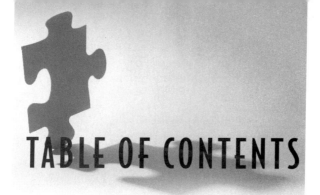

TABLE OF CONTENTS

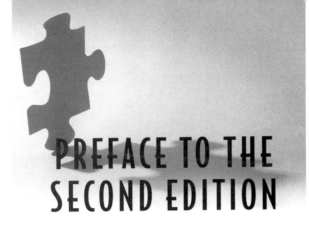

PREFACE TO THE SECOND EDITION

There have been many changes in health care since the publication of the first edition of *Ethics in Health Administration*. Technology astonishes us with its creations, and hospitals are considering patient-centered care as a way to increase profits. Universal health care is once again part of the national discussion and public health continues to be challenged to provide disaster relief. In addition, the changing economy creates challenges that would test the wisdom of Solomon.

Despite these changes, much remains the same. We are still expected to provide quality care for all those in need and our budgets are stretched by this mandate. Healthcare institutions are expected to hire highly qualified personnel and maintain exceptional levels of ethics-based operation practices. Administrators are still expected to be role models for ethics-based healthcare delivery. These expectations make an excellent argument for you to have a foundation in ethics and be able to apply ethics to your daily practice as an administrator. The chapters, cases, and readings in this second edition will assist you in becoming an ethics-based healthcare administrator.

Ancora Imparo

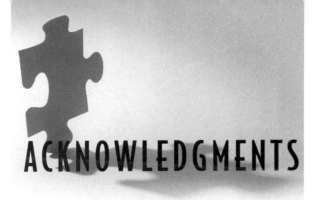

ACKNOWLEDGMENTS

I owe a great debt to my friends, family, and colleagues who served as sources of inspiration, guidance, and wonderful stories. I also want to honor all of my students who have taught me in more ways than they will ever know. Special gratitude goes to my publisher, Mike Brown, and to my editors, Catie Heverling and Kristen Spina, who gave me encouragement and assistance in making this new edition an even better learning tool.

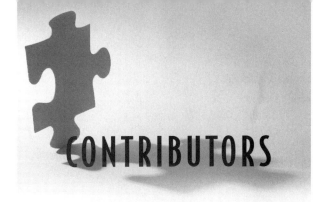

CONTRIBUTORS

The following individuals have contributed stories that were fictionalized to create the case studies in this text. The author is deeply grateful to each of them.

Karen Bawel-Brinkley, PhD, RN

Associate Professor of Nursing
San Jose State University
San Jose, California

Rohn Butterfield, MBA

Instructor of Health Administration
University of Southern Indiana
Evansville, Indiana

Kim Contreraz, RN

St. John's Hospital
Anderson, Indiana

Mario Contreraz, RN

University of Indiana Medical School
Bloomington, Indiana

Jan Gardner-Ray, EdD

Chief Executive Officer
Country Home Health Care, Inc.
Charlottesville, Indiana

Maudia Gentry, EdD

Community Coordinator
Parkland Hospital
Dallas, Texas

Ericka Lochner, MBA, RN

Chief Nursing Officer
West Valley Medical Center
Caldwell, Idaho

Elizabeth Morrison

Norfolk, Virginia

Oren Renick, JD, FACHE

Professor of Health Administration
Texas State University
San Marcos, Texas

Martha J. Morgan Sanders, PhD, RN

National Faculty
Nova Southeastern University
Fort Lauderdale, Florida

Michael P. West, EdD, FACHE

Executive Director
University of Texas at Arlington Fort Worth Center
Fort Worth, Texas

Colin Wren

Social Services Agency
Isle of Wight, England

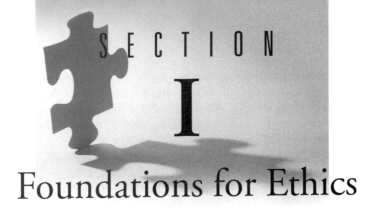

Foundations for Ethics

■ INTRODUCTION

"It was the best of times, it was the worst of times. It was the age of wisdom, it was the age of foolishness. It was the epoch of belief, it was the epoch of incredulity. It was the season of Light, it was the season of Darkness. It was the Spring of hope, it was the Winter of despair. We had everything before us, we had nothing before us. . . ."

This quote from *A Tale of Two Cities* by Charles Dickens (p. 1) could have been written about the healthcare system of today. It is truly the best of times and the worst of times. The American healthcare system is one of the most technologically advanced in the world. The potential to conquer diseases and extend life to almost biblical proportions seems possible. A system exists that once was just part of the imaginations of science fiction writers and dreamers. In many ways, this is the best of times in health care.

Yet, these same advances in the system pose enormous challenges in the human dimension and could lead to the worst of times. Members of the system and society at large are faced with decisions that would test the wisdom of Solomon. For example, one must determine the answer to the following question: "if we have the technology to create new forms of human life, does this mean we should use it?" From an organizational standpoint, how do we decide who benefits from technology and life-extending procedures, and who does not? Who will pay for optimal health care for all Americans? The tremendous progress in medical knowledge and technology makes it a difficult time for ethics and ethical decision-making.

What is the role of healthcare administration in all of this? We know that healthcare administrators (HCAs) do not provide the care, conduct the research, or design the technology. Yet, they are critical to the success of these functions because they provide the environment where the important work of health care can take place. Administrators are the creators of structure and support for the healthcare system. They are also the connection to the community and the stewards of the resources society invests in health care. Certainly, this is a grave responsibility.

How are you, as an HCA, supposed to meet this responsibility? The task requires a foundation in knowledge of system functions, human relations, finance, and leadership that you will gain through your formal education. It also mandates a deeper understanding of the principles of ethics and appropriate ethical behavior from the individual, organizational, and societal view. This foundation will provide you with the tools to make decisions that are not just fiscally sound, but also ethically appropriate. Ethics must be a way that you conduct the business of health care on a day-to-day basis.

A Word about the Text

Just like a healthcare organization, this book has a mission and a vision. Its mission is to give you solid preparation in both the theory and principles of ethics. More importantly, it will guide you to be able to apply ethics in the real world of health care. Scholarly textbooks exist on many forms of ethics and the knowledge they provide guided the creation of this text. However, theory alone is not enough. To fulfill this book's mission, it must also give you practical examples of how you can use ethics in your daily decisions as an HCA.

Therefore, this text combines theory and practice in a palatable format. Each chapter contains a feature called "points to ponder" that should help you to focus on the most important chapter concepts. It is a good idea to think about these questions as you read the chapter. There is also a "words to remember" section that features important words and phrases. You will find these words in bold print in the content section of the text.

In addition to information about the topic under study, each chapter contains case studies in the form of stories. These are fictionalized versions of stories contributed by healthcare providers from many different healthcare settings. They attempt to show you how the chapter information relates to the real world of health care. References are also included at the end of each chapter so that you can do additional reading if you choose.

The model seen in Figure I-1 guides the vision for this text. Because you do not make ethics decisions in a vacuum, the circles in this model represent the impact of influences on your ability to make ethics decisions. They start with the circle representing theory and principles that are the foundation of ethical decision-making. The next circle represents community areas that are external to the organization but have an impact on how you operate as an ethics-based administrator. The model also includes a circle for forces within the organization that can also influence your decisions and practices. Finally, the inner circle

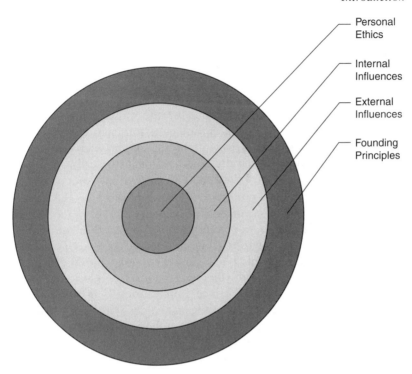

Personal
Ethics

Internal
Influences

External
Influences

Founding
Principles

Figure I-1. A System of Healthcare Administration Ethics.

represents how your own personal ethics influences what you do. Each circle should be part of your consideration as part of ethics-based administrator.

The chapters follow this model through sections that illustrate key issues within these circles. Section I, represented by the outermost circle, assists in establishing your foundation in ethics theory and principles. Chapter 1 explores founding theories of ethics that guide most of Western ethical thinking. Using this theoretical foundation, Chapter 2 explores autonomy, which is one of the four key principles of healthcare ethics. Chapters 3 and 4 deal with nonmaleficence, beneficence, and justice and represent the remaining key principles. In Chapters 2 through 4, you will also be able to read cases or stories that will allow you to apply these principles to real-world events.

Section II, the next circle, presents some of the external influences on ethics for the HCA. Chapter 5 provides information about how the community protects itself from the power of the healthcare system. Chapter 6 deals with the powerful influence of market forces, including managed care and alternative medicine. Chapter 7 also deals with external influences through a discussion of social responsibility and ethics. Finally, Chapter 8 presents an in-depth view of technology's impact on ethics. Each chapter also includes cases or stories that will help you apply what you are reading to practical ethical decisions.

The healthcare organization's influence on your ethical decisions is the focus of Section III. Chapter 9 presents the challenging area of how fiscal responsibility influences our ethical decisions. Chapter 10 examines the impact of organizational culture on ethics and features information on ethics committees and models for decision-making. Chapter 11 presents the issue of assuring the community that healthcare facilities are providing quality care. Finally, Chapter 12 addresses how the organization views patients and how it acts to meet their needs.

Section IV (the innermost circle) is designed to present a more personal look at your ethical foundation. Chapter 13 discusses the concept of moral integrity and its meaning for you as an HCA. Chapter 14 presents information about codes of ethics and the impact they can have on administrative practice. Chapter 15 discusses issues related to your day-to-day practice as an ethical HCA. Finally, because ethics is a dynamic area of health administration, Chapter 16 addresses issues that are in the immediate future and their ethical implications. It also provides an overall summary of the learning in the text.

Why bother reading this book? While it will not make you an ethics scholar, this book will assist you to become someone who is of great value in today's healthcare system. You will be of value because you can be an administrator who sees the world through "ethical eyes" as well as through financial ones. On the surface, this ability may make things more difficult for you because your decisions will not be simple ones. However, by being able to look at any situation holistically and make appropriate, ethics-based decisions, you can actually enhance the overall effectiveness of your organization. Because health care is a trust-based industry, you will be able to maintain the community's trust by helping your organization avoid actions that the community might view as unethical or immoral. In addition, you can enhance your own career by your reputation as an administrator who understands that ethics makes a difference.

Reference

Dickens, C. (1997). *A tale of two cities*. Mineola, NY: Dover Publications.

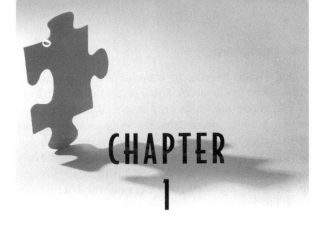

CHAPTER
1

Practical Theory

"A theory must be tempered with reality."

—Jawaharlal Nehru

Points to Ponder

1. Why does a healthcare administrator (HCA) need a foundation in ethics theory to be effective?
2. What ethics theorists are included in the Big 8, and what did they contribute to modern-day ethics?
3. What is my working definition of ethics?

Words to Remember

The following is a list of key words for this chapter. You will find them in bold in the text. Stop and check your understanding of them.

categorical imperative
conventional
eudaimonia
moral development
original position
premoral
practical wisdom
sense of meaning
utilitarianism

consequentialism
deontology
I-THOU
natural law
preconventional
principled moral reasoning
self-interest
social justice
virtue

■ INTRODUCTION

Becoming an ethics-based administrator begins with a foundation in the theory and practice of ethics. This foundation is necessary because your work will challenge you to balance the financial and human aspects of the healthcare business. These decisions are hardly ever black or white. In fact, their shades of gray might cause you some sleepless nights. Having a foundation in ethical theory and using it in practice should help you sleep better and be able to defend your choices.

Ethics has been a subject of study for many thousands of years and brilliant scholars have spent their lives exploring it. In this chapter, you will examine eight key theorists who were instrumental in creating the foundation of ethics for the healthcare setting. When students read these theorists' works in their original forms, they find them obtuse and uninteresting. Some have even complained that they found it hard to understand what these "old dead guys" were trying to say.

In order for you to view to see these theorists as people and not just "old dead guys," the chapter begins with a brief biography of each theorist. Each theorist created a large body of work and there are experts who specialize in each of the theorists cited here. However, a concept summary with the essence of each scholar's key points is included to help to have a working knowledge of their thinking. Finally, as Nehru suggests, their theories will also be "tempered with reality" through the inclusion of a section on application to health care.

The survey of theorists should lead you to the final section in the chapter that examines various definitions of ethics. After this review, you should be able to develop your own working definition of ethics. Your personal definition, based on the thoughts of experts, should serve as a solid foundation for your role as an ethics-based HCA. Therefore, the goal of this chapter is to give you a personal theoretical foundation and working definition of ethics.

■ WHY STUDY ETHICS THEORY?

Can you imagine being a surgeon and not knowing the anatomy of the human body? What if you were an accountant and did not know how to use a calculator? You might do the job, but the results would be a complete disaster. It is not any different for an HCA. You must have the basic knowledge, skills, and attitudes to do your work effectively and efficiently.

Why include a foundation in ethics as part of these basics? Health care is a dynamic environment where one area affects the other. Answers to problems that you will encounter may not be found in a textbook or on a balance sheet. They involve qualitative intangibles such as organizational mission, values, trust, human dignity, and service to community. Therefore, your decisions have to be made based on an accurate assessment of your financials and resources (quantitative information), in conjunction with qualitative intangibles. In addition, your patients, staff, organization leaders, and the community expect your decisions to be ethical. How can you make ethics-based decisions without a foundation in ethics?

The writers represented in this chapter are known as the Big 8: Aquinas, Kant, Mill, Rawls, Aristotle, Buber, Kohlberg, and Frankl. These philosophers created the ideas that led to the major principles of ethics found in Chapters 2, 3, and 4. The first group of philosophers— Aquinas, Kant, Mill, and Rawls—examined the global issues surrounding ethics and ethical decisions. The second group—Aristotle, Buber, Kohlberg, and Frankl—studied personal ethics and moral development. This chapter gives a summary of their works and provides an understanding of their contributions to healthcare ethics.

■ ST. THOMAS AQUINAS (1225–1274)

Biographical Influences on His Theory

Aquinas received his calling to the church early in his life, but his family did not support this vocation. They considered his choice to join the Dominican Order inappropriate because this order was too radical. In an effort to change his mind, his family actually held him prisoner for two years. They even tried to make him renounce his calling by tempting him with worldly pleasures (including women). Finally, the family relented and allowed him to go to Cologne, join the Dominican Order, and study with the major scholars of his day. Aquinas became a prolific writer; the greatest of his writings was the *Summa Theologioe*. Part Two of this work was devoted entirely to ethics and combined Aristotelian and Christian thinking. This work helped to establish the concepts of **natural law** that are part of Aquinas' ethics theory.

Concept Summary

Aquinas believed that God is perfectly rational and that He created the world in a rational manner (Summers, 2009). His design for the world included giving humans the ability to reason and to wonder about the cause of all things. Because humans have this gift of rationality, they are capable of choosing good and avoiding evil. Notice the word "capable"; it does not mean that people always do this. Rational people may violate natural law because they are also given the gift of free will. However, if people are true to their rational natures, they will listen to their consciences (i.e., the voice of God) and choose good over evil.

So what is goodness as defined by Aquinas? He believed that goodness preserves life and the human race. Something is good if it advances knowledge and truth, helps people live in community, and respects all persons. He also believed that to find happiness people must not look to pleasures, honors, wealth, or worldly power because these are not the true source of goodness. True happiness is only found in the wisdom of seeking to know God and the achievement of your highest potential. Truly understanding God is the ultimate good that is sought by all rational human beings.

Theory Applications

First, you must remember that knowledge of ethics builds on the work of previous scholars. Aristotle, Dionysius, and Christian doctrine heavily influenced Aquinas' thinking. How does his philosophy of ethics apply to today's world? If people choose to act against their "rational nature" (as defined by Aquinas), they can do things that are evil for themselves and others. Think of a modern day example. It is not rational to drink to excess and then get behind the wheel of a car. Yet, if people make this irrational decision, their actions can cause them harm or even death. This harm can also extend to others who have the misfortune of coming into contact with them in their compromised state.

In addition, Aquinas's idea of "basic good" seems on the surface to be simple. All you have to do is respect people and help them live in community. However, when you translate this into the healthcare system and its policies, it becomes much more complex. What does this system do about people who do not make rational choices for good—such as those who abuse alcohol or drugs? Do they deserve the same level of care as those who make rational choices? How can the business of health preserve the human race and still have enough money to keep its doors open? These questions relate to' the difficult choices (gray areas) that are part of today's healthcare system, where demand for care often exceeds finances.

■ IMMANUEL KANT (1724–1804)

Biographical Influences on His Theory

Although Kant became a dominant force in ethics theory, he rarely left his hometown of Königsberg, Prussia. He began his academic career by studying math and physics and proposed a theory of the formation of the solar system. However, he is better known for his work in moral philosophy. His writings in this area even came to the attention of King Fredrick William II, who accused him of corrupting young people through his writing and teaching. In fact, in 1792, he decreed that Kant could not teach or write about anything related to religion or ethics. While Kant honored the King's right to censor, he actually scolded the King (McChance, 2004)!

Concept Summary

Kant's work in metaphysics had a major impact on his work in ethics. His two most important works in this area were *Foundations of the Metaphysics of Morals* (1785) and *Critique of Practical Reason* (1787). He was a foundational theorist for an entire area of ethics called **deontology**, or duty-based ethics (Summers, 2009).

For Kant, everything in a society had worth based on its relative value. Therefore, nothing was good in and of itself. Everything could be used for good or evil. This is true because attributes (such as intelligence, physical beauty, or bravery) are gifts of your genetics or from your environment. They also have their source in your mind or perception, so you decide who is smart and who is not. Likewise, personal attributes that are valued by a society, such as influence, money, or even happiness, can be used for good or evil. For example, if you are highly intelligent or extremely wealthy, you might discover a cure for a terrible disease or create a heavenly symphony. You might also use that same intelligence and wealth to become a serial killer.

For Kant, the only good that can exist without clarification is something called good will. Good will meant that there was no ultimate end for the person who chooses it. In other words, acting with good will does not give you benefit. You just do it and it is valuable all by itself. Therefore, good will is not a means to an end; it just is.

In the Kantian view, all humans have absolute worth simply by the fact of their existence. People are not a means to accomplish an end or societal good. They are an end in themselves. What does this mean? It means that you cannot use people as a way to get what you want and remain ethical. You should honor them because they exist. For Kant, humans are subject to universal laws that are always in place. How does this translate today? It means that, when dealing with humans, you have a duty to choose to act as a moral mediator and base your actions on good will. Anticipated consequences or the end product of your decisions should not be a part of the decision-making process.

How do we know what is good? First, Kant acknowledged that all of us have the ability to think and make our own decisions. In fact, free will was essential to ethical behavior and to understanding what is good. Kant also provided a tool for understanding how to determine what is good. He called this the **categorical imperative**, which is a way to test your actions and help you make moral decisions. Decisions should be based on the idea that what is right for one person is right for all persons. You can ask yourself the question, "Would I want everyone to act as I just did?" If the answer is "yes," then it passes your categorical imperative and is a moral duty for you. In Kantian ethics, all humans have worth, so you are obligated to apply your decisions to all individuals in similar circumstances and to treat all people with respect.

Theory Applications

First, Kantian, or duty-based, ethics acknowledges the value of all human beings and gives you a rule to guide decision making regarding actions toward all. It tells you that, for moral decision-making, all persons in similar circumstances deserve the same treatment. Kant also presents the idea of a moral duty, which means that you have obligations to other people as fellow humans. All people you meet in your daily work-life—employees, patients, community members, etc.—have absolute value simply by the fact that they exist. Just because they can accomplish more or less in society's eyes does not change their value as human beings.

The categorical imperative can be useful for decision making when you are developing policy and procedures. For example, if you have to develop personnel policy, you can ask yourself, "Why am I really doing this? What is the reason behind it?" You can also try to discern if it can apply to everyone in the same way, or if the policy will treat some employees better than others. Finally, you can ask, "How would I feel if this were done to me?"

Despite its base in good will, you can see that being a strict Kantian might be a problem for the HCA. To follow Kant, you should make all your decisions based on good will and not on things like profit, legal mandate, or pleasing your stakeholders. This is not practical or even possible in the political world of health care. Kantian moral theory also tends to deal in absolutes and does not provide answers to all of the complex issues in today's healthcare system. Let us look at just one example. If a researcher uses human subjects in a study to help find the cure for cancer, is he or she not using them as a means to an end? Does this negate the worth of human beings and fail the categorical imperative test? You could say that it does, and yet there is potential benefit to a larger group from the knowledge gained.

■ JOHN STUART MILL (1806–1873)

Biographical Influences on His Theory

John Stuart Mill certainly had an interesting childhood. In today's view, it might be seen as abusive. He was an extremely intelligent child who was heavily influenced by his father's insistence on strict discipline in learning. At 15, Mill was already disagreeing with current moral theorists and began to write his own theory, which was influenced by Bentham's utility concepts. When he was 21, Mill suffered what was then called a mental crisis that was attributed to the physical and cerebral strain of his strict, self-imposed education. Later in life, he married Harriet Taylor, a feminist and intellectual, who came from a Unitarian background. She was an author in her own right and published articles advocating women's rights. They shared philosophies and collaborated on many articles. His major works on ethics include *Utilitarianism* and *The Subjection of Women*. Mill was ahead of his time in his activism in support of his beliefs. For example, he became a member of parliament to use his political power to help improve the status of women.

Concept Summary

Mill is one of the most influential theorists in the American view of applied ethics, especially in the area of health care. Based on the idea of Telos, or ends, his theory of **utilitarianism** has been used in the formulation of many healthcare policies that affect the American public today. Utilitarianism or **consequentialism** was founded on the idea that ethical choices should be based on their consequences and not just on duty. In this view, you weigh the consequences of actions and their affect on others. Then, you use this reasoning to make your decisions based on the good that they can achieve.

Something is good if it produces utility. Just what is that? Mill meant that it gives the greatest benefit (or pleasure) to the greatest number of those affected. It is wrong if it produces the greatest harm for the greatest number of those affected. The focus of an ethical decision is not on the individual person, but on the best outcomes for all persons. Mill discussed Christian theology as the best example of utility because the Bible asked people to live by the Golden Rule and to love their neighbors as they love themselves. In health care, you could say that the opportunity for the highest quality of life should be provided to the highest number of people in a community. Ashcroft, Dawson, Draper, and McMillan (2007) provide examples of the greatest good in health care, such as public health, quality of life efforts, and the work of healthcare economists.

Mill divided ethical decisions based on utility into two main groups. The first is to act from utility, which means that each decision is made based on its own merit. The consequences for that specific case are analyzed and a decision is made. However, to act from utility or make each decision independently is not always practical in health care because your decisions are numerous, complex, and often interrelated.

The second is to rule by utility. In contrast to the first group, this ethic uses the consequences of decisions to determine rules for action. These rules help guide decisions so that, on average, they produce the greatest good for the greatest number or cause the least amount of harm to the least amount of people. Rule by utilitarian decision-making appeals to HCAs because it allows for decisions that will be the best in most cases. It also is part of using the process of cost/benefit or gain/loss analysis to justify a decision.

Theory Applications

Many HCAs perceive Mill's utilitarian principles of ethics as a practical way to tackle difficult healthcare decisions. Because there is always a scarcity of resources, there has to be a way to make decisions based on universal benefit. Using the balance sheet approach of identifying consequences, determining merit, and making a decision that will benefit the most people who are affected should make ethical decisions easier. You will see evidence of this approach in later chapters where you will examine some ethics decision-making models.

One limitation of this theory is that it might be possible to ignore the needs and desires of the minority to provide the greatest good for the majority. The individual is not the focus of moral decision; the consequences of the action are the most important element. An example might clarify this point. Suppose you funded a screening program that served all the members of a community. This would seem to benefit the greatest number. However, by funding this program, you eliminated funding for a program that served a small group of uninsured patients who needed liver transplants. Your program might provide the greatest good for the greatest number, but those who were left untreated might have good reason to disagree.

■ JOHN RAWLS (1921–2002)

Biographical Influences on His Theory

As you can see by his birth and death dates, Rawls was a modern ethics theorist. He began his studies at Princeton and served in the military during World War II. While in the service, he witnessed the aftermath of the bombing of Hiroshima. It had such an impact on him that he declined a commission as an officer and left the Army. When he returned home, he finished a doctorate in moral philosophy at Princeton.

Rawls taught at Princeton, Oxford (Fulbright Scholar), and Massachusetts Institute of Technology. In his final academic appointment, he served as a professor at Harvard for 40 years. His work centered on defining what a moral society should be through social justice. Because of this work, he had a great influence on modern political and ethical thinking. He continued his work and study right up to his death in 2002.

Concept Summary

John Rawls was interested in defining what makes a moral and just society. He studied all of the philosophers who came before him and found that he both agreed and disagreed with them. For example, some of Kant's arguments appealed to him, but he was opposed to the position of utilitarianism. He formulated his own theory of justice that was based on the concept of **self-interest**. What did he mean? In order to explain his ideas, he set up a hypothetical scenario where all persons are equal to each other. An example of this scenario could be the very moment of birth. He called this the **original position**. He also asked that we assume the "veil of ignorance." This meant that we ignore the characteristics of the people who exist in our society. Given the original position and the veil of ignorance, we would act in our own best interests. What would be in our best interests?

Because humans generally live in social groups, they must set up rules that protect their personal interests and those of the society in which they live. To live in society with any kind of peace and justice, people must agree to these rules and practice them. He defined something he called the liberty principle (Cahn & Markie, 1998), which means that all people should have the same basic rights as all others in a society. For example, if the rich have a right to basic education, then so should everyone else.

In his view of **social justice**, people must make choices in order to protect those who are in a lesser position in society. This includes children, those in poverty, and those who have medical problems that affect their quality of life. This idea has been called the Maximin Rule (Cahn & Markie, 1998). Why would anyone choose to do this as part of his or her self-interest even when he or she is not in a lesser position in society? In Rawls's view, everyone has the potential to be in a lesser position, so acting to protect the rights of those who are less well off is actually based on self-interest. Further, the problems in a society tend to be suffered more by those who are in disadvantaged positions. For example, those in poverty are also more likely to be victims of crime or have more severe health problems. Finally, societies are often judged by how they treat those who are not well off or in optimal health. Again, using the Maximin Rule would be favorable for those who are in power, because they will be known as just leaders in a just society.

Does this mean that everyone in a society has to make the same amount of money and have the same circumstances? Rawls postulated that differences and advantages could exist in economic and social position in a society if they were used for the benefit of that society. For example, a physician is paid more than others in a society and has greater status. With this difference comes the responsibility of service to the community in which he or she lives. However, such positions of advantage have to be available to all persons in the society. So technically, in Rawls's view, anyone who has the ability should be able to attend a university or college and become a person of privilege.

Rawls also dealt with the idea of providing services or benefits for everyone. He felt that it was morally right to limit services when there is a greater need among certain groups. This can mean that not everything is available to everyone in every instance. For example, if you go to the emergency department with a sprained ankle, there are many services available to diagnose and treat you. However, you might not get immediate treatment or even all of the available treatments if there are people in life-threatening situations present. It is in the self-interest of all if those in greater need are treated first.

Theory Applications

Rawls has had a great influence on how leaders think about social justice in America. His ideas also influenced how America is judged by other nations. For example, how does America treat its poor or imprisoned citizens? This can be seen as a greater indicator of the nation's quality than its wealth. Rawls's thinking about social justice also influenced the introduction of such programs as Head Start and Medicaid/Medicare. His theory has ramifications for institutions such as education, public health, and health care.

Rawls presents a great challenge to the American market-based health care system. His theory asks that you consider more than the greatest good for the greatest number or the greatest profitability for the greatest bottom line. Instead, it asks that you address how you treat those in your community who have the least amount of financial resources to invest in health care. You are expected to provide for their needs and still maintain a bottom line that allows you to stay in the business. This certainly poses a great challenge for the healthcare system.

■ PERSONAL ETHICS THEORISTS

A few words of introduction are needed before you read about the next four theorists. Rather than look at the macro picture of the ethics, these philosophers addressed how people acquire their morality, ethical thinking, and decision-making. Aristotle was one of the most influential of this group because his work provided a foundation for many of the great ethicists who followed him. Martin Buber presented ethics in terms of moral relationships, while Lawrence Kohlberg investigated stages of moral development. Finally, Viktor Frankl addressed personal ethics and its relationship to the ultimate meaning of life. This section continues the previous format. You will learn about these writers' lives, basic concepts, and their influence on healthcare ethics.

■ ARISTOTLE (384–322 BCE)

Biographical Influences on His Theory

Aristotle's father was the physician for the king of Macedonia, which meant that Aristotle was a child of privilege. At 17, he was sent to Athens and studied under Plato. He continued this study by attending Plato's lectures for 20 years! Aristotle was also the tutor of Alexander the Great. His extensive writings included works in physics, logic, psychology, natural history, metaphysics, politics, and ethics. However, his fame did not protect him when the Macedonian government was overthrown. He had to escape from Athens to avoid prosecution for a charge of impropriety.

Concept Summary

Aristotle's work in ethics centered on how people can achieve the highest level of good or virtue. Just talking about what you should do or not do, as a moral person, was not enough. For Aristotle, you must build your character by taking action and practicing virtue. His book, *Nicomachean Ethics*, presented his views on virtue and the virtuous life (McKeon, 1971). It included the concepts **virtue**, **practical wisdom**, and **eudaimonia** that are presented in this section.

How did Aristotle describe the concept of virtue? First, virtue requires that you make choices that require action, not just discussion. You base these choices on your knowledge and experience and they must be made voluntarily. Virtues are witnessed through your character or the way that you consistently live your life. Examples of virtues include practicing temperance instead of being impulse-driven, and helping a friend when you get no reward. Other examples of virtues are courage, honor, and a friendly nature.

Since building a virtuous character requires action and choice, Aristotle also presented the concept of practical wisdom. You will always be presented with situations that are new to you. This means that you might not have an answer about what is right to do in these situations. Aristotle suggested that you engage in what he called practical wisdom. This means that you need to be stronger than your impulses and research your choices. You then assess these choices as good or bad and weigh them against each other. Your rational self would guide you to choose the best option for any situation that you face. This option is often the middle ground between the choices you considered. Practical wisdom can be also applied to groups or even whole societies as they attempt to choose the most virtuous action for any given situation. Aristotle reminded us that "it is not possible to be good in the strict sense without practical wisdom" (McKeon, 1971, p. 1036).

Aristotle also introduced the idea of eudaimonia. This concept has been translated as happiness or the idea of flourishing (Summers, 2009). However, Aristotle did not think of happiness in the modern sense. He meant that you could be happy if you chose to practice virtue in your life and worked to build your moral character. Such action requires the ability to contemplate and address difficult issues including how to live together in community. Therefore, eudaimonia is unique to humans because animals do not have the ability to contemplate.

Theory Applications

How can Aristotle's ideas apply to the modern HCA? The modern theory of virtue ethics has been derived from his works. This theory describes how we should evaluate actions based on what someone with moral character would do. It also asks that we think about why we are making a decision as part of our moral character. In addition, virtue ethics helps us define what character traits we should have as a person and as a professional (Ashcroft, Dawson, Draper, & McMillan, 2007).

You can see evidence of Aristotle's work in the process of professional socialization. Every profession defines a set of characteristics that describe its ideal practitioner. Defining these characteristics and assuring that they are present in professionals is part of the moral responsibility of the profession. In health administration, characteristics include honesty, trust-worthiness, compassion, and competence. The profession, through its educational process, then attempts to inculcate these character traits in its students through lecture, discussion, field experiences, and other methods. You could say that educators are encouraging their students to a life of eudaimonia. This goal makes sense because students become practitioners. As graduates, they represent both the profession and their alma mater to the community.

The concept of practical wisdom can be applied in your professional and personal life. When you are making a decision about what is the best choice to make, rely on your learning about ethics and lessons from experience to assist you. You can also use the wisdom of others such as teachers, clergy, and parents to guide your contemplation. If you make practical wisdom as part of your daily practice, you are well on your way to eudaimonia.

■ MARTIN BUBER (1878–1965)

Biographical Influences on His Theory

Martin Buber was born in Germany and was part of a family of scholars. He became a social activist and tried to help Eastern European Jews during World War I. In 1933, he served as the Director of the

Central Office for Jewish Education during a time when Hitler would not allow Jews to go to school. In 1938, he immigrated to Palestine and continued his writing. One of his most important works on ethics is called *I and Thou* (1996).

Concept Summary

Buber examined how people relate to each other and behave in moral or immoral ways. He organized a hierarchy of these relationships and showed how they move from what he considered the lowest to the highest ethical levels. At the very bottom of his hierarchy is the "I-I" relationship. In this level, a person is seen as merely an extension of another person. An example of this might be a child who is expected to become a physician because his father is a physician. The child is seen not as person, but as an extension of the father's ambitions. In severe cases such as a psychopathic personality, a person cannot see anyone except him or herself. The needs of others simply do not exist and neither does the responsibility of ethical behavior toward them.

Buber's next level is the "I-IT" relationship. In this case, people are merely tools to be used for a person's own benefit or for the benefit of the organization. People are not individuals; they are the vehicles for accomplishing some goal. Names are not important or even known; people are just "Its," or convenient labels.

For Buber, I-IT relationships are morally wrong because they fail to accept people as having individuality and value. People serve only as a means to an end for the person or the organization. Examples of I-IT relationships occur when an administrator uses the term "my people" to refer to the healthcare professionals. Another example could be if Mrs. Smith is referred to as "the colon in 405" instead of by her name. Still another example of an I-IT relationship happens when an administrator uses the expression "FTEs" in planning without any regard for the fact that a "full-time equivalent" is a person.

Next in Buber's hierarchy are the "I-YOU" relationships. In this case, people are recognized as individuals with value; they each have unique talents, gifts, and ideas. These differences are not only recognized, but they are also accepted and respected. An example of this type of relationship can be found in a well-functioning healthcare team when each member respects the contributions of the others. In health care, patients expect I-YOU relationships as a minimum level of performance from all employees. Employees also expect and appreciate this level of ethical relationship with their supervisors and with each other. When such an environment exists, staff members are more productive and exhibits higher morale.

The highest moral relationship that you can have is called "I-THOU." It is based on the Greek concept of agape (meaning love for others), which Buber viewed as the most mature human relationship. In an I-THOU relationship, each person is recognized as being different and having value. In addition, a choice is made to consider that person as beloved or special. Notice that the word "choice" is used in that last sentence. Making a choice requires many things from people who make the decision to consider someone beloved. These requirements include increased tolerance of differences, patience, and efforts to make that person's needs equal to their own. A person who is beloved is held in high esteem or unconditional regard.

I-THOU relationships do not exist with each person that you meet. However, in health care, patients assume that they are in an I-THOU relationship when you are providing for their health needs. They assume that you value their needs equally with your own because you chose to have a career in a service-based industry. Likewise, the community assumes that, as an administrator, you are acting with the highest regard for their needs and serve as a good steward of their resources.

Theory Applications

In this short summary, you have only looked at the basics of Buber's complex thinking about ethics and ethical behavior. However, his definitions of ethical relationships can be useful to you as an administrator. For example, when you are planning a new venture or evaluating a current program, do you think of employees as tools to get the job done or as people who can contribute through their talents? When you are in conference with a fellow employee, do you try to have at least an I-YOU relationship? Finally, when you choose to be in an I-THOU relationship, do you really put that person's needs and wants on equal footing with your own? Are you aware of how the community sees your relationship to them? These questions can be helpful in examining your personal ethical behaviors and relationships.

■ LAWRENCE KOHLBERG (1927–1987)

Biographical Influences on His Theory

Lawrence Kohlberg joined the Merchant Marines during World War II. At the end of the war, he was actively engaged in smuggling Jews through the British blockade for settlement in Palestine. Because of this experience, he began to think about moral reasoning and how ethical thinking is learned.

Kohlberg finished his doctorate at the University of Chicago and became a professor at Harvard University. He began to theorize that **moral development** happened in stages and researched this theory using children and adults. He used a qualitative research model based on categorizing responses to stories featuring moral dilemmas, such as the now famous Heinz's Dilemma. This story was used to evaluate a person's level of moral development based on his or her answers and the reasoning behind those answers. The responses to these stories and the reasoning behind them helped to formulate a hierarchy of moral development. His theory of moral development has been subsequently verified by studies in America and throughout the world. Kohlberg became an international name in the study of morality and ethics, but his death is assumed a suicide. He disappeared in January of 1987; his body was pulled from Boston Harbor by the police.

Concept Summary

How do you become an ethical person? To understand Kohlberg's answer to this question, you need some information about developmental stage theory (Kohlberg, 1984). In this theory, people must go through one stage before they can achieve the next highest stage of development. The movement through stages is not always chronological, but happens as you are challenged by life and attempt to find solutions for those challenges. Finding solutions helps you to advance in your moral development and reasoning. In addition, Kohlberg believed that you could not understand the moral reasoning that is too far beyond your own level. It is also possible to be grown-up physically, but not be morally mature. Kohlberg believed that only about 25% of people ever get to the highest level of moral development and that most people remain on what he called Level IV.

What are Kohlberg's stages and what do they mean? There are two stages (Level I and II) that Kohlberg calls **premoral** or **preconventional**. These stages exist before you have a true sense of moral decision-making. In Level I, you make decisions purely to avoid being punished or because a person in higher authority tells you to do it. Your decision is centered on what might happen to you and nothing else.

Level II is also premoral but is centered on the personal outcome of the action. In this case, decisions are made based on selfish concerns and the ability to gain personal reward. This is sometimes called the "What's in it for me?" orientation to ethical behavior or decision making. In this stage, people are valued for their usefulness to the individual and not for any other reason. Generally, Level I and II stage behaviors are common in young children, but they are also present in adults. An example of this behavior is if you choose to act ethically only when it benefits your own agenda.

Kohlberg's Levels III and IV are what he calls **conventional** or external-controlled moral development stages. In Level III, people make moral decisions based on the need to please people and to be seen as "good." The motivation for making ethical decisions is in trying to avoid guilt or shame. People who do what is perceived as good should be rewarded and those who do not should be punished in this view.

Ethical decisions for people in this stage are made so that they can be viewed as good employees, good parents, or good friends. They also want to avoid the stigma of being labeled as a "bad employee."

In Level IV, moral reasoning is governed by the need to respect rules and laws and maintain a certain order. In this stage, justice is being punished for disobeying the law. Ethics is seen as obeying the law and keeping order in society. Authority is usually not questioned; the idea is that if it is the law, then it must be right. This stage explains how Nazi soldiers could actively participate in the holocaust and consider themselves moral people. They simply claimed that they were being good soldiers, obeying a higher authority, and "carrying out orders."

Levels V and VI of the Kohlberg theory are designated as **principled moral reasoning** because decisions are based on applying universal moral ideas or principles. In Level V, ethical decisions are based on a set of rights and responsibilities that are common to all members of a group or community. These rights encompass the law but go beyond it. Moral decisions are based on respect for yourself and for the rights of others. Level V requires complex thinking about the social contract you have with others and not just about laws. When society-based decisions are made about healthcare resources, an element of Level V reasoning should be present.

Kohlberg's Level VI moral reasoning is based on ideas or principles that are universal. These principles are higher than the authority of law and include ideas of justice and respect for persons and their rights. Ethical decisions are made based on higher-level principles and not just for legal compliance. In addition, those who are functioning at Level VI assume that all humans have worth and value regardless of their societal status. Level VI ethical thinking occurred when Martin Luther King Jr. and others said that segregation, while legal, was unethical. Segregation violated a higher law than that which was created by the courts. They were willing to disobey the law to bring attention to this issue and to bring about change.

Theory Applications

Kohlberg's theory of moral reasoning helps to provide an understanding of why people make the decisions that they do. It might be helpful, as an administrator, to understand that not all persons have the same ethical reasoning. In addition, if there is too great a difference in the levels of reasoning, they might not even understand why you see your decision as ethical. Understanding Kohlberg's ideas can also help you analyze your own decisions and determine your moral reasoning behind them. This ability should prove useful when you are required to defend your decisions. Why did you decide to act as you did? What was your reasoning?

There is another implication for knowing and understanding Kohlberg's theory. The implication occurs in patient/system relations. Think about your role as a HCA in society's view. Society has granted that health care is a system of a high level of authority. Along with this authority comes an assumption of trust in the system. Patients must have faith that you are functioning at high levels (at least on Level IV) of moral reasoning when making decisions about their care and treatment. In other words, they expect you to have the ability to put their needs first and profit second. When evidence of actions that do not meet this standard is uncovered, the public can lose trust in the system itself. They can view the healthcare system, and you as its representative, of being unethical and untrustworthy. Once trust is lost, it is difficult to regain and can have a negative impact on the financial future of both your organization and the system in general.

■ VIKTOR FRANKL (1905–1997)

Biographical Influences on His Theory

As a young man, Viktor Frankl demonstrated wisdom beyond his chronological age. While still in high school, he began a correspondence with Freud, who published his work. He had the courage to draft a book on his own view of psychology early in his career. However, in 1942, Frankl, along with his new bride, brother, and parents, was arrested and taken to a concentration camp in Theresienstadt. His wife, parents, and brother later died in the camps.

Frankl survived the brutality of four different camps before his release. Instead of losing hope, he actually used this experience to test his theories of human motivation and conscience. His observations confirmed that those who had a **sense of meaning** and purpose kept their humanity even in this unbelievable suffering. His experience led to his lifelong work in what has come to be called meaning theory (logotherapy). He is author of many books, but the most well known is *Man's Search for Meaning*, which has sold over nine million copies and has been translated into dozens of languages.

Concept Summary

First, Frankl believed that you are not just a body or a brain. You are a total person who has a mind, body, and spirit. You are also unique in the entire universe and entitled to dignity. Your life has meaning no matter what your personal circumstances. As a thinking person, you are able to question and wonder about your purpose in life and what life means to you. Only humans can ask, "Why am I here and what am I supposed to do?" For Frankl, morality is also related to your sense of meaning. You make decisions to behave in moral ways for the sake of something in which you believe, to which you are committed, or because of your relationship to God (the ultimate meaning).

When you do not feel a sense of purpose in your life, you will have emptiness, or an existential vacuum. You might fill that void with, alcohol or drugs; while others might use work, food, or power. For Frankl, "A lively and vivid conscience is the only thing that enables man to resist the effects of the existential vacuum" (1971, p. 65). What is a conscience? It is your ability to go beyond a situation and find meaning in it. You can then make choices that are ethical and affect more than your selfish needs. Your conscience is not infinite; it does not have absolute knowledge. It tries to find the best action to take in a situation. Because your conscience is a part of you, you can choose to make decisions that honor those things you value and avoid those things that bring harm.

Theory Applications

Can you see a connection here? It almost feels like you have closed a circle that goes back to the writing of Thomas Aquinas and Aristotle. Conscience is again part of your consideration of ethics. In the case of Frankl's interpretation, you can use it to help you understand the meaning of your actions and choose the best action possible. Think about the word "choose." By using this word, Frankl implies that because you choose your actions, you are responsible for them. In health care, the statement has profound implications. Each day you make decisions that can affect the health and quality of life of both patients and employees. You should make these choices based on as much data as you can obtain and after serious consideration. Basing your decisions on the best data available is a choice that might take more effort on your part, but it also demonstrates your willingness to be responsible for what you do.

■ WHAT IS ETHICS?

Now that you have reviewed summaries of the basic concepts of the Big 8, you are ready to define ethics in a professional and personal sense. Again, many authors have attempted to define this word. If you refer to Figure I-1 in the Introduction, you can see that ethics can be theoretical, community-based, organizational, or personal. As an administrator, you must be knowledgeable about all of these forms of ethics. For example, from a theoretical base, you can define ethics in terms of a theory such as deontology or utilitarianism. You can also clarify your understanding of the basic principles of ethics (see Chapters 2 through 4) and use them to guide your decision-making.

Ethics can be defined as a way to examine or study moral behaviors. Of course, that definition is too general for your purposes and needs some clarification. Darr (2005) uses a complex definition that stresses that ethics is more than just obeying the law. Law is the minimum standard that society approves for actions or behaviors; ethics is much broader and often much more difficult to codify. So, you could behave legally, but not ethically. You can probably think of many examples where a law has not been broken, but the lack of ethics has caused problems for a person or an organization.

The community establishes its sense of what is appropriate ethical behavior, and that sense can vary within communities. Often, administrators are not aware of community standards and suffer career setbacks because of this ignorance. For example, if you are a hospital administrator in a large city, it might be acceptable for you to go to a bar after work and have a drink. In a small community, that same behavior might be seen as unethical, and even be reported to the Board of Trustees.

Summers (2009) discussed ethics in terms of knowing right from wrong and applying ethics theory to your life (normative ethics). He also stated that this type of ethics challenges you to find the correct moral rules to follow. Normative ethics are also concerned with a general ethics code or decision-making pattern for a group or organization (Beauchamp & Childress, 2008). Other authors call this organizational ethics, or "the way we do things here." This form of ethics helps people understand the standards for acceptable behaviors within an organization. Taking the time to establish basic ethical standards for a healthcare organization is of great importance because of its power and influence. However, healthcare organizations are made up of people who have differing ideas about ethics. Can you see why establishing normative ethics for an organization is so important?

These authors also talk about professional ethics, which is part of the innermost circle of Figure I-1. Guidelines have been developed by your profession to assist you in identifying expected ethical behaviors. For example, there are codes of ethics that have been developed for nurses, physicians, physical therapists, occupational therapists, and even massage therapists. In addition, as an HCA, you have guidance from the American College of Healthcare Executives on ethical behavior and policy development. There is even a self-assessment test to help you keep your ethics on track. You will be studying these codes later in this text.

Of course, ethics really comes down to you (the innermost circle in Figure I-1). You must be aware of theoretical, community, and organizational ethics as you make daily decisions. You also have to be in tune with what your profession or professions require of you. However, in your daily operations as an administrator, you are ultimately the one who must choose the actions that you take. You might ask, "Isn't ethics just doing what is right at the right time?" The answer is "yes, but. . . ." In healthcare organizations, what is right is not a simple matter. This is why you must develop your "ethical bottom line."

First, think about the community in which you live and what it expects from you as a person in the healthcare system. You must also become more aware of the mission and values of your organization and explore the code of the profession or professions with which you are affiliated. Finally, you must think about your own values and ask yourself, "What is my true ethics bottom line? On what issues would I be willing to act even if it meant quitting my job?" This thought process should lead you to design a personal ethics statement that can assist in making the difficult decisions. The chapters in this book will help you to do this and to apply your ethics to your daily decision-making. Your ethics actions must match your ethics words or you face being seen as a hypocrite.

Summary

This chapter should help you better understand the theory behind ethical decisions. You will see how these theories translate into principles in Chapters 2 through 4. In addition, you should be able to recognize the influence of these theorists in other chapters of the book as you explore how the community and organization view the practice of healthcare ethics. It is hoped that you will also integrate some of their thinking into your own ethics decision making as a practicing HCA.

Web Resources

The following are Web sites that provide additional information about the theorists in this text.

St. Thomas Aquinas
http://www.utm.edu/research/iep/a/aquinas.htm

Immanuel Kant
http://www.utm.edu/research/iep/k/kantmeta.htm

John Stuart Mill
http://www.utm.edu/research/iep/m/milljs.htm

John Rawls
http://www.iep.utm.edu/r/rawls.htm

Martin Buber
http://plato.stanford.edu/entries/buber/

Lawrence Kohlberg
http://www.iep.utm.edu/m/moraldev.htm

Viktor Frankl
http://logotherapy.univie.ac.at/

References

Ashcroft, R. E., Dawson, A., Draper, H., & McMillan, J. R. (2007). *Principles of health care ethics*. West Sussex, UK: John Wiley & Sons, Ltd.

Beauchamp, T. L., & Childress, J. E. (2008). *Principles of biomedical ethics* (6th ed.). New York: Oxford University Press.

Buber, M. (1996). *I and thou*. New York: Touchstone.

Cahn, S. M., & Markie, P. (1998). *Ethics: History, theory, and contemporary issues*. New York: Oxford University Press.

Darr, K. (2005). *Ethics in health services management* (4th ed.). Baltimore: Health Professions Press.

Frankl, V. (1971). *Man's search for meaning: An introduction to logotherapy*. New York: Pocket Books.

Kohlberg, L. (1984). *The philosophy of moral development: Moral stages and the idea of justice*. New York: HarperCollins.

McChance, D. (2004). *Medusa's ear: University foundings from Kant to Chorla L*. Albany, NY: SUNY Press.

McKeon, R. (Ed.). (1971). *The basic works of Aristotle*. New York: Random House.

Summers, J. (2009). Theory of healthcare ethics. In E. E. Morrison (Ed.). *Health care ethics: Critical issues for the 21st century*. Sudbury, MA: Jones and Bartlett, pp. 3–40.

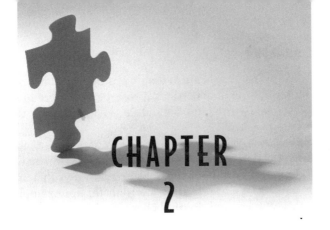

CHAPTER 2

Autonomy

He alone is free who lives with free consent under the guidance of reason.

—Spinoza

Points to Ponder

1. What are the key issues for the healthcare administrator (HCA) with respect to informed consent?
2. How does HIPAA change the way you view confidentiality?
3. Is it ever appropriate to withhold the truth from a patient?
4. What is the significance of fidelity to the success of HCAs?

Words to Remember

The following is a list of key words for this chapter. You will find them in bold in the text. Stop and check your understanding of them.

authorization
disclosure
informed consent
veracity

competence
fidelity
reasonable person standard
voluntariness

■ INTRODUCTION AND DEFINITIONS

Autonomy is one of the four major principles of healthcare ethics that are derived from the theories you studied in Chapter 1. In this chapter, you will explore the meaning of this principle and its application to healthcare practice. Current concepts of autonomy stem from its Greek definition as self-rule and self-determination (Beauchamp &

Childress, 2008). The healthcare system's position on this principle is supported by Kant, Frankl, and others who believe that because people have unconditional worth and should be given respect, they also deserve self-determination.

To be applied, the principle of autonomy must assume that you are free from the control of others and have the capacity to make your own life choices. You also must have the right to hold views that are incongruent with those of the healthcare establishment. For example, if you are a Jehovah's Witness and do not believe in blood transfusions, you have the right to refuse such treatment even when your physician recommends it. The word "choice" is a key element in this principle. How does this relate to your position in health care? As an administrator, you must understand that people should be free to choose whether to be compliant with their physician's instructions or not. They must also be able to make informed decisions about signing consent forms for surgery or other procedures without undue influence or punitive repercussions from medical staff. You will learn more about the complexities of autonomy as informed consent later in the chapter.

Autonomy is more than just making informed choices. It is also concerned with how individuals are viewed and treated within the healthcare system. If autonomy is an ethical principle for your organization, then certain standards should prevail. In this chapter, you will explore some of these standards including autonomy as confidentiality. You will also examine how the Health Insurance Portability and Accountability Act of 1996 (Title II) (HIPAA) rules have increased the awareness of the need to protect this area. Autonomy as truth-telling is also included in this chapter; you will learn what telling the truth means in healthcare situations. Finally, you will explore autonomy as expressed as fidelity and learn what it means to keep your word to patients and employees. A summary will be included to reinforce the key concepts of the chapter. You will then be able to apply your knowledge of this principle to two cases that are based on real-world healthcare incidents.

■ AUTONOMY AS INFORMED CONSENT

Legal and ethical considerations come together when applied in the area of **informed consent** for treatment. Through case law and legislation, informed consent has come to be seen as the duty of physicians or their designees to obtain the patient's permission for treatment. This permission should be given only after the patient understands the treatment and supports its implementation. Failure to obtain permission can constitute negligence or even lead to medical malpractice actions. From a larger view, informed consent is an ethical issue because it requires respect for the autonomy of individuals and their right to choose what is done to their bodies.

Autonomous consent is implied through a person's actions. For example, if you make an appointment with your dentist and keep that appointment, it is implied that you consent to treatment. However, if a procedure must be used that is not routine, then there is an ethical (and often legal) duty to obtain specific written consent.

What is meant by informed consent? Beauchamp and Childress (2008) present a model that clarifies this term and serves as a basis for discussion. This type of permission to treat contains the preconditions of **competence** on the part of the patient to understand the treatment, and **voluntariness** in his or her decision-making. It also requires disclosure on the part of the physician of material information including the recommended treatment plan. Finally, consent means that the patient is in favor of the plan and gives his or her **authorization** to proceed.

The idea of competence is not a simple one in health care. In general, it is assumed that adults are competent to make decisions about their health but that children are not. However, adults can be in situations where they are not deemed competent. This includes incidents when they are unconscious, mentally ill, or under the influence of drugs. There are exceptions to the child rule, too. Children can be deemed competent when they are legally emancipated from their parents. In these nonroutine circumstances, healthcare professionals can need additional guidance about informed consent, and the physician's responsibilities through policies, procedures, and training programs that are provided by the institution in which they practice.

Voluntariness means that the person is not under the influence or control of another person when making a decision. This means that he or she is not threatened or forced into treatment. While this sounds bizarre, there are occasions when patients can think they are being forced into treatment by healthcare professionals or other parties. In even more rare occurrences, the patients are actually threatened to undergo treatment by physicians presenting dire consequences if they do not. Whether the situation is actual or perceived, these patients do not freely choose to participate in the treatment. The use of threats or the perception of a threat means that an autonomous decision by the patient is not possible.

Similarly, if a healthcare professional tries to manipulate a person into consenting to treatment, this negates autonomy. For example, suppose a researcher needs a certain number of subjects in order to maintain funding for his study. This researcher finds a suitable subject and promises him or her that there are benefits for participation in the study. The subject then signs a consent form, without knowledge of the researcher's true agenda. This manipulation of study information is unethical and removes the voluntary element from the process of informed decision-making.

Disclosure is a major element in both legal and ethical aspects of informed consent. It can appear to be a very simple thing to disclose information about a patient's condition, the methods of treatment, and alternatives for that treatment. However, this does not always happen. Many states now require what is called a **reasonable person standard** with respect to what should be disclosed in order to obtain consent. This means that there is an obligation to present enough information so that a "reasonable person" would be able to make an informed decision about the procedure. Adhering to this guideline poses some ethical issues, particularly in sophisticated and often expensive research studies. If a researcher is too zealous in making statements about the anticipated benefits versus the risks of the study, the subjects might choose not to participate. This could lead to expensive searches for subjects or even a loss of funding for the research.

In order for patients to make an informed decision about their healthcare options, a recommendation must be made by the health professional. Recommendations must include all of the options available for the patient and the practitioner's best assessment of the best choice. Even this part of informed consent is not without difficulty. For example, there are alternative treatments, such as the use of herbs or holistic medicine, that have proven to be effective but are not approved by the Food and Drug Administration or fully recognized by the medical community. If the physician does not support the use of such forms of treatment, he or she might not present these options to the patient. Another complexity of disclosure occurs in the case of managed care. The physician's recommendation cannot be based solely on the covered treatments in the plan. The patient should be informed of the costs of other existing treatments so he or she can decide if he or she is able to pay for them if the treatments are not covered by his or her health maintenance organization.

Making efforts to ensure the patient understands the disclosures and the treatment plan is an ethics obligation if you are seeking informed consent. News about a medical condition and required treatment can evoke an emotional response on the part of the patient that affects his or her ability to make sound decisions. Therefore, requiring a signed consent too soon after such news might not be appropriate action. Ignoring the patient's human reaction to his or her state has the risk of obtaining uninformed consent. However, delaying consent too long can impede treatment and potentially cause a negative outcome.

Achieving understanding also requires comprehension of what is being presented. This is a challenge because consent forms are often full of legal and medical jargon and are written at a college reading level. Because the average reading level of Americans is between sixth and eighth grade, a true understanding of such forms might not be possible. Again, HCAs have the responsibility to put policies, procedures, and forms in place that encourage understanding as a way to meet the competence aspect of autonomous consent. Checking the readability of such forms and having qualified personnel available to answer any questions is both good business and good ethics.

Finally, you must consider the patient's decision to implement the plan and the appropriate authorization. This final step can require the use of additional personnel to verify that the patient fully understands the form and the procedures described therein when he or she gives consent to proceed. Even though nonphysician personnel are used during the process of obtaining informed consent, ultimately, the responsibility for this consent lies with the physician. Therefore, he or she must be willing to verify informed consent with the patient.

As you can see from the discussion, the issue of autonomy as informed consent is a complex one for the healthcare system. It is important for you, as an administrator, to know your level of responsibility for ensuring that forms used to gain consent are understood, questions are addressed, and procedures are followed during this process. You also might be required to maintain proof of consent in various formats and to ensure that this proof is kept confidential and secure. You must also keep up to date on any changes in the HIPAA laws and maintain compliance with these changes.

■ AUTONOMY AS CONFIDENTIALITY

Autonomy is also practiced when information about a person's identity, family, health status, and treatment procedures is kept private. This aspect of autonomy also extends to information that you know about employees and their families. As an HCA, you have many duties when it comes to confidentiality, some of which extend into the legal realm because of the HIPAA laws.

When patients enter the healthcare system, what is their expectation of confidentiality? Most believe that they have a right to privacy or to have control over access to their physical bodies, their health information, and their decisions. When patients choose to surrender some of their privacy, they expect that what they say or what is done to them will be kept confidential (Beauchamp & Childress, 2008). This expectation goes all the way back to the time of Hippocrates when physicians were cautioned not to disclose what was said to them in confidence.

Is there absolute confidentiality in health care settings? The truth is that it can often be necessary to share private information about patients to treat their conditions. Nurses, physical therapists, radiation technicians, and many others might need access to a patient's information in order to treat him or her appropriately. HIPAA allows types of communication with those involved in the patient's care and even family and friends under certain conditions. However, patient consent or agreement is required and professional judgment is required in specific cases (Office for Civil Rights, 2008). Only those who have a legitimate need to know the information should have access to the patient's medical record. Safeguards need to be in place to ensure that medical information is protected from access by those who do not have a need to know.

On the surface, this sounds straightforward, but safeguarding confidentiality in today's healthcare system is not as simple as a locked file cabinet. With the advent of the electronic record, the risk of inappropriate access to confidential information has greatly increased. This is part of the reason for the enactment of certain provisions of HIPAA. These provisions standardize the electronic record and provide safeguards for confidentiality. While none of these policies is foolproof, they demonstrate that efforts are being made to protect confidentiality.

There are additional problems involved in safeguarding confidentiality beyond those surrounding electronic records. Within the structural procedures at a hospital or clinic, there are practices that can automatically threaten the patient's confidentiality. For example, before HIPAA, it was customary to post patients' names and procedures on a white board outside of outpatient surgery. While this might have been standard procedure and convenient for the staff, it could be devastating for patients when they realized that anyone who saw that board knew their impending procedures. If this action were to occur today, it would be a violation of HIPAA. What about discussing the patient's medical condition when he or she is in a semiprivate room? Only a curtain separates the patient from the other occupant of the room, so confidentiality is not protected. Every effort needs to be made to ensure that confidentiality is respected, but it can be difficult to accomplish.

Actions in the informal organization that can threaten confidentiality can be even more subtle. If your staff is not trained on how to manage patient information effectively, discussions about interesting cases can occur in the hallways, elevators, break room, or the cafeteria. Such conversations, while not intended to do harm, can be overheard by anyone, including the patient's family. It is your responsibility as an administrator to reduce the likelihood of such staff actions through appropriate policies, procedures, and training. In addition, you can conduct informal observations to evaluate how such training is being utilized; this has often been called "management by walking around."

Patient confidentiality is not an absolute even with appropriate practices and procedures in place. There are occasions when the law or ethical practice makes such action necessary. Legally mandated exceptions to confidentiality include such things as reporting certain diseases, traumatic events such as gunshot wounds, and incidents of child abuse. In the case of mental health providers, there is a duty to warn others if a client threatens to be violent. This position is supported by the utilitarian theory that you have studied; it is based on the consequences of keeping that confidence versus the benefits of breaching it.

Other issues of confidentiality pose even more complex ethical challenges. For example, should employers have a right to your medical records? If so, can they use what they find in them to avoid hiring you if you have an expensive pre-existing condition that will drive up their insurance costs? What if you are diagnosed with a genetic condition that could affect the health of your family members? Should the physician tell your relatives even if you do not want it discussed with them? These questions are just a few examples of how complicated confidentiality can be when considered in its full ethical context. The decision of a patient to withhold information from his or her family can create some true dilemmas for the practitioner and the organization. As an administrator, you have to understand that such decisions are not always black and white. An ethics committee (to be discussed in Chapter 10) can assist you with determining appropriate action in these cases.

There is another area to consider with respect to confidentiality. This concept goes beyond the realm of patient care. Depending on your position in the health facility, perhaps you have access to very private information about your employees and their families. It is imperative that you recognize the need to maintain confidentiality with this information and not to share it with those who have no need to know. Because you are in a position of authority, violation of employee confidentiality might not only be a breach of trust, but might also cause you to lose your job. Therefore, it is vital for you to be aware of the need to keep private information private.

■ AUTONOMY AS TRUTH-TELLING

Should you always tell the truth? Kant includes truth-telling as meeting the categorical imperative. The truth should be given to everyone. Beauchamp and Childress (2008) consider it one of the obligations of health care. "Society cherishes truth telling because it is the glue of human community. . . " (Boyle, Dubose, Ellingson, Guinn, & McCurdy, 2001, p. 14). Can you imagine trying work as an HCA if you could not assume that people were telling the truth? You would drown in "proof paperwork." Contracts and verbal agreements would be all but impossible to negotiate.

Therefore, truth-telling or **veracity** is a key part of the business of health care. When patients interact with a person in the healthcare system, they have an assumption that they are being told the truth. Likewise, the practitioners must assume that truthful information is being given to them by their patients. Confidence in truthfulness is the basis of trust that underlies decisions for effective treatment.

Given this patient right to truthfulness, you could assume that it is always ethically correct to tell the truth. However, health care presents situations where an absolute position on truth-telling might not be the best position. The utilitarian position on truth-telling is that you should always weigh the benefit against harm before disclosing the truth. Once this assessment is done, it might be more ethical to be cautious about disclosure or to tell the truth in pieces over time. What exactly does this mean?

Professionals in health care often have to give bad news and even news of impending fatality to patients. The full information about this news and the timing of full, truthful disclosure can be influenced by the age and emotional state of the patient and the family's desires for such disclosure. For example, if a 90-year-old patient has been diagnosed with end-stage cancer, the family might not want her to know the full truth. They might feel that it is more ethical to deceive this patient and have her enjoy what time she has left. If the physician is aware of the family's request, it can pose an ethical dilemma. Does the physician tell the family and not the patient? What does this mean to the patient's right to know and to choose what she wants to do with her remaining time? Will the family feel that their trust has been violated if the physician tells the patient the truth?

There can be different standards about the scope of truth-telling when dealing with the diagnosis and the subsequent prognosis of a condition. Perhaps a patient can be given the full truth about his or her condition and treatment options. However, when it comes to what happens under treatment, practitioners can choose to give information in pieces over time to avoid overwhelming the patient (Beauchamp & Childress, 2008). This decision is justified as ethical because no one ultimately knows how well a person can do under treatment. Treatment results may deal with statistical data and not human determination. In dealing with the truth in stages, providers do not erode the patient's hope—which in and of itself can be a great motivator for treatment compliance and even healing. This type of truth-telling has the potential to challenge the trust between practitioner and patient, but compassion is the motivation behind it.

Truth-telling is not limited to the clinical aspects of health care. As an HCA, you are in a position of power. Your power can affect those with whom you work, the patients whom you serve, and the larger community in which you live. Power carries with it the ethical responsibilities of truth-telling. In fact, the American College of Healthcare Executives Code of Ethics (Hoffman & Nelson, 2001) specifically addresses this issue and makes it part of your responsibility to your organization. This code is described in detail in chapter 14.

On the surface, this seems like an easy thing to do. However, there can be times when it is extremely difficult. For example, when there is a possible need to downsize the staff at your organization, do you tell the whole truth? If you do, there is a possibility that your best staff will seek employment elsewhere rather than go through the stress of this process. It is also possible that senior executives do not want anything disclosed to protect their fiscal interests. Therefore, you might also find yourself engaged in stages of truth-telling, just like the clinical staff.

Even in daily interaction with staff, you must remember how powerful your words are and be careful in how you use them. Truth can destroy or enhance performance depending on how it is delivered. Consider your words carefully. This applies to both spoken and written communication. Words can have great emotional impact on others, but written words can come back to haunt you. Be sure to consider the text of your e-mails when considering truthful communication. In the business world, e-mail is not just a friendly exchange; it can be evidence of your truthfulness on any given issue.

Your silence can also provide a certain truth because it implies your consent. You must have the courage to speak your thoughts about an action or a decision, even when it might challenge your career status. Finally, you must be aware that lying, while expeditious now, might cause the end of your career. You have to keep track of lies and tell others the same lies to cover them up. Eventually, a lie can lead to a loss of integrity and even to the loss of your position (Dosick, 2000).

While truth-telling seems, on the surface, to be a straightforward aspect of autonomy, you can see that, with regard to health care, it is much more complex. There is power in the truth and you will be tempted to use that power in both positive and negative ways. It is wise to remember that the way in which truth is delivered (the message) is often as important as the facts (the content). Think carefully about the methods of telling the truth before you deliver the truth.

■ AUTONOMY AS FIDELITY

Fidelity means keeping your word to others, or promise-keeping. In ethics, it fits the Kantian view of the categorical imperative because it is universal. People want to have their promises kept by others, so they should, likewise, keep their promises to others. Buber agrees with promise-keeping as part of autonomy because it respects the I-You relationship. Because you respect the individuality of people, it is ethical to honor them by keeping your promises. Even the utilitarians agree with this aspect of ethics because it can provide the greatest good for the greatest number or avoid the greatest harm.

In business, the idea of fidelity has long been an ethics standard. It used to be said that a man was as good as his word. Business deals could be accomplished with a handshake and only scoundrels failed to uphold them. Even in today's business settings, fidelity is important because there is an assumption that contracts, both oral and written, will be honored. This assumption permits services to be rendered and payment to be made without undue concern about fraud and abuse. The vendors with whom you do business count on your fidelity as part of their business.

You are acting in a trust-based business. This means that fidelity is expected by the community as well as your business contacts. The community considers it a norm that you will keep your word to treat patients with dignity and fairness, and provide care that is appropriate and effective. The *Patient Care Partnership* documents created by the American Hospital Association (2003) reflect the promises expected by patients. They assert that fidelity is not only an ethics duty, but it is also a right for all patients and that you will honor this right.

This ethical imperative is also part of your mission statement that can be used by the community as an indicator of your business position. For example, if you use your mission to advertise your services, you have an obligation to honor those promises. For example, suppose a hospital uses the mission statement "Grant Hospital: Demand Excellence" in its television, print, and radio campaign. The employees at Grant Hospital might well be inundated with patients "demanding" all kinds of services and special treatment based on these advertisements. Perceived promises would not be kept and employees and patients would feel deceived.

This obligation of fidelity means that you must create a mission statement that is specific enough that you can actually meet it but not so crass as to offend your community. Therefore, you would not want to have a mission statement that says "Profit Is Number One" because the community thinks that they, the patients, should be your number one concern. Likewise, your mission statement should not be something vague like, "Optimum Health for All People" because it is a promise that cannot be met. Remember to review your mission statement frequently so that it truly reflects your commitment to service and ethical behavior. In addition, you are obligated to make sure all employees understand what fidelity toward this mission means in their daily work behaviors.

Fidelity is also an ethics obligation to your employees. If you make promises about any aspect of the employment relationship, you must honor those promises. Be careful about perceptions versus actualities. Your words are powerful and can easily be viewed as a promise by employees. This is why you need to be aware of what you say and when you say it. For example, if you are discussing benefit changes with employees, you must have correct information on what those benefits will be, what they will cost, and when they will be in effect. Misinformation can lead to situations where trust can be broken. This is especially true when major changes are occurring, such as during a merger or buyout. You must be able to act on any promise that is made, so use your words appropriately.

As you have seen in earlier sections, maintaining autonomy through fidelity is not a simple matter in health care. Violations of promise keeping occur for many reasons. Perhaps the most obvious is the potential conflict of keeping your word to the patient while also being loyal to third-party payers' demands. Are you loyal to those you serve or to those who pay for services? In health care, these are often two different groups. Payers might require gate-keeping and other functions to provide appropriate levels of care at the least amount of expense. However, when managed care organizations pay bonuses to physicians for controlling this access, an ethical problem can occur. Would the physician be tempted to cut corners on treatment when 10% to 20% of his or her salary is at stake? Should the physician disclose the bonus arrangement to the patient? Gate-keeping and other fiscal arrangements are appropriate for the bottom line but could present real ethics problems for patient fidelity.

There are other incidents where fidelity to patients can be challenged. For example, when a healthcare professional works in a prison setting, there can be conflict of fidelity between the interests of the patient and those of the institution. Certainly, when the legal system is involved, there might be a need to violate patient fidelity because of a subpoena or other action. In areas of public health, such as in the prevention of epidemics, fidelity to the overall community can take precedent over fidelity to the individual. This is also true in the military where different rules exist for physicians and other healthcare professionals. Using knowledge and skills to keep soldiers "combat ready" and regarding them as "government property" can appear to be an issue of fidelity to the organization over that of the individual.

What is your responsibility for fidelity as an administrator? Certainly, you need to be aware of the impact of mission on fidelity and do what you can to see that the promises of your mission are fulfilled. This can entail periodic reviews of the mission statement, training efforts, and observation to see if the mission is being met. You also have an obligation for fidelity where any contract is concerned. This means that you should understand the word and the intent of the contract before you sign it. You must also be able to communicate the features of the contract to those that the contract will affect. In the case of third-party payers, this communication effort includes patients as well as employees. Finally, using the Kantian question of, "If I were the patient or the employee, would I want this promise kept to me?" can guide you in making appropriate decisions about the fidelity aspect of autonomy.

Summary

Autonomy as a principle of ethics assumes a certain level of respect for persons and their ability to take actions that affect their health. It includes issues of informed consent, confidentiality of information, truth telling, and promise keeping. On the surface, autonomy seems to be a basic principle that should remain inviolate; however, in health care it is never this easy. There are situations and relationships that challenge the principle of autonomy and make it difficult to follow on a consistent basis. Your responsibility is to be aware of these challenges within your organization and to do whatever you can to maintain the right of autonomy. The community and your employees expect this of you.

Cases for Your Consideration

The Case of the Misguided Relative

As you read this case, consider the following questions. Responses and commentary will follow the case.

1. What aspects of autonomy were violated in this case?
2. Why did Ms. Jamie Jenson make the telephone call?
3. What was the impact of this action on the family?
4. What action could the family take?
5. If you were the administrator of this clinic, what action would you take?

Case Information

The Scene: The office of Dr. Randy Williams, internist, in Smalltown, USA.

The Situation: Mr. Basil Carpenter was suffering from problems with urinary insufficiency and frequent urination so he went to his physician, Dr. Williams, for evaluation. Dr. Williams performed an ultrasound in the office and saw a shadow in the kidney area. He explained to Mr. Carpenter that this might be a tumor and that he needed a consultation with an urologist. An appointment with Dr. Samuels would be made as soon as possible.

While Mr. Carpenter was not thrilled to hear this news, he knew that further tests were needed before he should be worried about his situation. He accompanied Dr. Williams to the front office where instructions were given to Ms. Jamie Jenson, the receptionist. She was to make an appointment with Dr. Samuels so that he could evaluate Mr. Carpenter. She also needed to make a follow-up appointment for Mr. Carpenter. After reviewing the chart, she made the call to Dr. Samuels, scheduled the follow-up, and gave Mr. Carpenter his appointment card.

However, Ms. Jenson was the cousin of Mr. Carpenter's ex-wife and this news was just too good to keep. As soon as Mr. Carpenter left the office, she called her cousin and told her that Basil had a kidney tumor and it might be cancerous. On hearing this news, Basil's ex-wife called their son, Hamilton, and told him that there was a problem with his father; he had cancer of the kidney and might not live.

Hamilton decided to get further information about his father's status and called Basil's current wife, Sandra. His first question to her was, "Does Dad have his will and finances in order?" Sandra responded, "Why are you asking this?" Hamilton told her that that Ms. Jenson from Dr. Williams' office said that Basil had kidney cancer and was terminal. Sobbing, Sandra hung up the phone just as Basil walked in the door. Only 30 minutes from the time he left Dr. Williams' office, he walked into hysteria of unknown origin.

Responses and Commentary on Questions

1. What aspects of autonomy were violated in this case?

   It should be noted that this case occurred before the HIPAA rules were in effect. However, it clearly is a case of breach of confidentiality by a nonmedical staff member. Because Ms. Jenson needed to provide referral information, she had the right to access the chart. However, information that she found, no matter what the relationship with the patient, should have been kept confidential.

   Kant would be very upset by this situation because it violated the categorical imperative for confidentiality. Imagine if this same incident happened to Ms. Jenson instead of Mr. Carpenter. How would she feel? Yet, she did not even consider this question before she called her cousin. The utilitarians would also find this action inappropriate because it had the potential to cause the greatest harm to the greatest number if it were to become a routine in this practice.

   Comment: The self-profit motive enhances the temptation to violate confidentiality when there is access to confidential records. Suppose the patient was a major celebrity and the condition was erectile dysfunction. The temptation to leak this information to the press for profit might sway a person's sense of ethical obligation. This might sound like an exaggeration, but similar incidents frequently occur.

2. Why did Ms. Jenson make the telephone call?

   Several things could have motivated Ms. Jenson in this case. Perhaps she saw herself as altruistic by giving the family important information that might not be shared by the new wife. Perhaps, she saw it as an issue of family loyalty and a duty to honor the family's right to know. She might not have even realized that she was violating Basil's right to confidentiality because no one ever told her not to do this. Of course, the motive could have been more purulent and she could have succumbed to the need to share gossip that was truly juicy.

Comment: It is important, as an administrator, to consider that everyone who has access to the medical record is important to the chain of confidentiality protection. Often persons who are not on the clinical side of patient treatment are forgotten in this important area. Receptionists, office managers, and even custodians might have more access to sensitive materials than you realize. Training and monitoring of policies and procedures is necessary.

3. What was the impact of this action on the family?

In this case, the family includes an extended network of individuals. First, you need to consider Ms. Jenson—who just put her job in jeopardy to inform her cousin of some family news. We will deal with her consequences in later responses. You must also consider Basil's ex-wife, who was upset enough to contact their son, Hamilton. How do you think she was feeling? Basil is her son's father and his loss could be very painful. Of course, you might also wonder why she called Hamilton when she did not have the whole story about Basil. Perhaps less than altruistic motives were in place.

How about Hamilton's role? He received this shocking news from his mother. Perhaps he was upset and concerned about his financial future. Of course, he too had the option of waiting for the full story before he called Sandra. You might wonder about his motivation and his response to the news, but you cannot deny that he was affected by this misinformation and added to the chain of grief that it caused.

Poor Sandra. She waited for Basil's return from Dr. Williams' office and was worried about his health. Then she got that telephone call from Hamilton. The news shocked her but also made her furious. How did Basil's ex-wife know about his condition before she did? What right did Ms. Jenson have to share this information with Basil's ex-wife before she even knew it? Just how bad is the situation? Will she lose her husband and the father of her children? It is no wonder she is crying.

What do you think about Basil? Can you imagine walking into this situation? He had been given potentially frightening news but decided to put it in its proper prospective until more information was known. He knew that he would have to tell his family but did not want to upset them too soon. Despite his sensible nature, he must have had some fears in the back of his mind. He wondered,

"What will happen to my family if I am not around?" He walked in the door to chaos. Sandra was crying and he did not have a clue why. Imagine how angry and upset he was.

Comment: Sometimes it is difficult for healthcare personnel to understand how much of an impact their actions have on others. This case is an example where an entire family was affected by the actions of one healthcare team member, but there are many incidences where whole communities can be affected. Healthcare professionals must always be aware of their power and use it ethically.

4. What action could the family take in this situation?

    Minimally, Basil should contact Dr. Williams personally and inform him of what took place. This would allow the physician to take appropriate action in his practice and deal with Ms. Jenson. Dr. Williams could also apologize to Basil for what happened and assure him that it would never happen again. If Basil was so inclined, he could contact his attorney to see if there were grounds for suit.

    What actually occurred in this case was very interesting. Sandra accompanied Basil to his appointment with the urologist. She told the specialist that she did not want the records released back to Dr. Williams. She also asked that they be stamped as confidential. When she was asked the reason for her request, she informed the urologist of the events. He was upset for the family and promised to honor Sandra's request. He also spoke to Dr. Williams about the situation. Shortly after this, Basil received a telephone call of apology and numerous statements in the mail about new protection of confidentiality policies in Dr. Williams' office.

5. If you were the administrator of this clinic, what action would you take?

    First, the minute you received the information about what transpired, you would have the obligation to investigate. You would document what the family told you about the situation. It would be important to remain calm, listen attentively, and provide assurance that action would be taken. Next, you would need to speak with Ms. Jenson privately to hear her account of what happened. You might also want to contact your legal counsel to get his or her advice on the best course of action. Once all of the information has been obtained, you would have to confer with Dr. Williams about the situation. He could decide on immediate termination or some other form of action with regard to Ms. Jenson.

    This action would deal only with the immediate situation, however. To prevent future incidents of this nature, you would have to review your current policies and procedures to make sure they are clear about confidentiality. You would also need to review all

HIPAA rules and regulations to be sure that you comply with those standards. New policies or clarifications would have to be written if they are needed.

In addition, you would have to determine that the current staff understands the policies and how their implementation. You might want to have an in-service education meeting to review confidentiality procedures with staff. In addition, you might consider doing some nonintrusive observations to see if procedures are being implemented. These actions would help you to prevent any future legal actions regarding the violations of confidentiality.

The Case of the Valiant Skateboarder

As you read this case, consider the following questions. Responses and commentary will follow the case.

1. How does this case illustrate the concept of patient autonomy?
2. What are some ways to protect Aidan's autonomy?
3. If you were the administrator of St. Mark the Ascetic Hospital, what action would you take?

Case Information

"It hurts! It hurts! Nothing has ever hurt like this!" Twenty-one-year-old Aidan Emerys attempted a frontside boardside on his skateboard. When there was a problem with his Ollie, his fall caused a break in his kneecap and he was admitted to Saint Mark the Ascetic Hospital for knee surgery. Before going to his room, he needed to have blood drawn for laboratory tests and an intravenous line (IV) placed. At St. Mark's, these procedures are done in the intensive care unit (ICU).

At the ICU, Aidan noticed a group of people standing around. A nurse told him that she needed to start an IV as part of the preparation for his surgery. He knew the stick might hurt, but he could take it. He was a man. However, the nurse said, "I can't get this in. I'll have to try again." The next stick hurt even worse, but Aidan thought he could take the pain if this was the last one. However, he did not appreciate having an audience of people watching his ordeal.

The nurse said, "You have bad veins so I am going to have to get someone else to try this." From out of nowhere another nurse appeared. This nurse tried to insert the IV in another spot, but again it did not work. She said, "I just blew this vein." All Aidan knew was that it hurt beyond his ability to "suck it up." He began to feel nauseous and someone handed him a basin. He was sick in front of the whole audience in the room. However, he was not finished. A new face appeared. This man said, "I am from the lab and I need to have some blood for your tests." He inserted yet another needle in Aidan's arm.

Before leaving the ICU, a nurse told him that she would send another nurse to his room to insert his IV. This person was known for his ability to insert IVs in difficult patients. Aidan was still terrified. He also felt humiliated that he was sick in front of all those people. He thought, "How can I survive in this torture chamber?"

Responses and Commentary on Questions

1. How does this case illustrate the concept of patient autonomy?

   First, you must understand that informed consent means that patients give permission for procedures that may invade their privacy and their bodies. These procedures are needed for treatment and healing. However, informed consent still requires us to respect patients' autonomy as much as possible.

   Think about Aidan's situation. First, there were three attempts to find a suitable vein for an IV. Each attempt was more painful than the previous one and Aidan was to blame for the lack of success! No one asked him about his level of pain or provided any acknowledgement of his personhood. He was just another case, expected to take the pain and remain cooperative. In addition, he was required to submit to these attempts in front of witnesses. No one told him who these people were or why they were present. How do you think he felt about his ability to exercise self-rule? Did he have any autonomy?

   In addition, Aidan was told that he had to supply a blood sample for the lab before he could be taken to his room. Imagine how embarrassed he was. He was exhausted from the pain and smelled awful, yet he was supposed to submit his body to more pain for the sake of the laboratory. This was just expected; no compassion or explanation was given. Again, you can see a lack of respect for his autonomy. It is no small wonder that he sees St. Mark's as a torture chamber.

2. What are some ways to protect Aidan's autonomy?

   First, remember that Aidan is just another patient and this is just another day in the ICU. The nurses have had difficulty with IVs before and they have seen people vomit from pain before. This is nothing new. However, this is Aidan's first experience with any hospital procedure. For him, this is not just another day. Could his autonomy be protected in this situation?

   Even though he signed an informed consent form at admission, Aidan did not know the specifics of what would happen on admission. The first thing that should have happened in the ICU was some introductions. Simply explaining to him who was in the room and why they were there would have reduced the anxiety of being observed by an unknown audience. Then, the nurse could have explained why she was inserting an IV and what she was going to do. This would have given Aidan the opportunity to understand why the pain was necessary.

When the nurse was not successful on her first try, she could have called in her back up. This person should have been the nurse who was especially trained in inserting IVs. Explaining the need to do this without blaming Aidan for having bad veins would have protected his dignity and decreased his unnecessary pain. In fact, he may have even been spared the embarrassment of being nauseous in front of everyone.

You should also consider the laboratory technician who watched Aidan's ordeal and insisted on getting his samples. He could have taken the time to explain why this additional pain was necessary and been compassionate in his attitude toward Aidan. For example, he could have assured him that he would get the sample as quickly and painlessly as possible so Aidan could be taken to his room for rest. Even a minor attempt at honoring Aidan as a person and preserving his self-respect could have gone a long way.

3. If you were the administrator of St. Mark the Ascetic Hospital, what action would you take?

This case shows the need for policies and procedures that go beyond informed consent. Of course, Aidan did provide written permission for the procedures to be performed, but he did not consent to the treatment that went with them. As administrator, you can work with the appropriate clinical staff including the director of nurses and clinical laboratories to define protocols. For example, one protocol could be only the necessary personnel are present when a patient has a procedure and that all persons in the room are introduced to the patient.

There also needs to be protocols for what happens in a difficult case. How many times should a patient be "stuck" in order to insert an IV? Is three times an acceptable number? At what point should the backup IV expert be called? At a minimum, there should be more communication with the patient and more compassion shown.

This case also makes a great argument for continuing education. The ICU nurses are generally experts at insertion of IVs. However, it does not mean that periodic sessions to renew and sharpen skills are not needed. More importantly in this case, an increased awareness of patient autonomy and the need for communication and compassion is needed. Perhaps some case studies and discussions or even role-plays about how patients feel and how they should be treated would prevent the torture chamber image of St. Mark's in the future.

Web Resources

The following are Web sites that provide additional information about areas in this chapter.

HIPAA Information
http://www.hhs.gov/ocr/hipaa/

Patient's Care Partnership (AHA)
http://www.aha.org/aha/issues/Communicating-With-Patients/pt-care-partnership.html

References

American Hospital Association. (2003). *The patient care partnership: Understanding expectations, rights, and responsibilities* [Brochure]. Chicago: Author.

Beauchamp, T. L., & Childress, J. E. (2008). *Principles of biomedical ethics* (6th ed.). New York: Oxford University Press.

Boyle, P. J., Dubose, E. R., Ellingson, S. J., Guinn, D. E., & McCurdy, D. B. (2001). *Organizational ethics in health care: Principles, cases and practical solutions*. San Francisco: Jossey-Bass.

Dosick, R. W. (2000). *The business bible: Ten commandments for creating an ethical workplace*. Woodstock, VT: Jewish Light Publishing.

Hoffman, P. B., & Nelson, W. A. (Eds.). (2001). *Managing ethically: An executive's guide*. Chicago: Health Administration Press.

Office of Civil Rights. (2008). *Understanding HIPPA privacy*. Available at: http://www.hhs.gov/ocr/privacy/hipaa/understanding/index.html. Accessed May 16, 2009.

CHAPTER 3

Nonmaleficence and Beneficence

Love and kindness are never wasted. They always make a difference.

—Barbara De Angelis

Points to Ponder

1. How does the principle of nonmaleficence affect the healthcare administrator's (HCA) role in the organization?
2. How can you avoid causing harm to employees?
3. What does the principle of beneficence have to do with operating a healthcare organization?

Words to Remember

The following is a list of key words for this chapter. You will find them in bold in the text. Stop and check your understanding of them.

beneficence   nonmaleficence

■ INTRODUCTION AND DEFINITIONS

This chapter presents two parallel principles of ethics: **nonmaleficence** and **beneficence**. Some ethics writers view these principles as inseparable cousins. Others argue that nonmaleficence is the strongest obligation of the two. Whatever the relationship, these two areas are central to a trust-based healthcare system because they are assumed by society and individuals to be its pillars of practice. This has been the case as far back as Hippocrates, who recognized these duties in his oath of practice.

Just what do these words mean? Nonmaleficence involves an ethical and legal duty to avoid harming others (Beauchamp & Childress, 2008). It is based on the Latin maxim primum non nocere or "First, do no harm." This principle involves areas of healthcare practice including treatment procedures and the rights of patients. In addition, it has an impact on how you treat employees in your practice as an HCA. You will read more about these applications in this chapter's section on nonmaleficence.

In health care, you go beyond avoiding harm to people. Your obligation is to create benefit and contribute to optimum health for individuals and the community at large. This obligation is called beneficence. Beneficence includes the obligation to help those in trouble, protect patients' rights, and provide treatment for people who need it. Kantians agree that these obligations exist because you are dealing with the basic needs of humanity and because all people have value. However, in day-to-day healthcare decisions, the utilitarian view of beneficence is often used. This involves balancing benefits of a healthcare decision against its harms. Avoiding the absolutes of Kantian logic, practice or policy decisions are made on this reciprocity. You will read more about beneficence and its implications for you as an HCA later in this chapter.

■ NONMALEFICENCE IN HEALTHCARE SETTINGS

First, do no harm. How can this be part of the principles of ethics in today's technology-centered healthcare system? Do you not have to cause patients pain and suffering to cure them? Should you not use invasive diagnostic tests and blood work to provide optimal care? Should we consider the emotional pain of receiving a diagnosis? Certainly this "first, do not harm" concept does not mean that you cannot ever cause harm to patients in order to treat them. Sometimes harmful action is necessary, but it should never be automatic. The benefits that you provide through your procedure should outweigh the suffering that you cause.

Nonmaleficence has been upheld in both the ethical and legal practices of health care. Using utilitarian logic, the benefit of procedures is balanced against the harm. If there is greater benefit, the act is viewed as an ethical one. In fact, you have a duty to provide appropriate care to avoid further harm to the patient under what some legal texts call a due care standard. This basically means that you have taken all necessary action to use the most appropriate treatment for the condition and have provided that treatment with the least amount of pain and suffering possible. From an administrative standpoint, the care should be provided by professionals with appropriate levels of education and training. Policies for safety and protection of the patient's physical health and dignity are applied to avoid harm. Infection control and other environmental practices are also part of the process of providing care and avoiding harm. Therefore, your patients receive care with a trust that it will not cause them harm even if some pain and suffering is involved.

Like many other areas of health care, nonmaleficence is complicated when advanced technology is part of the regimen. Issues around withholding or withdrawing life support, extraordinary measures, and death with dignity involve decisions about avoiding further harm to the individual. For example, healthcare professionals and family members seem to be more comfortable with withholding (i.e., not starting) treatment than withdrawing it. Somehow, what has come to be called "pulling the plug" seems more harmful to the patient than not starting the technology to support life. The line between extraordinary and ordinary care has become murkier with the advent of advanced life-sustaining technology. The now classic Terri Schiavo case is an excellent example of this level of complexity. It used to be that health care did not go to extraordinary efforts when there was no hope of benefit. However, family members, educated in the marvels of modern medicine, changed this view. The family might see what used to be called extraordinary measures as ordinary and appropriate for their loved one. Even some physicians who see death as a failure might advocate for care that prolongs some form of life but increases the suffering of the individual.

How does your work affect nonmaleficence for patients? Of course, you are not actually treating the patient, but you create an environment where this principle can be applied. For example, if advance directive policies are not in place and are not clearly written, you may be involved in policy development or refinement. If they are in place, you certainly will be involved in making sure that they are implemented appropriately. This responsibility will include periodic staff education so that staff members are clear about their responsibilities and actions. In addition, you might be working closely with an ethics committee who can advise you when challenging situations occur.

Nonmaleficence and Staff

The application of the principle of nonmaleficence is not restricted to patient treatment. It also must be considered when dealing with any member of the healthcare staff. You have an ethical obligation to provide a working environment that is safe and does not harm your employees. Such an environment allows for discussion of concerns without fear of reprisal. It should also be a positive environment where values are respected and employees can do their best work on behalf of the patients they serve (this is the I-YOU relationship). This environment should be free of harassment, imposition, and discrimination for all employees, regardless of their status in the organization.

Creation of a positive environment or climate of trust can go a long way to ensure the implementation of the principle of nonmaleficence for employees. However, situations can occur that are potentially a violation of this principle. Certainly, downsizing has a potential to cause the staff great personal and professional harm. How can you implement a layoff plan and cause the least amount of harm to employees? The American College of Healthcare Executives (ACHE) gives you some assistance through its *Policy Statement—Ethical Issues Related to a Reduction in Force* (ACHE, 2005). This statement urges you to consider both the long- and short-term impact of this decision, not only on those who will lose their jobs, but also on those who will remain in the organization. Survivor guilt can often be destructive to a positive workplace and productivity.

The ACHE also stresses the need for frequent and accurate communication with all those involved in the layoffs and the provision of as much support as possible for those who lose their jobs. Often, administrators try to avoid communication about layoffs because they fear disruption and loss of productivity. In keeping information from affected employees, they are trying to balance their view of benefits versus harm. Knowledge of what is to happen is kept to a select group. Inevitably, the rumor mill will take over for the void in accurate communication and make the situation worse. Even though it might seem to make your burden easier in a difficult situation, silence is truly not golden and can cause unnecessary harm.

It is equally important to remember those who remain after a layoff. There can be an administrative attitude of "You should think yourself lucky to have a job" and a lack of empathy for the feelings of survivors. This attitude causes unnecessary harm because it fails to acknowledge the human reaction of "Why them and not me?" or survivor guilt. Care should be taken to acknowledge what has occurred and allow time for processing the feelings associated with it. This can be done through several channels of communication including meetings, newsletters, and e-mails. In addition, communication needs to be ongoing regarding workload expectations and the potential for any future reductions in the workforce.

As an administrator, you will be dealing with diversity on many levels. Your staff are educationally diverse in that they represent a range of credentials from a GED to an MD/DO. They are also professionally diverse because they come from many different professional backgrounds, each with its own culture. They can also be ethnically diverse because they represent different cultural traditions and experiences.

Your ability to recognize this diversity, honor its differing values, and still administer a cost-effective organization will certainly pose a challenge. In order to create a culture of inclusion, you must review your policies and procedures with respect to diversity and make sure that they are designed to protect differences and decrease the potential for harm. For example, you need to make it very clear that discrimination, harassment in all forms, and sexual imposition are not tolerated. Appropriate steps need to be in place and enforced when violations occur. Looking the other way when violations occur seems easier in the immediate present, but it has a great impact in the end. Staff will come to believe that you condone behaviors that cause harm by your silence and lack of action.

Workplace bullying is another staff issue related to nonmaleficence that you must consider. Workplace bullying is a form of psychological violence that can cause great harm to staff and their families. Bullying involves aggressive behaviors toward employees including spreading untruths, social isolation, constantly changing work expectations, assigning unreasonable workloads, publicly belittling the opinions of others, and engaging in intimidation. Bullying manifests itself when there is a pattern of such behaviors (Barton & Morrison, 2004).

American employees do not have any legal protection against this form of aggression as they do with racial and age discrimination or sexual harassment. In fact, they might even see this as "business as usual," because the majority of bullies are bosses. Bosses might see this as good management or a way to get rid of those who do not agree with their management style. A lack of understanding of effective management behavior is part of the reason why bullying is so prevalent. Some experts believe that one in five employees will experience it in the workplace.

The impact of bullying on staff can be profound. First, employees sometimes take responsibility for the bully's behavior. They work harder, put in longer hours, and try to prove that they are valuable. This leads to increased stress levels and can take its toll on overall family life. However, these efforts usually fail to stop the aggression and can actually make the bully feel more powerful.

Next, targets may begin to experience psychological symptoms such as loss of confidence, depression, and helplessness. Physical symptoms may also occur including headaches, panic attacks, and hypertension. If targets question or take action concerning their treatment, they are accused of insubordination. Fellow employees try to avoid being associated with a target, so that they do not become the bully's next victim. They can even join in the aggression to stay on the bully's best side.

As you might imagine, the workplace soon becomes unhealthy and productivity is decreased. Targets of bullying absent themselves from work more frequently because of physical problems or the need to avoid the bully. They can lose their motivation to provide high quality service and just go through the motions. These actions contribute to a loss of productivity. Morale is also decreased as others see the bully's actions and wonder if they are next. Finally, turnover rates can increase as the targets choose to resign and move to another job to avoid the situation.

A stereotype of the phenomenon of workplace bullying is that it occurs only in male-dominated professions or corporate settings. However, research has shown that the top three professions for this behavior are the female-dominated fields: nursing, education, and social work (Barton & Morrison, 2004).

What should your role be in preventing workplace bullying and the harm that it causes? First, assess your own actions and communications with staff. How do you treat people whose personalities do not agree with yours? What do you do about any needed disciplinary action? Do you keep information confidential or are you part of the gossip mill? These questions and others need to be answered to be sure that you are not a bully boss.

You should also be committed to a safe and healthy workplace for all employees. This means that you need to have established policies that make it clear that all types of aggressive behavior are inappropriate in your workplace. This includes the range of behaviors from bullying to sexual harassment and physical violence. Education is critical here so that administration and staff can identify these behaviors and know what to do if they occur. Providing examples through case studies or even role-plays helps to clarify. There should also be a confidential way to make a complaint about bullying without fear of reprisal. All complaints should be taken seriously and investigated as promptly as possible to avoid revictimizing the target.

■ BENEFICENCE IN HEALTHCARE SETTINGS

Beneficence is another principle of ethics that is expected to be a given in a healthcare setting. Patients assume that you are there for their benefit and will act with charity and kindness toward them. Without this element of trust, it would be very difficult for individuals to be treated by practitioners, especially when such treatment often requires embarrassing, painful, or even life-threatening procedures. However, practicing beneficence means that healthcare personnel must make an active decision to act with compassion. This decision requires that they go beyond the minimum standards of care and consider the patients' needs and feelings. It also requires that they communicate compassionately with the patient about what is going to happen and why the treatment is necessary.

In healthcare settings, practicing beneficence is often challenging. You must deliver bad news, but you do not have to be brutal. Even a small act of compassion will be remembered. For example, active beneficence can be as simple as holding a patient's hand during a painful procedure. It can also require more effort such as taking the time to go beyond what is necessary and assure that patients receive appropriate care postdischarge. It can also involve the entire organization through community service projects that have nothing to do with profit, but everything to do with compassion for the community.

Making the decision to be actively beneficent fits well with Buber's I-YOU and, even in some cases, I-THOU relationship. It acknowledges that each patient as a unique individual who has worth. From a business standpoint, it increases the organization's positive image and level of trust in the community. However, it is not without a price. It is not easy to practice this principle on a daily basis because it requires a spirit of giving that is not always rewarded. Think about the real business of health care. You often see people at their worst, when they are in pain or deep grief. You also see things happen to people that others in the community never see and do not understand. Suffering and dying are part of your professional life. You need to decide how much you can give to patients and retain balance in your life (Tong, 2007).

The real beneficence challenge is consistently treating patients with compassion even under stressful circumstances. Effort and training are required to accomplish this goal on a daily basis. Often personnel are emotionally exhausted at the end of the day and experience what has been called compassion exhaustion or burnout. They feel like they simply cannot give any more. Yet, the next patient still expects the same level of caring received in the previous encounter.

It is important to remember the effort required to provide active beneficence and do what can be done to foster it among staff. It can be as simple as telling staff members how much you appreciate their efforts. It might include publishing in the newsletter (with the patient's permission, of course) a thank-you note from a patient or the family written to the staff. It can also mean watching the amount of overtime hours worked and allowing staff enough flexibility to use their vacation time for vacation. Some institutions even use rewards programs with various titles like "Caught You Caring." They provide cash rewards to staff who have done something that demonstrates active beneficence. Their photographs can be placed in the lobby. (A word of caution: While some of these ideas sound like great ways to boost staff morale, they are not always well received by patients. Some patients feel that staff should not have to be "caught caring." They assume the staff will be caring at all times.)

Beneficence also should also be included in the organization's planning function conducting a cost/benefit analysis for decision-making. In this model, there is an attempt to balance community or business benefit against potential harms. It seems to be useful for many types of healthcare organizations with differing financial structures and including public health organizations. This system would certainly be supported by utilitarians, who see ethics as the greatest good for the greatest number. However, cost/benefit analysis as a decision-making model is sometimes difficult to implement effectively. It requires time for accurate data collection, openness to discussion, and the application of the principles of ethics to final decisions. Generally, this extra effort is well worth it because the organization can justify its actions to its board and community at large. You will learn more about beneficence in decision making in a later chapter in this text.

Beneficence and Staff

As an administrator, you should strive to have a climate of caring in both your formal and informal organization. While you cannot guarantee that your employees will always practice active beneficence, you can work to create a culture where this behavior is reinforced. The way in which employees are treated in the organization can do much to create this culture of compassion.

A compassion deficit can occur when patients are provided active beneficence, but employees are not. The message taken by employees is that they do not matter in the organization. They can be replaced at any minute. It is easy to see that this impression does not foster the motivation to go beyond the minimum requirements in caring for patients or for each other. The organization becomes a place to do one's time and hang on until retirement.

Your behavior and attitude as an administrator can help you prevent such attitudes from having a negative impact on your organization. You can use your power to increase the dignity and growth of staff. For example, you can choose to praise your employees in public for the work that they do, rather than just assume that it is their job to do well. If corrections need to be made, you can choose to do this in private and in a constructive manner. By practicing respect and honoring an individual's work, you help to foster a climate of caring (Dye, 2000).

Being an administrator in a culture of compassion requires more than knowledge of budgets and strategic planning. You must practice "stewarding with respect" (Dye, 2000, p. 33). This means that you use your influence as an administrator to ensure completion of the necessary work, but you do it in a manner that promotes self-esteem and demonstrates respect. There are several ways to do this but they require some degree of effort. For example, you can choose to seek out information and ideas from staff before you make decisions. While you do not have to use every idea that is offered, asking and considering others' ideas is part of respect. Offering guidance to employees when tasks need to be done rather than "barking orders" also shows respect. This can also be cost effective because the time spent in clarification can prevent costly errors or resentful, passive aggressive behavior. Not only should you show appreciation for your employees and their work, but you should also be appropriately enthusiastic about the work that you do. In addition, you can demonstrate enthusiasm for the mission of your organization and department. If you cannot, perhaps it is time for a job search.

Last, but not least, you need to think about being a good steward to yourself. You need to practice frequent self-assessment so that you can build on your strengths and work on your weaknesses. You need to be willing to own your mistakes and apologize when necessary. As an administrator, you need to consider yourself a lifelong learner and be open to new knowledge and practices. Because all of these ideas will take effort on your part, you need to practice self-protection through whatever means works best for you. This can mean planning quiet time in your day, taking time out for exercise, remembering that family counts too, and planning real vacations for self-renewal. These actions are not only a benefit to you, but actually assist the organization. You will have greater energy to provide the kind of leadership that encourages a culture where active beneficence is the norm, rather than the exception.

Summary

Nonmaleficence and beneficence are often viewed as paired principles because they seem to be linked together. Actually, nonmaleficence requires only that you prevent individuals from being harmed. This act of prevention can involve creating an environment where treatment can be practiced in a safe manner and where employees can be free from harassment in its many forms.

Beneficence requires that you go beyond prevention to ethical action. You work to respect the individuality (I-YOU relationship) of all employees and find ways to nurture them. Making the effort to be a steward of resources and talent is, in itself, a virtue but it can also have a positive impact on your bottom line. It is much more cost-effective to do the small things that are necessary to build employee morale and retention than to pay the price of constant recruitment and rehiring.

Cases for Your Consideration

The Case of the Academic Bully

As you read this case, consider the following questions. Responses and comments will follow the case.

1. Why did Ms. Nodons treat Dr. Xenia differently than Dr. Kado?

2. What was the impact of her actions on the overall morale of the department?

3. Why did Dr. Xenia resign and what was the impact of this action?

4. What could have prevented this situation?

Case Information

This case occurred in an academic healthcare setting, but the behaviors seen here are typical of bullying in hospitals, clinics, and other environments. After 20 years in nursing and hospital administration, Ms. Nodons was appointed the director of the health studies program at St. Dismas University. With her leadership, this program had grown to over 200 undergraduate students. She received approval to begin a master of health studies (MHS) program. With this approval came authorization to hire two doctoral-prepared faculty, and Ms. Nodons was excited about the prospect. After conducting a national search, Dr. Kado was hired. Dr. Kado was a recent doctoral graduate and was given a position as an assistant professor. Ms. Nodons also hired Dr. Xenia as an associate professor.

Ms. Nodons immediately charged Dr. Xenia with the task of designing the curriculum for the new MHS program. Dr. Xenia clarified her responsibilities and formulated plans for data collection, objective writing, and curriculum design. She then presented a draft of these ideas at a faculty meeting for consideration. However, Ms. Nodons's reaction to Dr. Xenia's work came as a total surprise. She began to attack Dr. Xenia verbally, asking her, "Just who do you think you are?" She followed this up with the abrupt statement, "I am the boss here, and I make the decisions, not you." The other faculty members just sat in silence. Dr. Xenia was shocked and tried to explain that she was only trying to come up with a plan for the project. She also apologized for any misunderstanding that she might have caused.

From that time on, Ms. Nodons's negativity toward Dr. Xenia became even more evident. Dr. Kado was granted special travel money to attend meetings, allowed to have flexible work hours, and given high visibility committee assignments. Dr. Xenia was chastised if she was not at work at 8:30 A.M. or used sick leave. She was denied travel funds for meetings and had to use her own money to finance these trips. Faculty meetings became excruciating for Dr. Xenia because any comment she made was immediately attacked. In contrast, all of Dr. Kado's ideas were applauded as brilliant.

When she made an appointment with Ms. Nodons to discuss the situation, she was accused of being paranoid and insubordinate and was called a failure as a team player. The meeting also led to retaliation from Ms. Nodons in the form of increasingly personal comments about Dr. Xenia at faculty meetings. Ms. Nodons also began to complain about Dr. Xenia to her fellow faculty members, accusing the associate professor of "not knowing her place." These faculty members reported the comments back to Dr. Xenia to "help her" but did nothing to defend her, either publicly or privately.

Dr. Xenia tried to maintain high standards of teaching despite all the strain of preparing her courses, the lack of collegial support, and the increasing intensity of bullying behaviors by her boss. While she had been an award-winning teacher in the past, she began to doubt her ability to teach. She also experienced physical symptoms including headaches, acid reflux disease, and panic attacks while driving to work. Her blood pressure increased dramatically and she was placed on medication to control it.

Trying to be a problem solver, Dr. Xenia considered making an appointment with the dean to discuss the situation. However, the dean was a friend of Ms. Nodons. In fact, they had been friends for 20 years and regularly played tennis and golf together. When she discussed her situation with the human resources department, she was told that there were no grounds for any inquiry. The advice she was given was just to live with the misery until Ms. Nodons retired or quit. Her administrative assistant promised to warn her when Nodons was having a "bad day" so that she could stay clear. Dr. Xenia assessed the situation, began a job search, and resigned.

Responses and Commentary on Questions

1. Why did Ms. Nodons treat Dr. Xenia differently from Dr. Kado?

   There could be any number of explanations for difference in treatment between the two faculty members. First, it is possible that Ms. Nodons simply did not like Dr. Xenia's personality. There could have been something about Dr. Xenia that "rubbed her the wrong way." Of course, she did not acknowledge this even to herself. Second, the difference in treatment could have been because Dr. Kado was male and Dr. Xenia was female. Ms. Nodons, through her life experience and education as a nurse, could have been taught to defer to males. Dr. Kado was also a brand new doctorate, so perhaps he posed less of a threat to Ms. Nodons than Dr. Xenia did.

   Whatever the reasons behind the behavior, Ms. Nodons's actions certainly fit many of the signs of bullying described earlier in this chapter. However, she probably did not see herself as a bully. She was used to unquestioned obedience in her former nursing and administrative positions. She ran a tight department with large class sizes and low faculty-to-student ratios. Although she had never had a female faculty member, she felt competent to handle women in general. She wanted to teach Dr. Xenia to know her place and not cause any problems.

   Comment: Remember that bullying behavior is sometimes perceived as good management, especially when it has been reinforced in the past. In Ms. Nodons's previous work experience, she was probably rewarded for "keeping her nurses in line" so that the work of the hospital was accomplished with minimal interference. In her academic career, she was the sole source of power, so any form of questioning was not even in her experience. She also viewed any questioning of her actions as a lack of obedience and insubordination. A collegial model is usually found in an academic setting but it was not part of her administrative background. Ms. Nodons's administrative style should certainly not be emulated but should make you stop and think about your own interactions with staff.

2. What was the impact of her actions on the overall morale of the department?

When you think about this question, try to view the big picture. Was Dr. Xenia really the only one affected here? How about Dr. Kado? Initially, it must have been great to be the "golden one" and have all of your ideas praised. It also must have been nice to have special benefits that others did not have. However, a golden status can be fleeting. What happens if he does something that has a negative impact on Ms. Nodons? Will he face the same treatment that was afforded to Dr. Xenia? Of course, if he was functioning at the Buber I-You level of ethical relationship, he might not be happy with the treatment he sees Dr. Xenia getting. He might also consider a job change to avoid her fate.

How were the rest of the faculty and staff affected? You can well imagine that this is not a healthy workplace when the administrative staff has to figure out if each day is a bad one or a good one. Can you imagine how unpleasant faculty meetings are for everyone? The lesson taught, through the treatment of Dr. Xenia, was to keep your mouth shut unless you want the same treatment. Obviously, a flow of creative ideas did not occur, and the potential was great for stagnation and high turnover.

There was also no discussion about teaching assignments in this department. Faculty taught what they were told to teach even when they did not have sufficient expertise in the area, or time to develop that expertise. Maybe Ms. Nodon purposely made class sizes extremely large to boost her to high productivity statistics within the institution. The result was either a high potential for faculty burnout, or the provision of low quality instruction, or both. Overall, this was an unhealthy environment, with some of the faculty just biding their time until they retired—or until Ms. Nodons did.

3. Why did Dr. Xenia resign and what was the impact of this action?

Dr. Xenia resigned because she had no power to counteract the environment in which she found herself. After attempting to address her concerns with Ms. Nodons without success, her next step should have been to make an appointment with her dean. However, the close personal relationship between the dean and Ms. Nodons made this seem futile. The human resources department was not even aware that bullying in the workplace was an issue, so they were not of any assistance. Faced with an unfixable situation and increasing health concerns, Dr. Xenia made a decision that was appropriate for her.

This decision had impact on many aspects of the program. Immediately, Ms. Nodons sent out an e-mail to all faculty stating that Dr. Xenia had resigned because she was a poor team member and did not fit well in the department. However, faculty who knew Dr. Xenia well questioned this and began to wonder who would be next in the "pecking order." Fearing that the work environment would only get worse, Dr. Kado also began a search for a new position, even though he had been afforded special treatment.

Adjunct faculty had to be hired to take over Dr. Xenia's heavy course load. This required four different adjuncts a semester and added additional expense to an already tight department budget. A national search, with all of its expenses, had to be conducted to find a replacement. This took over a year and was not successful.

Students in the graduate program were particularly affected by this resignation and began to question the stability of the new MHS program. Several of them chose to transfer to a competitor institution that was perceived to be more stable. The loss of student base threatened the future of the program and its expansion.

Comment: The important thing to remember here is that keeping a healthy workplace that is free from bullying and other forms of aggressive behavior is much more cost-effective than losing staff. Think about all of the unnecessary harm that happened to the survivor faculty, students, staff, and—yes—even to Ms. Nodons. Certainly, her days are now more stressful because of the additional burden of making sure classes are taught and searching for replacement faculty. Much of her stress could have been avoided by exercising a different administrative style.

4. What could have prevented this situation?

How could St. Dismas University have addressed or prevented harm caused by bullying? The first action that should have been taken was to increase awareness of this issue. No one at St. Dismas University had even considered bullying to be an issue for academe. Awareness might need to start at the University level, rather than the school or department, by having significant and influential personnel receive training in the recognition of bullying and its effects. Information on appropriate policy development should also be a part of this training opportunity.

Once trained, the group could work with the human resources department to develop policy and procedures to inform all faculty and staff about acceptable and unacceptable behaviors. Procedures about complaints and investigations would be delineated. Of course, once this policy is developed, additional training would be required, starting with the administrative level. In addition, the organization must be willing to enforce the policy even if it means the dismissal of department heads or deans. Failure to take action when a proved case of bullying exists means that such behavior is acceptable, if not encouraged.

The Case of the Beneficent Boss

As you read this case, consider the following questions. Responses and comments will follow the case.

1. Why did Ms. Dee choose to take the actions that she did in Cindy's case?
2. What was the impact of her actions on the staff?
3. What was the impact of her actions on Cindy?
4. What was the impact of Ms. Dee's actions on the bottom line of the New Hope Community Program?

Case Information

Ms. Teresa Dee was a human resources director for a small nonprofit organization called the New Hope Community Program (NHCP) that was funded through United Way and other community sponsors. Its mission was to decrease the relapse rate of substance abusers by providing the knowledge and skills needed to obtain and keep jobs. Using effective prevention methods to reduce treatment costs for these individuals was also part of the NHCP mission.

Once a client was employed after completing her program, Ms. Dee had the responsibility of serving as liaison between the employer and the client. This required frequent follow-up contacts with both parties. Follow-up duties could be delegated to appropriate staff, but she tried to do her fair share so that they were not overwhelmed.

One Monday morning, Ms. Dee walked out of her office and saw a thin, young, blond, unkempt woman waiting in the reception area. A review of the referral form from St. Dismas Drug Rehabilitation Center revealed that the client's name was Cindy Rumford and that she had only six months' sobriety. She was only 17 years old but had already had six arrests for prostitution. Ms. Dee's experience told her that Cindy had an uphill struggle ahead at best.

The initial interview was not a positive one. Cindy's appearance and demeanor showed almost no self-confidence and her responses were barely audible. Ms. Dee was able to determine that she had not finished high school, had no discernible job skills, and did not know what she wanted to do with the rest of her life. When asked if she was serious about staying sober, she quietly replied, "Well, I guess I can. I want you to help me make it." Such a response was not a good omen for a positive result for this client. Yet, Ms. Dee sensed something in Cindy that warranted further attention. After all, helping people like Cindy was the mission of NHCP.

From that initial intake visit, she took particular interest in Cindy. She held a staff meeting to design a plan to meet Cindy's immediate needs for safe housing, clothing, food, and transportation to the program office. After settling on a plan, the staff worked with Cindy so that these basics could be met. Next, she explained NHCP's Work for Recovery Program to Cindy. She could sign a contract with the Program to attend classes to complete her GED and learn basic work habits like applying for jobs, maintaining a good business appearance including dress and makeup, and learning skills to interview and communicate appropriately. Once she completed her classes, Cindy was required to work at the Program Office for three months.

During Cindy's training period, Ms. Dee took special interest in her progress. At first, she seemed to be a passive learner who barely made eye contact with the staff. She did show some interest when an employer came to talk to the class about what he expected from his employees. The day she passed her GED seemed to begin a real turnaround for Cindy. It was the first time Ms. Dee saw her smile.

Cindy's three-month trial employment at the program began with housekeeping activities. Ms. Dee made a point to tell her how well she was doing with her attendance and attention to detail. Gradually, she increased Cindy's responsibilities to include reception and office work. Cindy's confidence seemed to grow with each new responsibility. By the end of her contract-training period, she had become a more confident person with a professional appearance and a ready smile.

Ms. Dee contacted those employers whom she knew would be open to giving Cindy an opportunity to continue to build her work skills. After only one interview, she was hired by a small company as an office assistant. Ms. Dee decided to follow up personally on her placement rather than to delegate it to the staff. Although there were a few rough times, Cindy maintained her sobriety and her position. Ms. Dee still gets Christmas cards from Cindy thanking her for caring and the difference she made in her life.

1. Why did Ms. Dee choose to take the actions that she did in Cindy's case?

   Ms. Dee had seen many "Cindys" in her position as human resources director. Some of them completed the program and went on to become sober and productive citizens. However, many of them chose to drop out when it became too difficult. Still others completed it but relapsed when faced with the pressures of the real world. Experience should have made Ms. Dee cynical about Cindy's chances. Yet, she chose to act with beneficence. Perhaps she saw something in her demeanor that others did not see. Perhaps it was just her nature to refrain from generalizing from previous experiences to the current one. Whatever the reason, Ms. Dee decided to act with kindness in this case and remain hopeful.

Ms. Dee was also being true to the mission of her organization and her position as an administrator. If you consider its purpose, all of NHCP's activities were rooted in the principle of beneficence. As an administrator, she had the obligation to demonstrate its mission in action. Her decision to live the mission rather than just post it on the walls might have added to her already busy workload, but the time she spent with Cindy seemed to make the sacrifice worthwhile. In addition, Ms. Dee had the personal satisfaction of knowing that her actions made a difference.

2. What was the impact of her actions on the staff?

As an administrator in a small organization, Ms. Dee was highly visible to the staff. In addition, her multiple roles ensured that she was not "office bound" but had the opportunity to interact with them on many occasions. Because of this situation, she served as a role model, not just for Cindy, but for the staff as well. When she took extra time to praise Cindy for her efforts, it was noticed. When she followed up on her status when she was not mandated to do so, it was noticed. When she remained positive about Cindy's future in spite of her odds, it was noticed. She did not have to preach about the mission of NHCP and what it meant; she exhibited it through her interactions.

Her behavior toward staff compared well to her actions toward clients. She listened to their concerns, acted on suggestions that were appropriate and feasible, and gave credit to the staff members who suggested them. She always made a point to acknowledge the work of her team. When there was a staff issue, she held a frank and documented discussion with the individual including the development of an action plan for improving the situation. She lived the mission with her staff and her clients.

Because actions really do speak louder than words, Ms. Dee set the norm for the organization. Staff members tried to emulate her behaviors and in turn used active beneficence in their dealings with their clients. While the relapse rates for all of their clients did not change dramatically, there was a shift to the positive in their yearly statistics. In addition, overall morale seemed to be much more positive and clients seemed more appreciative. The result was that, on most days, the staff was happy to do their meaningful work, and the clients reaped the benefits of their attitudes and actions. Turnover was very low, which saved the organization thousands of dollars in lost productivity, recruitment, and re-staffing funds.

Comment: You should remember that as an administrator what you do is noticed. This should not make you paranoid, but should help you to motivate your staff. A variation of The Golden Rule works here. Do unto your staff well, and by your example, it is more likely that the staff will do their jobs well. Therefore, this means that you must at least understand the jobs that your staff do and be willing to "pitch in" when necessary. On a daily basis, if you want an environment where beneficence is the norm, then you must choose to practice it in your actions toward others.

You also should remember that when you treat a client with beneficence but deny it to your staff, you are creating an environment of inconsistency. The morale of your department can quickly deteriorate when you see the staff's efforts as "just doing their jobs." They will get the message that they can be replaced at any minute with anybody. This lack of active beneficence will reinforce an I-It relationship with you. Because no one really wants to be replaceable, morale will decrease even among your most dedicated staff. Your potential for high turnover and its associated costs will grow, as will your negative reputation with the higher echelon.

3. What was the impact of her actions on Cindy?

Certainly, this decision to practice the principle of beneficence made a difference to Cindy. Maybe this was the first person who took a special interest in her well-being. Cindy responded to even the smallest positive comment from Ms. Dee. The encouragement bolstered her own determination to stop her cycle of addiction and its consequences.

In addition, Ms. Dee made a point to have Cindy's first real world work experience be with a person who practiced active beneficence. Her new employer continued to foster Cindy's confidence and self-esteem. She was not treated as a charity case but as a true employee of the firm and offered the same level of respect. While there were times when she made errors, she was given assistance to correct any problems. Because of the training and affirmation she received from Ms. Dee and the staff, Cindy was able to become a valued employee in her new position. Having a job and the income it provided gave her the opportunity to live a different and healthier lifestyle.

4. What was the impact of Ms. Dee's actions on the bottom line of the New Hope Community Program?

Certainly, one person cannot make or break an organization, but he or she can have a positive impact. In the case of Cindy, Ms. Dee and her staff were able to see that practicing beneficence brought both personal and organizational rewards. While NHCP's success rates were not perfect, the overall environment of beneficence toward clients and staff did produce less staff turnover and better client results. It is true that this decision took more effort and time than "business as usual," but the reward of a positive work environment offset the investment, making it a positive return on investment.

Comment: Sometimes, the small stuff makes a difference or makes a statement. For example, a chief executive officer (CEO) of a major hospital makes a point to pick up any trash seen each morning on the way in from the parking lot. This is a small action indeed, but it carries a large message about pride in an organization. When employees observe or hear about this behavior, they think "If the CEO can pick up trash, then maybe I should care about this place, too."

Beneficence is cost-effective because actions of charity and kindness well outweigh the costs of time and effort. It seems so easy to do on the surface, yet you will all get busy with your daily efforts and crises and forget that there are humans behind those full-time equivalents. Therefore, the practice of active beneficence requires a daily decision to act within Kant, Frankl, and Buber principles. The organization, your employees, and your career will gain the benefits of this decision.

Web Resources

Classic version of the Hippocratic Oath
http://www.pbs.org/wgbh/nova/doctors/oath_classical.html

Bullying in the Workplace
http://www.safety-council.org/info/OSH/bullies.html
http://www.ccohs.ca/oshanswers/psychosocial/bullying.html

References

American College of Healthcare Executives. (2005). *Policy statement: Ethical issues related to a reduction in force.* [Electronic version]. Chicago: Author.

Barton, G. M., & Morrison, E. E. (2006, January/February). What happens when harassment is personal? *Journal of Medical Practice Management*, 21(4): 1–4.

Beauchamp, T. L., & Childress, J. E. (2008). *Principles of biomedical ethics* (6th ed.). New York: Oxford University Press.

Dye, C. F. (2000). *Leadership in healthcare: Values at the top.* Chicago: Health Administration Press.

Tong, R. (2007). *New perspectives in healthcare ethics: An interdisciplinary and crosscultural approach.* Upper Saddle River, NJ: Prentice Hall.

CHAPTER 4

Justice

I know, up on top you are seeing great sights,
But down at the bottom we, too, should have rights.

—Dr. Seuss

Points to Ponder

1. What is patient justice? Why is it difficult to practice?
2. What are the different positions on distributive justice?
3. How does distributive justice affect a healthcare organization?
4. What does it mean to be a just administrator for staff?

Words to Remember

The following is a list of key words for this chapter. You will find them in bold in the text. Stop and check your understanding of them.

distributive justice
justice
staff justice

ethicist
patient justice

■ INTRODUCTION AND DEFINITIONS

Before you deal with the application of the principle of justice, it is important to understand what it means in healthcare settings. When dealing with people, whether they are patients or staff, **justice** is concerned with doing what is perceived to be fair or deserved. This implies an active ethical response in each situation so that people in equal situations are treated equally. However, justice does not apply just to individuals. The term **distributive justice** is used when considering what is fair and appropriate to protect the rights of a community or society with respect to its resources. Since groups in American society view distributive justice very differently, this is an area of great controversy for both society and the healthcare system. As an administrator, you will struggle with different societal and organizational views and will have to come to a viable compromise for your organization. In this chapter, you will learn more about this form of justice. In addition, you will explore aspects of **patient justice** and **staff justice**.

■ JUSTICE FOR PATIENTS

When people enter the healthcare system at any level, they believe that they will be treated with fairness and that their needs will be met expeditiously. They believe that they will be treated with respect regardless of their lifestyle or financial circumstances. Egotistically, patients believe that you will do everything you can to heal them. Their primary view is that healthcare organizations are places where healing is the mission. Television and advertisements can reinforce this view. Health care is often presented as a place where restoring or protecting health is the primary mission. Seldom is there any mention of the business aspects of health care or the resources needed to stay in business.

The American healthcare system might not be able to live up to this idealized patient view. From a treatment standpoint, there can be times when a patient does not get the full attention of the system no matter what his or her financial circumstances. For example, in a busy emergency department (ED), a screaming child with an earache might have to wait far longer than his parents view as fair. This "unfairness" happens when people with more severe emergencies enter the ED at the same time as the child. While this system of prioritizing is necessary, unless it is explained to the parents, it can be viewed as unjust.

While patient justice seems to indicate that all patients who have the same healthcare issues should be treated the same way, it is not an easy principle to maintain. First, health care truly is a business and not all patients have the ability to pay for its services. Depending on what statistics you read, there are 47 million uninsured people in the United States. Who will pay for their care when it is needed? Because insurance is linked to access, these individuals might not receive the same level of care as those who are well insured (Shi & Singh, 2008). You will learn more about this issue in the section about distributive justice.

Even if they can pay for services, some patients stretch the professional's ability to apply the principle of patient justice. The personality or life choices of a patient might offend the professional's personal values and sense of professionalism. Yet, these health professionals are expected to act with justice even when patients demonstrate unpleasant behaviors, are filthy, or verbally abusive. They must also be just when patients are arrogant and demanding.

Such behaviors should not affect patient justice, but they do. The daily exposure to demanding, unpleasant, or challenging patients puts a definite strain on the ability to act with justice. Some professionals react to the strain by using labeling and dark humor as a protection. For example, you can find the term GOMER (get out of my emergency room) used instead of a patient's name. People become "Its" instead of humans when justice is strained.

Active patient justice requires positive consistency. This means that you strive to treat each patient with dignity and justice, as Kant and others would advocate. It also requires careful observation and discernment to determine the best way to act with justice for each person. For example, one patient might find a simple touch on the shoulder reassuring, while another might find it offensive. Your goal should be an I-THOU relationship while you are in the patient's presence. In other words, he or she should be the most important thing to you at that moment.

However, the ability to use careful observation and positive consistency in behavior is not innate. It must be taught in schools by focusing on the human elements of care and not just clinical skills. It has to be reinforced in the workplace through role modeling, in-service education, and frequent reminders. Work practices such as shift scheduling and taking meal breaks can decrease "compassion fatigue" and increase the likelihood that patient justice will be the norm in your facility.

■ DISTRIBUTIVE JUSTICE

Definitions

The principle of distributive justice involves the appropriate and fair distribution of the benefits offered by a society. It also includes the distribution of the burdens for these benefits (Beauchamp & Childress, 2008). Just what does this mean? In health care, the available benefits are not limitless and many resources are scarce. Distributive justice reflects how society decides who gets the benefits of health treatment, how much they get, and who pays for them.

Distributive justice in health care seems simple on the surface. People who need medical services should get them, and those with the same diagnosis should be treated equally. However, the United States is a market-driven economy; how it defines who needs assistance and the mechanisms for providing such assistance are not that simple. For example, if people have risky lifestyles and do not take good care of their health, should they be given free health care? In a market driven economy, this simply does not make good business sense. On the other hand, is it just to allow people to suffer and die prematurely because they did not follow all of the rules for good health? The answers to these questions are even more confounded by the knowledge that determinants of illness are complex and not always linked to personal lifestyle choices.

In the United States, access to health care is linked to the insurance coverage. While government is becoming increasingly more involved in the financing of health care, the backbone of the system is still the employer-provided insurance system (Shi & Singh, 2008). Approximately 63% of the American population has this coverage, but it varies in its benefits. Another 25% of the population has private or publicly supported insurance. However, there are people who have no coverage for a variety of reasons, including those who have a high-risk status or conditions that are excluded from policies, who work for companies that do not offer plans, or who are unable to pay for private coverage. This group of over 47 million Americans includes over 9 million children. While access to health care alone does not guarantee health, some would argue that the problem of the uninsured constitutes a failure of distributive justice.

Theories of Distributive Justice

Why is health care for all Americans not provided through the government as it is in many other industrialized countries in the world? Would that not be distributive justice? A discussion of the differing views of distributive justice and rights prevalent in American thinking might help you better understand this quandary. Each of the views on this topic is founded in principles based on societal and ethical arguments and traditions. In this section, you will examine the basic concepts of the views that commonly apply to health care. This should assist you in understanding why "just pay for it" might not be the best answer for the U.S. healthcare system.

First, think about the utilitarian position. Utilitarians tend to view justice in health care as taking actions that can provide the greatest amount of benefit to people or prevent the greatest amount of harm. They favor public health activities such as sanitation, air pollution control, and protection against epidemics, which would improve the health for the entire population. They also find the provision of basic services to all as a form of distributive justice.

However, in the purest form, the utilitarian position might support denying access and treatment to the frail elderly, or the most gravely ill. In this view, these population groups use a disproportionate amount of scarce healthcare resources and tend to have poor treatment outcomes. The money spent on them might be better used to benefit society through prevention programs and prevent the greatest harm to the greatest number of people. However, this analysis certainly does not appeal to the families of individuals in vulnerable situations or to those who are forced to deny them care.

The free market or strict business approach to distributive justice takes the position that health care is a business and not a right. In a business, providers of goods and services should be able to provide them or deny them in order to make a profit. In addition, those who work and earn income should be able to purchase goods and services in accordance with their wealth. When this is translated into health care, those who have the funds have the right and the freedom to purchase the health care that they choose. Physicians and other healthcare providers also have the right to provide such care or to refuse it based on the individual's ability to pay. There is no moral obligation to provide health care any more than there is a moral obligation to provide any other commodity (such as a home, a coat, or a hamburger).

The market position on distributive justice makes sense when you consider the bottom line in running any business. Payroll and expenses must be met and stockholders or the community must receive a fair return on their investment. To survive in a competitive environment, there must also be a sound fiscal foundation. While you might feel compassion for people and their situations, you still have to keep the doors of your facility open. This concept is where the phrase "no margin, no mission" has its origin.

Because American culture is based on its capitalist success, on the surface, this approach makes a good deal of sense. However, in the court of public opinion, a healthcare institution would not fare well if it applied this concept of distributive justice as its operational definition. If your mission statement reads "Profit Is Number One," the media would certainly portray your facility as "Scrooge Hospital." Certainly, the government would not look favorably on your denying access to patients and might try to deny you payment or close you down. Therefore, the market view of distributive justice, while it has some merit, cannot be the only principle for decision making about the use of health resources.

Rawls would argue that distributive justice means that people need to have fair access to health care when they need it. However, not all persons have the same ability to access healthcare services because of economic or other barriers. Society has an obligation to do what it can to eliminate or reduce those barriers. By meeting this ethical obligation, it would allow people to increase access to care. Restoring and maintaining health also allows each person to be a full member of society (Beauchamp & Childress, 2008).

However, this position does not mean that all people should be given everything that the healthcare system has available. It does not mean that, just because you want a "tummy tuck," you should get one free of charge. What it does mean is that, regardless of your social or insurance status, you should have access to adequate basic health care. Those who have insurance or the financial means should be able to purchase services beyond this basic level.

Already you can see a problem with this position. The term "adequate basic health care" is incredibly vague. Just what does this mean? People of high ethical thinking and an understanding of the American economic system have argued this for years. Often this argument leads to a discussion about what basic health care is not, rather than what it is. The state of Oregon attempted to identify basic health care for its Medicaid patients by using an elaborate system that included citizen input. While this attempt was laudable, it caused some real public relations nightmares for the state. However, even if it is not popular, this issue will not disappear. If anything, the need to grapple with it will increase as the boomers come of retirement age and use more of the nation's healthcare resources. Who will be entitled to services and how will Americans finance it?

Issues for Healthcare Organizations

The application of distributive justice can bring many concerns at the organizational level. Each organization has to create its definition of justice or fair treatment for patients. This definition should consider the positions that you have just examined. What is the organization's obligation to its community for just care? How will it balance its fiduciary obligation to its stockholders, payers, and others with this obligation? How does your organization define basic health care for those it serves? Should care be different based solely on the ability to pay or will other criteria determine this? These questions should not be taken lightly. They require an investment of time and resources to formulate an ethically sound position. You might even need to use an **ethicist** or specialist on ethics on a consultant basis to assist in defining your position on these issues. If you serve in a religious-based facility, the answers to these questions can form a major part of your mission statement.

Distributive justice on an organizational level is more than theory, discussion, and mission statements. For example, your facility might have invested a good deal of capital and staffing on its oncology services. It might pride itself on this effort and even advertise them on radio and television. However, your advertisement campaign can backfire if too many of these high-risk patients use your services. What if their needs are not fully covered by insurance or, even worse, what if they have no insurance at all? The community expects that you will provide the just and compassionate treatment that you have advertised. However, you still must maintain your bottom line (Pearson, Sabin, & Emanuel, 2003).

What does this mean for the practicing healthcare administrator (HCA) when both high-risk and high-profit patients are served? First, the organization must construct its definition of just treatment in this case. For some organizations, each service is a business entity, so it must make a profit like all other entities. In this case, you would have to balance the number of Medicare, Medicaid, and charity care patients against those who are well insured so that you do not have a profit drain. You might have to limit the number of these cases to preserve your profit status.

Another way for the organization to deal with this issue is to limit its service area so that only those high-risk patients in this defined area are served. While this can mean turning some people away, it could allow you to concentrate on providing quality care to those who are in your service area. The disadvantage of this approach is that it limits you from expanding your service area into more lucrative markets.

For some facilities, the service of high-risk patients is the mission. This is typically found in faith-based facilities. Their mission emphasis means that they must concentrate more on the ethics side of the equation rather than just the business side. However, they must still find the funds to treat these individuals. Care for high-risk patients becomes part of their business and fundraising strategies in the community.

Whatever approach is taken in planning for high-risk patients, Pearson, Sabin, and Emanuel's (2003) research provides some solid information to guide you. First, it is important to assess your community and its high-risk patient potential. You must use whatever data are available through state and local sources to get a snapshot of your community's health status, its resources, and its culture. This assessment of both medical and social health will give you the ability to plan your programs with more realistic detail. In thinking about this population and its needs, provide ways for easy access to your system to address questions and concerns and to educate. Time spent on this effort can potentially save you from costly treatments later.

They also stress the need for timely access to your services in the broadest definition of that word. High-risk patients can face many barriers to using your services including transportation, language difficulties, and a lack of insurance coverage or inadequate understanding of coverage. You might need to be very creative to be able to provide true access for these patients, including coordinating or even providing transportation, helping with insurance coverage, and providing adequate patient education. If your mission includes services to this population, this extra effort can benefit both the patients and the organization by making sure services are used and funded appropriately.

■ STAFF JUSTICE

The concept of justice is also about fairness and equity for employees. You should begin your understanding of staff justice by realizing that, as an administrator, you have both title power and subtle power. First, you have a title and all of the responsibilities and accountabilities that go with it. This alone gives you a certain amount of authority or you could not do your job. However, perhaps even more important, you have subtle power. How you present yourself, what you say, and how you say it can be perceived as fair and just—or just the opposite.

Of course, your title alone does not make you a model for ethics in your department or area. How you treat staff determines the climate for what is expected and how people will treat each other. You need to be concerned that your behaviors enhance fairness and decrease the likelihood of inequity. For example, even though you like some staff more than others, you should not have lunch with them every day to the exclusion of the others. Exclusionary lunches with you are more than burgers and fries; they provide a connotation of favored status. Whether this is true or not does not matter. The image is set and inequity is perceived.

Think about when perceived injustice has happened to you in a job. How did it make you feel? Certainly, you saw this taking place in The Case of the Academic Bully from Chapter 3. For no easily discernible reason, Ms. Nodons (the boss/bully) gave Dr. Kado preferential treatment, and Dr. Xenia was victimized. It seemed that Ms. Nodons preferred Dr. Kado's personality, style, and even his gender over that of Dr. Xenia. Ms. Nodons also mistreated her support staff. It was fine to abuse them verbally, she thought; they were not faculty. However, Ms. Nodons never saw herself as an unjust administrator. She believed that she was top-notch, ran a tight ship, and kept her people in line. However, contrary to her belief, she was the administrator of a hostile work environment, with a department of low productivity, and the potential for a serious employee retention problem.

What can you do to be a just administrator? Can you use your subtle power as well as your position power to create a just work environment? First you must read. Policies and procedures are not just pieces of paper; they can be used to form an agreement about how business is done in your department. Therefore, you will need to review them to refresh your understanding. Are they clear? Are they fair? Do they function to make things work more smoothly? Do your staff members know what the policies are?

˚ How can you know the answers to these questions? You could do something radical (or sometimes radical in a healthcare setting) and ask the staff. If you have a climate of trust, they will tell you what is working and what is not. You can also do some "management by walking around" and observe work processes. Some healthcare facilities even have the administrators spend one day doing their employees' jobs (nonclinical, of course) so that they truly understand policy in action.

If the answers to these questions do not turn out to be positive, then you must reword or even discard those policies and procedures that do not meet the criteria. Again, staff input can be used to assist you in reviewing drafts for clarity and practicality. You can schedule a policy review meeting so that everyone is up-to-date and understands how they are supposed to work.

Next, you must plan. While you often have to make "right now" decisions, they should not be your entire administrative style. Immediacy is necessary but it does not afford you the time to think about the justice of what you have ordered. You want to consider the big picture when making your decisions. This is quite a challenge, but you are prepared for it.

How about a practical and quick planning example? When you hold a meeting, think about more than the agenda. Consider what you are going to say and what impact it will have on others. Consider how you can give bad news or even good news in a way that is fair to all. Remember that you are sending a message that goes beyond your words. While you do not want to look like you are making a speech during your meetings, having "talking points" to remember to emphasize certain words is a good idea. You can even do a mental rehearsal of what you will say so that you appear confident and prepared. As you saw earlier, your image is part of your message.

Next, you must write well. When you communicate in writing, how will it be interpreted? Do your written decisions convey just treatment? If there is a need for some people to be treated differently, is there an explanation? Providing a reason, rather than just issuing an order, is more likely to be viewed as just by your employees. Your written words should be tools for efficiency and not creators of problems in staff relations.

Is your writing unambiguous without being terse? Remember that any document is a permanent record of your decisions and applications of policy. While you do not want to be paranoid, you also do not want to write words that could be interpreted as being unjust to your staff. In times of crisis, such as a downsizing, your written words become even more important. The environment can be emotionally charged, so you need to be aware of what you are writing and how it can be interpreted under those circumstances.

When you consider your writing and how it can be just or unjust, do not forget e-mails. This is becoming a society of "right now" communication. While that has its advantages, it also has some real drawbacks and can lead to unjust behavior. Suppose you arrive at the office late after a bad start to your morning and an even worse commute. You open your e-mail and find a message that "irritates your last nerve." One temptation is to fire off an immediate response that reflects what you think of this person or his or her message. Be careful.

First, because e-mails can be read and interpreted in so many ways, the e-mail that bothered you might not have been intended to be negative. Even if it was, you are supposed to be able to avoid getting to the level of pettiness and retribution. Maybe the best executive decision is to "take ten" and get a cup of coffee before you respond. Maybe you could telephone this person and get clarification before you "jump to administrative conclusions." Because your e-mails can be kept as a record (i.e., a paper trail) of just or unjust communication with your employee, you always want to use care in responding.

Even the time of the distribution of your words can be just or unjust. For example, if you were the one who was being laid off, when would you want to receive your written notice? Would you want to know at 8:00 A.M. in front of all your peers or just before leaving work on a Friday? If this had to happen, would you want it to be on the day before Christmas Eve or after the holidays? Better yet, would you rather receive it after a discussion with your administrator so that it is not an unpleasant and public surprise? While deciding when to give bad news might not always be in your hands, you should try to do it in the most just way possible through your timing and verbiage.

Finally, you must become a keen observer. Management by walking around is not just a catch phrase for the HCA; you must know what is really happening in your department. It is also helpful to identify some-one who is already a just administrator. Observe how he or she deals with difficult situations when they occur. In addition, you might ask this person to serve as an informal mentor for you. Having a person who will serve as a sounding board to help you think aloud can assist you in making just staff decisions.

Reading, planning, writing, and observing are not the only skills that you need to exhibit as a just administrator, but they form a solid foun-dation for the application of this principle. They can be coupled with periodic self-assessment to assist you with staff justice. When decisions must be made that have an impact on your staff, ask yourself, "Do I have the facts?" and "Am I being fair to those involved?" You also have to be willing to explain your decisions, rather than using "Because I say so" as a justification. Certainly, the role of a just administrator is not an easy one but it does make for a more positive and productive workplace.

Summary

As you can see, justice is not an easy concept to implement in a health-care setting. While it is certainly laudable, many societal and business factors make its consistent practice difficult. As an HCA, you face the challenge of balancing mission and margin in an era of increasingly com-plex and costly technology coupled with changing patient and family expectations. Certainly, practicing justice will require more than just having a policy on the books.

You should not forget the import of your position and role on staff justice. Even small things when done carelessly can be seen as unfair. Staff should receive the same level of fairness that you afford to patients. Otherwise, the inconsistency can lead to costly issues of retention and lowered productivity.

Cases for Your Consideration

The Case of the Dipsomaniac Veteran

As you read this case, consider the following questions. Responses and comments will follow the case.

1. Why did Dr. Smythe include a Not for Resuscitation (NFR) notation for Mr. Dipsoma?

2. What should the staff have done about this notation and why did they fail to act?

3. How does this case demonstrate the failure of patient justice?

4. If you were the administrator, what would you have done in this situation?

Case Information

The actual story on which this case is based occurred outside of the United States, but it could have easily happened in any U.S. hospital, especially before the advent of Do Not Resuscitate (DNR) orders. Sam Dipsoma, a 44-year-old veteran, was a frequent readmission to the Clarion County Hospital (CCH) for treatment of cirrhosis and other complications. During his most recent readmission, he exhibited the symptoms of alcohol withdrawal delirium and liver problems. His medical history contained many incidents of alcohol abuse.

After Dr. Alistair Smythe reviewed Mr. Dipsoma's chart, the staff noticed that the medical notes had been appended with the abbreviation NFR. This meant that if he "crashed," or had a heart attack, or went into respiratory arrest, he should not be resuscitated. The staff knew that Mr. Dipsoma had not been told about this medical note, nor had any of his relatives. However, none of the staff questioned it or said anything to the patient or his family. Fortunately, he did not have a medical crisis during this admission but that did not take away the seriousness of his situation.

If he or any of his relatives had known about the note, they could have had a serious case for legal action. The irony of this situation was that this same hospital had just been in the news for its treatment of a major celebrity who suffered severe injuries when he wrecked his Mercedes while driving under the influence of alcohol and marijuana. Dr. Smythe had been part of a news conference to update the press on the quality treatment that the person received at CCH. Maybe wealth really does have its privileges.

Responses and Commentary on Questions

1. Why did Dr. Smythe include an NFR notation for Mr. Dipsoma?

   Perhaps Dr. Smythe had treated Mr. Dipsoma on several previous occasions and was disgusted with his repeated bouts of alcohol

abuse. Maybe he felt that Mr. Dipsoma was putting an unfair burden on the resources that could be used better for other patients
whose lifestyle was more socially acceptable. After all, he was accu-
mulating bills that, given his lifestyle, would probably go unpaid.
This could negatively affect the bottom line of CCH. Therefore, it
made sense in the physician's mind to include an NFR note in the
patient's chart. As for informing Mr. Dipsoma about this fact,
what good would that do, the physician thought. He probably
could not understand what it meant anyway.

Of course, when it came to the celebrity, Dr. Smythe had a different
view. While his alcohol and drug abuse was unfortunate, he was able
to pay his account in full. In addition, the care this celebrity received
was generating positive press for CCH. There might even be a major
donation made to the hospital when this person recovers. Dr. Smythe
saw no connection between this case and that of Mr. Dipsoma. The
doctor's review reflected his market approach to health care.

2. What should the staff have done about this notation and why did
    they fail to act?

First, the supervisory nurse should have politely questioned Dr.
Smythe to see if the note had been placed in the chart in error. This
would have afforded him the benefit of the doubt and allowed him
to amend it without penalty. If this were not the case, the nurse
could have asked Dr. Smythe if Mr. Dipsoma and his family should
be apprised of this note. If this second step did not resolve the issue,
the supervisor should report this situation to the Director of Nursing. The director would then alert the Chief of Staff or other appropriate authorities. Failure to address this issue of patient justice
could place CCH in legal jeopardy.

Perhaps the staff failed to take action because they felt they had no
power to contradict Dr. Smythe. After all, he was almost a celebrity
himself, especially after participating in the news conference where he
stressed the quality of care provided at CCH. Fortunately, there was
no true medical emergency during this admission of Mr. Dipsoma.
However, the staff's lack of attention could have placed the hospital
in the middle of a legal action. This example makes a case for having
a clear policy about the just treatment of patients.

3. How does this case demonstrate the failure of patient justice?

This case illustrates the need for a clear understanding about policy
related to patient justice. Sometimes people become frustrated with
the cost and care needed when an individual's lifestyle contributes to
his or her condition. The burden of providing such care often strains
the financial resources of the hospital. Nevertheless, there is no policy for differential treatment when someone's disease or condition is

a result of lifestyle behaviors. You are expected to treat people to the best of your ability regardless of their economic circumstances or life choices. Certainly, in this case, you can see that having economic resources made a great difference in the attitude and treatment of the two patients. This is the opposite of patient justice.

4. If you were the administrator, what would you have done in this situation?

Clearly, this case illustrates the need for policies and procedures related to NFR orders and the treatment of individual patients. You should have policies in place that define just patient treatment. Policies can be reviewed with all staff so that they are clear. They can also be part of the patient information packet during admission so that individuals and their families are informed. A patient bill of rights is often included in this packet.

In this case, you can assume that such policies were not in place or that they were violated. Once you are aware of the situation, even if it occurred after Mr. Dipsoma's discharge, you should confer with your Chief of Staff. He or she would then have a discussion with Dr. Smythe about staff attitudes and actions. Such a discussion might lead to a suspension of privileges or some other action. In any case, as the "informant" you should be careful to document your actions and even consider a telephone conference with your hospital attorney as a precautionary measure.

The Case of the Just Downsize

As you read this case, consider the following questions. Responses and comments will follow the case.

1. How did Mr. Muggs prepare to handle the situation with justice?
2. If you were a staff member, how would you feel about Mr. Muggs's actions?

Case Information

Jerry Muggs, director of a public health program called the Youth Anti-Smoking Project, had a staff of five extremely dedicated people. They were so dedicated to the prevention of smoking behaviors in young people that they often worked long hours without even a thought of overtime. Even the administrative assistant did extra duty by traveling to program sites to provide support to the three health educators. Unfortunately, the state health department had just decided that a reduction in force was required for all programs. Mr. Muggs would be transferred to another position, but his whole department was to be eliminated. The work being done in his program was to be added to existing staff in other departments. How could he deliver this news and keep his sense of justice? How could he prevent any unpleasant or even violent reactions from the staff?

First, Mr. Muggs was somewhat relieved by the fact that this decision would not be a total surprise for his staff. He kept them informed of the communications from the state and their deliberations about downsizing. Still, he knew that hearing that they were the ones to be downsized would be painful. Therefore, he immediately contacted the state offices to get up-to-date information on their elimination plans. He asked about the timetable, benefits, and salary packages to be given. He received information on the possibility for staff to transfer to other departments. Mr. Muggs wanted to be fully informed so that he could provide current and accurate information to the staff.

Knowing that not all of the members of his staff were financially independent, Mr. Muggs wanted to see what else he could do before he broke the bad news. He researched community agencies that might be of help and even contacted the local university to see if their career center could provide a consultant for outplacement services. Because he could anticipate that everyone would be upset by the news, he created information packets so that they could have reference materials to use after the meeting. After several sleepless nights, Mr. Muggs scheduled a staff meeting.

During the meeting, Mr. Muggs remained calm as he told the entire staff the news and expressed his sadness about it. He allowed some time for reaction before he gave them information about their options. Because he was prepared, he was able to answer their questions and give ideas for additional resources.

During the weeks that followed, he worked with each staff member to assist in any way that he could. The staff, while upset at their change in circumstances, told him how much they appreciated his efforts. Even though this was one of the most difficult times of his administrative career, Mr. Muggs felt that he did everything he could to handle the situation with justice.

Responses and Commentary on Questions

1. How did Mr. Muggs prepare to handle the situation with justice?

    First, Mr. Muggs provided information to his staff before the elimination decision was even made. They were kept informed about downsizing discussions to keep the secrecy issue to a minimum. While this was somewhat risky on his part, Mr. Muggs knew his staff's level of dedication and trusted them. The decision to create a flow of communication in this important area actually made Mr. Muggs's job easier when he had to break the bad news. While it was unwelcome, it was not a total shock.

Mr. Muggs also went beyond what he had to do to comply with the wishes of the state. He actually planned his words and actions to anticipate the needs of his staff. Certainly, he was not required to try to get outplacement assistance for them, but he did. Because of Mr. Muggs's altruism, the staff was better able to adjust to what they had to do and appreciated his efforts on their behalf. They did not blame him or the state for their fate, but understood that they were part of a larger situation. His preparation made a difficult situation much more palatable.

2. If you were a staff member, how would you feel about Mr. Muggs's actions?

First, it must be remembered that losing your job is one of life's most stressful events. Even though you were kept informed of the state's plans, you really did not believe that downsizing would happen to you. You might wonder if there was something wrong with your performance in the department that influenced the state to choose your department from all of the others. Your reaction might mirror the stages of grief identified by Kubler-Ross (1997) and others. Therefore, you might experience denial, bargaining, anger, sadness, and finally, acceptance. For the short term, you would be miserable.

Yet, you would have to respect Mr. Muggs's efforts on your behalf. Because he had earned your trust in the past and formed a strong working relationship with the team, you believed him when he explained the circumstances of the elimination. You wanted to be angry at him, but somehow you just couldn't blame him for the decision. You would then be able to try to make the best of a bad situation and move on to the next stage of your career and your life.

Web Resource

Information on the Oregon Health Plan
http://www.dhs.state.or.us/healthplan/overview.html

References

Beauchamp, T. L., & Childress, J. E. (2008). *Principles of biomedical ethics* (6th ed.). New York: Oxford University Press.

Kubler-Ross, E. (1997). *On death and dying.* New York: Scribner.

Pearson, S. D., Sabin, J. E., & Emanuel, E. J. (2003). *No margin, no mission: Health-care organizations and the quest for ethical excellence.* New York: Oxford University Press.

Shi, L., & Singh, D. A. (2008). *Delivering health care in America: A systems approach* (4th ed.). Sudbury, MA: Jones and Bartlett.

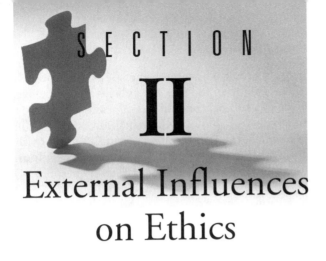

SECTION II

External Influences on Ethics

■ INTRODUCTION

To paraphrase John Donne, no healthcare facility is an island. It is part of the larger entity known as a community. This community includes people who represent a myriad of health issues and cultures; issues that affect the community also affect healthcare facilities. For example, if the healthcare facility exists in an urban area where social issues of overcrowding, crime, and poverty exist, these circumstances add to its treatment burden. If it exists in a remote rural area, maldistribution of professionals and distance add to its treatment challenges. Yet, each of these facilities markets its mission as serving the community's health care needs and creates expectations that its mission will be accomplished.

Because healthcare institutions exist in a community, they are subject to the values and standards of acceptable behavior defined by that community. Their ethics are judged partially by their ability to meet or exceed these standards. Standards influencing the practice of health care are articulated by local and state governments and by various branches of the federal system. They are also created by external agencies such as the Joint Commission on Accreditation of Healthcare Organizations or the National Committee for Quality Assurance. Standards also come from other businesses such as managed care organizations or business cooperatives. These standards are concerned with, among other things, the provision of care, patient rights, acceptable business practices, credentialing of healthcare professionals, payment for services, and ethical and legal issues. They are often copious, conflicting, and arcane.

Like all businesses, healthcare entities are also expected to be self-regulating. Therefore, they are assumed to have their own internal standards that serve to articulate appropriate behavior within the organization. These standards are often developed to comply with those defined by external evaluators, but should not be limited to these sources. Therefore, the healthcare business must be profitable amid a sea of external regulations and internal policies and guidelines.

Already, you can see that the business of health care is like no other. In this section, you will study how external forces have an impact on ethics policy and behaviors of healthcare entities. You will also see how the community affects your day-to-day practice as a healthcare administrator. In Chapter 5, you will address the Latin question: "Quis Custodiet Ispos Custodes? Who Will Guard the Guardians?" You will examine the rationale for external controls in health care and some examples of how those controls influence ethical practices. In addition, you will study the issue of advocacy as a part of the guardianship role of health care. Finally, you will investigate the ethical issue of maintaining competency as a part of your ethics obligations to the community.

In Chapter 6, you will explore how market forces influence the ethics of healthcare administration. This chapter includes a major section on managed care, which is now a key influence on all of healthcare practice. In addition, you will be introduced to issues related to the consumer-led movement toward integrated medicine (IM). IM, or as it is also termed, complementary/alternative medicine, holds great potential, but presents unique ethical issues for the system.

In Chapter 7, you will examine the need for social responsibility in the healthcare system. This issue concerns health care because, while health care is a business, the community expects it to have a greater emphasis on social justice than other businesses. In this chapter, the difficult issues of resource allocation and efforts to address access to health care are also explored. You will also analyze the idea prevention services as a social responsibility. Public health and its emphasis on social justice and prevention will also be discussed. The chapter will help you decide what your relationship with public health should be and just how much you should be part of the prevention of disease. Social responsibility will also be examined in relation to issues of patient safety and quality of service. In the end, you will be able to develop your own answer to the question: "Are we our brothers' (or sisters') keepers?"

Chapter 8 presents the most challenging issues in the External Influences Section. It gives a brief overview of some of the current and anticipated advances in technology. A discussion of ethical implications for each of these modern miracles follows. You will come to understand that technology brings great promise to health care. However, you will also see that health care is not always able to match its ethics with its technical achievements.

This section addresses many external forces that affect the practice of health care. These forces are complex and can even conflict with each other. Because you are working in a business in which trust is the main commodity, you cannot ignore or de-emphasize the influence of your community. Yet, you are expected to run a business that provides a high quality product to meet community needs. How do you do that? While this section does not provide all of the answers, it will increase your understanding of these forces and challenge your thinking as an ethics-based health administrator.

CHAPTER 5

Quis Custodiet Ispos Custodes?

Who Will Guard the Guardians?

Everybody's for democracy in principle. It's only in practice that the thing gives rise to stiff objections.

—Meg Greenfield

Points to Ponder

1. Why is health care subjected to so many rules and regulations?
2. What do healthcare regulators say about ethical practices?
3. What can you do to practice ethics-based administration in light of multiple regulations?
4. How can you be an ethics-based advocate for health care?
5. What is your responsibility to ensure staff competence?

Words to Remember

The following is a list of key words for this chapter. You will find them in bold in the text. Stop and check your understanding of them.

ACHE	AHA	BFOQs
dogma	HIPAA	JCAHO
MGMA	NCQA	poka-yoke

■ THE AGE OF ACCOUNTABILITY

JCAHO, CMS, NCQA, HEDIS, FDA, EEOC, AHA, AMA, HIPAA, IOM: these are just a few of the agencies that want to know how you conduct the business of health care. You can add numerous state and local agencies to this list. Add also the various managed care organizations (MCOs) with which you have contracts. Do not forget consumer groups such as the American Association of Retired Persons. When you consider the enormity of the burden of accountability, it becomes almost overwhelming. As a healthcare administrator (HCA), you are expected to meet the requirements and standards of this plethora of agencies and still maintain a profitable enterprise. This section of the chapter will assist you in understanding why the burden of accountability is so great and provide some examples of these multiple accountabilities. In Chapter 11, you will read about this issue and the effort to go beyond compliance to quality care.

The reality of healthcare organizations is that they work under the microscope and magnifying glass of both macro and micro accountability. On the macro level, you are accountable to external regulators such as federal, state, and local governments. You are also responsible to your accreditation body or bodies. On the micro level, you are accountable to your patients, their families, and certainly, your superiors. In his classic work, Worthley (1997, p. 147) provides a set of questions to guide your assessment of your responsibility. He asks, "As health care professionals to *whom* are we accountable? For *what* are we accountable? *How* are we held accountable? *Why* are we held accountable? And *what results* from all of this?"

To answer his questions, you must understand the public's view of the healthcare industry. To paraphrase an old song, "There's no business like the healthcare business." No other business has the amount and type of power over its clientele. It can literally kill its customers or heal them. It can cause them unnecessary suffering or relieve their pain. In addition, many of the practitioners in this business hold a monopoly on the ability to provide their services through certification and state licensure. This means that not only is the business of health care the most powerful one in the United States, but individuals within this business hold power over others.

American society has learned to have a certain level of mistrust for anyone or anything that wields such absolute power. History shows how such power can be abused by those who have less than altruistic motives to the detriment of the population. Therefore, society must protect itself from the professional power held by health care by taking certain actions. First, society must try to limit such power by limiting its boundaries. You can see this action evidenced in external controls such as accreditation by the Joint Commission on Accreditation of Healthcare

Organizations (JCAHO) accreditation (more on this later), Medicare/Medicaid regulations, and state laws that govern various medical practices. In addition, lawsuits and adverse publicity through the media can sometimes limit the power of organizations and individuals within those organizations. Consideration of the impact on an organization's reputation and marketplace confidence should cause an organization to rethink its position.

Society can also protect itself from the power of health care by trying to structure it. It establishes certain regulations regarding payment for services that also control demand and supply. In turn, these regulations influence the structure of the system itself. For example, because certain areas are covered by insurance, they are more likely to be provided by the healthcare system and are included in its design. This puts some limits on what the system can do and serves to control its power through its bottom line. Some would maintain that without such controls, the healthcare system could become even more expensive and demand even more of the U.S. gross national product. Another example of control is the need for clinical trials and proof of effectiveness before drugs are released to the public. While this is not a foolproof system, it does try to curtail the absolute power of the drug industry.

Society also attempts to limit health care by checking the power of individual practitioners. It should be noted that legislation on practice, continuing education requirements, accreditation of undergraduate and graduate programs, and to some extent, enrollment requirements all assist in limiting professional power. On the micro (i.e., organizational) level, strict standards on employment practices including background checks, verification of credentials, formal policies on employee ethics, and serious investigation of employee actions that appear to violate the organization's policies all serve to protect the public. Maintaining staff competence is also part of the organization's responsibility to the community and will be discussed later in this chapter.

Shortell and colleagues (2000) provide additional reasons for the demand for accountability. The United States has a long history of valuing individual rights and the ability of professionals to make decisions about health care. However, the changes that have occurred in the healthcare industry have caused a greater demand for more community accountability. They include managed care, knowledge about the quality of health care and its problems, and information technology including the Internet. In addition, public awareness of how health care works has increased because of news coverage and television programs. Today, consumers can actually be "in" the operating room and watch what is happening through entertainment programming. They see the hospital in action through "reality" and fictional programs. These up-close views of health care, whether accurate or not, influence the demand for accountability for both the outcomes and the costs of healthcare practice.

The demand for accountability in health care has also been increased by public attention to ethics violations in other industries. When you turn on the television or read any print news source, you cannot help but wonder what has happened to corporate ethics in general. You see chief executive officers (CEOs) testifying in Congress about their misdeeds and domestic divas facing time in prison. People have lost life savings through corporate scandals involving creative accounting and other practices. While these cases have ended up in the legal system, they began with the lack of ethical standards and practices in large corporations. The public is beginning to wonder if anyone in business has any ethics. Are the business ethics courses provided in MBA programs useless? The overall climate of trust for business in general is eroding.

Large healthcare systems are not exempt from this situation and have had their share of executives in disgrace. It is not surprising then, that the public wants more information about what is happening in health care. The potential erosion of trust is particularly bothersome for you as an administrator because, as Annison and Wilford (1998) have stressed, you are involved in a trust-based business. Without a high level of trust from the community, your bottom line can erode or even disappear. Imagine the level of accountability you would face if that trust were lost.

Given this concern from the public, whether it is a government agency, business contractor, or private citizen group, it is not surprising that you live in an environment of high accountability and constant scrutiny. You must be prepared to operate a profitable business entity despite this sometimes-cumbersome environment. The first step in this challenging process is to know your organization. You will learn more about establishing a mission, vision, and values statement in Section III. However, you should keep in mind that knowing your organization assists you in meeting the compliance challenge. Once you understand who you are, you will need to establish both formal and informal structures and practices that will keep you accountable for your espoused values.

In addition, you must know your confronter. In other words, you must understand the standards that govern your business practices and what they mean in your particular organization. This can entail many hours of tedious reading, telephone calls for clarification, and meetings with staff for interpretation and practice applications. However, because knowledge truly is power in this case, the payoff is worth the effort. Some examples of the standards you will need to know and how they specifically pertain to ethics will be discussed in this section. Standards relating to staff competence will be featured in subsections of this chapter. While it is not possible to detail all of the articulated ethics standards, you will learn about major external influences including JCAHO, AHA, HIPAA, and NCQA.

The Dogma of JCAHO

Healthcare ethics is governed by **dogma** (or strongly held standards) that has its source in laws and regulations. One of the most prominent sources of such standards is the Joint Commission on Accreditation of Healthcare Organizations (JCAHO). This organization began in 1951 and originally focused on hospital accreditation. Currently, in addition to hospitals, it accredits long-term care facilities including assisted-living centers. It is also involved in the accreditation of ambulatory care facilities, clinical laboratories, rehabilitation facilities, and behavioral medicine organizations including residential treatment centers and foster care. JCAHO provides accreditation for home health agencies and healthcare networks. It also certifies disease-specific programs and disease management companies. Although participation in the JCAHO process is voluntary for facilities, it is often viewed as essential for healthcare organizations. In addition, Medicare recognizes its inspections as a substitute for its own process. Accreditation in this case is tied to funding. In addition, many state agencies contract with JCAHO to review MCOs. JCAHO also publishes performance reports that the public can access through its Quality Check™ program. Because of its scope and depth of involvement in healthcare accreditation, this organization has great influence on both the practices and ethical standards for the industry.

There are sets of standards, which can number into the hundreds, for all of the facilities that are accredited by JCAHO. Each organization has a detailed manual that is designed to guide the compliance with these standards and documentation of compliance. There is also an attempt to increase the performance-measures in that supplement the accreditation process through the ORYX® initiative. In addition, to the written reporting of compliance, there is an onsite visit of JCAHO-appointed evaluators.

This visit is expensive and requires many months of preparation. There used to be a time when a site visit meant that you made sure the carpets were cleaned, the walls were painted, and your documentation was complete. JCAHO accreditation used to be viewed as just meeting the minimum written standards. Now, the emphasis of a site visit has shifted to be more about the delivery of care and continued quality improvement. There are interviews with your staff, patients or clients, and their families. In addition, you might be selected for unannounced visits. This feature of the accreditation process is supposed to keep you vigilant in maintaining the standards.

JCAHO has specific standards that relate to your ethics. For hospitals and other healthcare facilities, this standard set is called Patient Rights and Organization Ethics. The abbreviation RI is used for all of these standards. There are separate standards dealing with ethics in patient care in general, respect for the rights of patients in treatment, and patients' involvement in their own care. Informed consent is stressed including separate standards dealing with participation in research. Standards are presented that stress the family and their right to be informed about care decisions and potential outcomes, and to be involved in decision-making. Advance directives, withholding resuscitation, withdrawing life support, and end-of-life treatment are all included in the standard set. The patient's right to pain management has also been assigned a separate standard. Organ donation and procurement also have a standard.

In addition, JCAHO addresses respect for confidentiality, privacy, and security in separate standards. Pastoral care and spiritual needs are included. The hospital itself must demonstrate that it works under a code of ethics and that its code deals with its marketing, admission, transfer, and billing practices. Clinical decision-making must be protected regardless of the financial compensation system used by the facility.

These are just some of the standards developed by JCAHO. You might think that they include all of the facility's ethics requirements, and your work is done if you comply. After all, they seem to comply with your previous reading about the principles of ethics including respect for autonomy, beneficence, and nonmaleficence. However, your thinking would not be correct. First, the standards themselves can be vague. For example, Standard RI.01.01 states, "The hospital respects the patient's cultural and personal values, beliefs, and preferences" (JCAHO, 2008, p. 7). This standard is open for many interpretations. Developing or implementing indicators that can be used to prove consistent compliance can be difficult.

Second, even though these standards are helpful in ensuring some level of ethics for patients in hospital settings, they certainly do not encompass all ethics concerns. No specific mention is made of the ethical treatment of employees or of the employers' treatment of vendors and contractors. Third, just meeting the standard does not constitute ethical behavior; you must go beyond the letter of the law. There is much more than can be done in this area and JCAHO continues to have initiatives to improve these and other standards.

The Dogma of AHA

Another agency that has influence on the hospital and its ethics practice is the American Hospital Association (**AHA**). This organization represents the interests of hospitals and other organizations in national policy development. It has been an organization since 1917 and still addresses healthcare issues today. According to its Web site, the AHA is involved in many issues that affect hospitals including readiness for disasters, HIPAA, issues relating to Medicare, and patient communication.

With respect to ethics, the AHA has published information about patient's rights since 1973. This document is now called *The Patient Care Partnership* and is available through AHA Web site in multiple languages. The current iteration contains includes information about the right to considerate care and accurate information about treatment, and the ability to make informed decisions. It also addresses issues of personal privacy and confidentiality of records, and continuity of care. Billing and assistance with insurance claims is also discussed (AHA, 2003).

This document tries to help patients understand their rights in the often-alien environment of the hospital. It addresses many of the principles that you have studied such as autonomy, beneficence, and non-maleficence. However, it can also pose problems because it can be misinterpreted by the patient. First, he or she might not even read the document and just assume that certain procedures will be done. Because the language is not concrete, even if he or she does read it, there is no guarantee that it will be fully understood or correctly interpreted. Many healthcare facilities choose to adapt the AHA document to provide additional clarity. No matter which format is used, it is imperative that you make sure that your staff knows how to interpret its meaning correctly for your patients.

Just having a document about patients' rights does not mean that these rights will be ensured. Continuing education, monitoring, and other administrative actions will still be needed to ensure the practice of patient-centered ethics. Just as you saw with JCAHO, AHA does not address all of the ethical issues you face as an HCA. You still must work to ensure the ethical treatment of staff, vendors, contractors, and the community at large.

The Dogma of HIPAA

In 1996, Congress passed the Health Insurance Portability and Accountability Act (**HIPAA**) as an attempt to engage in healthcare reform and to deal with new issues facing the industry. The act had several objectives including assurance of health insurance coverage when there was a job change or when pre-existing conditions existed, reduction of fraud and abuse, standardizing health information, and ensuring security and privacy of health information. The legislation had several titles to address all of these objectives. The Administration Simplification provisions dealt with rules for compliance with this act and addressed electronic claims submission, including standards of privacy, confidentiality, and maintenance of health information.

This legislation has an impact on almost all healthcare institutions and vendors who serve those institutions. Even educational institutions that had any contact with those institutions were affected by HIPAA. You can imagine how confusing the initial communications about the law and its mandates were. However, there are now numerous documents to advise you on HIPAA compliance. In fact, a whole industry has been created to assist you to maintain it. Remember that your staff has to be educated on both the provisions of the fraud and abuse and privacy aspects of the law; this training must be documented. The costs for coming into compliance are estimated to be in the billions, and the law offers no mechanism for recouping these costs.

The positive features of the law are that electronic transfers are becoming much easier and more cost effective. Security upgrades are beginning to improve the confidentiality of patient data. These efforts protect patients' right to know who has seen their medical records, and how their personal information is used within a healthcare organization. In addition, there is an increased awareness of the potential for violating confidentiality. Confidentiality is better protected through procedures for taking health histories, protections about in appropriate conversations about patients, and methods to prevent marketing firms to access patient names and addresses. Ethics aspects of autonomy and respect for patients can certainly be seen in the provisions of HIPAA.

What does this mean to you? Of course, you will be responsible for making sure that your organization does whatever is needed to be in HIPAA compliance. You may be spending long hours reading the many publications that relate to this law and keeping up with its revisions. You also have to ensure that training and its documentation are correctly done through either in-house programs or contracts with vendors. When site visits are held to confirm compliance with HIPAA standards, you may be part of the team that responds to the visit. HIPAA will certainly be a part of your life as an HCA now and in the immediate future. While it can cause you stress and additional expense, you should be better able to cope if you understand that its intent is based in ethical practices when dealing with health information and electronic records.

The Dogma of NCQA

The National Committee for Quality Assurance (**NCQA**) is a not-for-profit organization that was founded in 1990. Its purpose is to improve the quality of care provided by the managed care industry including health plans, MCOs, preferred provider organizations (PPOs), and disease management organizations. Data is collected through quality indicators called the Health Effectiveness Data and Information Set or HEDIS®. These indicators are improved each year and health plans must report their performance on at least two-thirds of the standards to quality for consideration for the NCQA Seal of Approval (NCQA, 2008).

Accreditation at this point is voluntary. However, according to its Web site, many employers rely on NCQA's quality assessments when choosing their employee managed care options. To assist in this process, NCQA maintains an informational Web site where employers and employees can access report cards on specific organizations. It also publishes a report (which can also be found on its Web site) called The State of Health Care Quality. The report provides information based on data derived from its Health Effectiveness Data and Information Set performance standards.

How Does All This Affect You?

We have examined just a few of the agencies that have standards of conduct to try to limit the power and influence the ethical practices of the guardians of health. Sometimes these standards seem overwhelming and they can be contradictory. They can make you feel that you are operating your business in a fishbowl. You are examined by so many external sources and so busy with such long paper trails that you can feel more like a paper pusher than an administration professional. On a visceral level, this multiple accountability can be almost painful. However, you must consider it part of the overall cost of doing business.

In the immediate, you must be able to juggle these responsibilities and still maintain your positive staff relations and attention to the bottom line. You also must take an active role as a continuous learner to keep up with any changes in current standards or the addition of new ones. In the next section of this chapter, you will learn how to have a greater impact on what laws are passed and how they influence you and your organization. In Chapter 11, you will learn how to go beyond just meeting standards toward the goal of consistent quality.

■ THE ETHICS OF ADVOCACY

How can you run your business in spite of all of this external control? How can you be proactive rather than reactive? Certainly, no one would argue that regulations, standards, and indicators are costly in both time and in the fiscal resources required to address them. However, none of this will change if you remain passive or just react to every new obligation.

First, you must understand that the larger community might not have a good understanding of the business of health care. You have already learned that individuals and lawmakers have differing views of what health care is and what it should be. Therefore, if you expect positive change in the future, you must be willing to assist in increasing understanding of the true nature of the healthcare business. You must become an ethics-based advocate for your particular organization, your part of the industry, and for your profession. The advocate role will require you to be aware and informed, involved in the community and in legislation, and model the behavior that you expect of others ("walk the walk, not just talk the talk").

Being aware and informed first requires that you research the current state of legislation in your area. This includes not only pending federal legislation but also state and even local laws. You also need to maintain currency in the main healthcare issues facing your community. Numerous databases are available that capture findings about the prevalence of healthcare issues. It is also smart to maintain a connection with your local public health department because it has information about state and local issues that are current or that might surface in the near future. Of course, journals abound with information about national trends in health including health problems, ideas for dealing with these problems, and pending legislation about these problems. For example, the media has publicized the rapid increase in childhood obesity and diabetes. A prudent HCA might consider that, when the awareness of this issue reaches sufficient strength, there will need to be programs to address it. If appropriate, a treatment program for this problem can be something that an organization should consider as a new revenue stream.

Being an advocate also means getting involved. You already saw the need to have contact with public health to maintain your knowledge. It is also proactive to examine the idea of joint initiatives to increase the likelihood of preventing expensive health problems. These might include community health assessment projects, health fairs, school programs, and other prevention-centered activities. You also might consider becoming an active member of the various groups and associations that represent your particular part of health care such as the local, state, or national chapters of the hospital or long-term care associations. Being an active member means more than just going to meetings. It would involve being on committees, giving presentations, or even holding office to support your part of health care. Finally, you should also consider being an active member of your professional association. For many who are administrators in the clinical side of health care, this includes tie-ins with organizations devoted to nursing, respiratory therapy, dentistry, mental health, or medical education, among others. A great many opportunities are available for advocacy in the local, state, and national chapters of the American College of Healthcare Executives (**ACHE**) and the Medical Group Management Association (**MGMA**). Their Web sites have been included in this chapter for your information.

You may be saying, "How can I afford the time to do all of this and still have a life?" This question is very appropriate. However, consider the cost of noninvolvement. It can mean that you and your organization are left behind when trends occur that can be either beneficial or detrimental to your healthcare business. You also might consider that, as an HCA, you are expected to be on top of things. If you maintain currency, you will become the go-to person for information and ideas about new initiatives. If you are prepared, this could be a true career builder. Finally, in order to "have a life" you should choose your advocacy opportunities wisely. You do not have to do everything, but contributing, reading your literature, scanning the Internet, and maintaining liaisons with public health offices can go a long way to keeping you "in the know" about current problems, pending legislation, and future business initiatives. Certainly, there will always be paperwork and long hours. However, by participating in legislation, community activism, or associations of professional interest to you personally, you will find that you do, in fact, have a life.

■ THE ETHICS OF STAFF COMPETENCY

When patients or clients enter the healthcare system at any level, they make at least one assumption—that those who are treating them know what they are doing. This assumption of competence is essential to the foundation of trust on which health care is built. Because healing is not just based on drugs or surgery, but also on faith in the healers, it can be said that this assumption is crucial to healing itself.

As members of a business that is charged with guarding the community's health, you must take the ethical responsibility to ensure the competence of all staff who provide or influence patient care. Obviously, this includes those who provide direct patient care such as physicians, dentists, nurses, and counselors. However, it also includes anyone who supports the facility such as supervisors, information services technicians, and housekeeping staff. In short, anyone who works in the healthcare setting should be competent to perform the tasks of his or her position. In this section, you will learn about practices and issues related to the ethics of ensuring staff competence.

Practices for Competency Assurance

The classic text in healthcare human resources by Fottler, Hernandez, and Joiner (1997) devotes several chapters to staff competence through human resources functions. The ethical responsibilities related to staff competency assurance actually begin with the analysis of the job itself. You need to be accurate and honest in determining just what is needed in each position and in assessing the level of required education and credentials. Your initial analysis will form the basis for the other human resources tasks of recruitment, selection, training, and performance appraisal.

Each of the stages of staff acquisition and retention has its own ethical responsibilities and challenges. For example, in the recruitment stage, you should have a thorough understanding of the type of professional you want to recruit. This should include the job analysis mentioned earlier but should go beyond the basic job description. Be aware of any specific requirements for the position, also called Bona Fide Occupational Qualifications (**BFOQs**) so that you can be accurate and honest in your recruiting efforts. When hiring healthcare professionals, regardless of their job title, you must also consider more than just their knowledge and skills. Attitudes, professional ethics, and ability to work with team members are equally important. It is also important to determine the kind of person that you want to hire. Be sure to also have a plan for recruitment and check all advertising and application materials ahead of time for concurrence with the Equal Employment Opportunity Commission rules, the organization's mission statements, and ethical practices.

During the selection process, many ethics issues can arise. First, you must be very careful to treat all applicants fairly and with respect. Even if the applicant in no way meets the position criteria, he or she should be treated with courtesy. You might have to discuss telephone protocols and review correspondence for ethics assurance. You are the organization to this person, so you want to be seen as friendly but professional.

You can choose to conduct telephone or in-person interviews on an individual or group basis. Be very careful about the way that you ask questions. Try to link your queries to the job analysis, allow time for responses, and remember to let the applicant ask questions. Be sure to provide honest and fair answers about your organization. Remember that interviews have many sources for bias, including the first impression of the interviewee, responses from candidates who preceded him or her, and physical appearance. Remember also that the interviewee is trying to be on his or her best behavior, but can also be very nervous. Obviously, you are not getting a complete picture of the candidate.

Checking references and credentials has become a key ethics responsibility in ensuring staff competence. In the past, people have engaged in such fraudulent practices as writing their own reference letters, altering transcripts, and forging licenses. Reference and credential verification, while expensive and time consuming, is essential for preventing such irregularities. Remember that a reference letter can be politely, but not entirely honestly, written. If you choose to follow up a reference letter with a telephone call, be prepared in advance with your questions so that you do not waste the person's time. Allow time for response and listen to both the words and the tone of the response. You can learn a great deal from the conversation. Be sure to make careful notes so that you can provide an accurate account of the conversation. This will help in later decision making about choosing the best fit for the position.

With respect to credentials, be sure to inform the applicant about what documentation is necessary. You should stress that he or she must be able to document a current licensure, educational background and training, and certifications if needed for the position. The applicant must also be informed that these proofs will be checked. In large organizations, the human resources (HR) department will assist you in the verification process, but in smaller organizations, you might be responsible for it. Be sure to ask that official copies of transcripts be sent directly from the colleges or universities involved. You will also need to verify current licensure and check for any suspension, modification, or termination of license. Be sure to get copies or verification of all licenses because the individual can be licensed in several states. This becomes an issue because the license in your state might be current but the person perhaps has a suspended license in another state.

You definitely need to check for citizenship and authorization to work in the United States, and for any felony convictions. Many organizations conduct a thorough background check to protect the organization. If appropriate, liability coverage should also be verified. You can see that this is a time-consuming process but one that is necessary to ensure staff competency in the hiring stage. Be sure to be current on all policies and procedures relating to employee selection so that you do not overlook important information. For example, some organizations require a physical exam, testing on Occupational Safety and Health Administration or HIPAA requirements, and drug testing before an offer for a position can be given.

After the employee is hired, your responsibility for ensuring staff competence has not ended. First, you must provide an orientation to introduce your new staff to the values and standards expected in the organization. This process can be somewhat lengthy depending on the complexity of the job responsibilities and the level of the new hire. For instance, a novice employee might require much more time for orientation and supervision than will an expert one. Some organizations function on a mentor system where the new employee is matched with an appropriate mentor. Usually the mentor is two or more levels higher than the protégé. If this system is used, care must be taken in matching up the two people, because the mentor will most definitely serve as a role model and have a great influence on both the practices and attitudes of the protégé.

The organization also has an obligation to provide job-related in-service education that goes beyond orientation. During these in-service sessions, specific training can be provided, such as the use of new equipment. Providing onsite training is also helpful to ensure consistency in the level of professional competence. Be sure to document competence in the required skills and maintain those records. In addition, in-service time can be required to keep staff informed about specific policies and procedures, and define attitudes that are required for the positions. For example, if the mission of the organization has been revised or a new program has been introduced, a staff in-service program might be required. It is your responsibility to ensure that staff is kept informed regarding job requirements and responsibilities. The process you use to deliver this information will vary depending on the size of your organization. If you have an HR department, it can help you make information delivery decisions.

There are differences of opinion regarding the organization's role in maintaining professional currency and continuing education requirements for licensure. Some organizations believe that it is the professional's responsibility to maintain his or her own license and do not offer any assistance with this process. Other organizations feel an ethical responsibility to cover the cost of continuing education units (CEUs), because they require a current license for employment. Many organizations use some combination of the two and provide released time for continuing education, some coverage for fees, or assistance with travel expenses.

If you choose to support continuing education for your employees, you must practice the principles of fairness in your policies. Be wary of "meeting hogs" who want more than their share of the travel budget, while less aggressive employees seldom get support. You will need to have clear policies about what kind of meetings and continuing education events will be covered, the amount, and type of support that is offered, and who is eligible for this benefit. Some departments have chosen to award a flat amount per employee per year for CEU efforts. Your message should be that all employees are equally valued and that you are interested in keeping them current in their field. You might even have to encourage some employees to take advantage of the CEU benefits. However, positive and fair policies in this area can go a long way toward maintaining department morale. Remember to keep accurate records of who is attending CEU programs and what they have attended so that you can demonstrate your stewardship of scarce CEU funding. Be sure to consider all staff in your plans for employee development support and not just the clinical professionals.

Experts in business encourage investment in training and employee development as ways to reduce turnover, increase morale, and stay competitive in hiring the best staff (Fottler, Hernandez, & Joiner, 1997). However, there is a risk in being too generous with staff development and CEU benefits. Less than ethical employees might choose to gain advanced degrees and credentials through your facility's generosity and then resign for a higher paying position. To avoid this ethics-based problem, many organizations require a signed contract from those who avail themselves of this benefit. The contract might stipulate that they will serve a certain amount of time after achieving their goals, or reimburse the facility for the costs of their education if they leave early. Of course, any such contract would have to be evaluated by the legal and human resources staff before it is even discussed with employees.

Ethics and Incompetence

What happens when a staff member demonstrates a lack of competence? This is one of the most difficult and emotionally draining problems for the HCA. First, you must understand that incompetence can be due to several reasons, including impairment from psychoactive drugs and health and personal issues. While many people in the United States take psychoactive drugs such as alcohol, caffeine, or tobacco, using them can interfere with professional judgment or patient safety. If there are signs of this, action must be taken. In the early stages of impairment, the symptoms might not be recognized by individuals or their coworkers. In addition, well-meaning coworkers sometimes enable the behaviors by making excuses, covering up mistakes, and privately complaining but taking no public action. They might choose to remain silent because they have engaged in the same behavior themselves, do not want to be a snitch, or be responsible for another's loss of livelihood. Some even fear retribution if the impaired person is seen as having power in the organization.

What should the ethical HCA do about such problems? First, you should remember that it is always better to be proactive than reactive. Policies should be in place that spells out acceptable and unacceptable behaviors. For example, it used to be acceptable to have an open bar at organization functions. While it was not a solid career move to overindulge in alcohol at such affairs, many did so without repercussions. In today's healthcare environment, a policy to look the other way would be highly unusual. It is best to avoid serving alcohol at functions or, at the very least, to limit its potential for misuse.

Education is always a good idea as a proactive strategy. You can educate staff on the policy, and on the signs and symptoms of impairment. Be sure to include information about resources that are available to assist the impaired person. For example, many states have special programs for impaired physicians and nurses. Your HR department can be a great source of information on this topic. In addition, if your organization is large enough to have an Employee Assistance Program (EAP), be sure to consult with them regarding available services.

Check to see that you have appropriate policies in place for reporting suspected impairment with protection for the person doing the reporting. Remember that failure to report can be viewed as negligence, especially if a patient is harmed. However, do not jump to conclusions if a report is made. Not all reports are true, so spend time investigating, and obtain the assistance of the HR department in this effort. When you do confront an impaired employee, be prepared for denial and hostility.

It is wise to have an expert from HR or your EAP to assist you and serve as a witness. Always remember your principles of ethics and duty to the patient when dealing with any impairment situation. Using appropriate counseling and interventions can prevent future problems and save someone's career.

Finally, you should be aware that a lack of competence is not always caused by substance abuse. Sometimes the aging process, early symptoms of Alzheimer's disease, or other health issues will cause impairment in the ability to treat patients effectively. Emotional problems such as going through a divorce or the death of a loved one can temporarily impede the ability to make sound judgments. If you have created a working environment of respect and trust, individuals can self-report such problems. If this happens, you should take time to counsel the employee and refer him or her to the appropriate source of assistance such as compassion leave, EAP services, or HR. If the change in behavior is reported by staff, you should investigate, while doing what you can to preserve the individual's self-respect and dignity. Again, be prepared for a strong reaction when you confront behaviors. This part of your work as an HCA is not easy. However, doing it well, with regard for both the staff member and the employee, you will increase your value to the organization and honor your role as guardian of patient safety.

What About Your Competence?

Steven Covey (1989) in his now classic work, *The 7 Habits of Highly Effective People*, stresses it. Carson Dye (2000) devotes a whole chapter to it in *Leadership in Health Care: Values at the Top*. What is it? It is the necessity for self-evaluation and assurance of your own competency. If you are an ethics-based HCA, you do not wait until your annual evaluation to appraise your level of competency. You should choose to engage in consistent self-assessment and in the process of lifelong learning.

How does this translate into your daily routine as an administrator? First, in keeping with what you learned from Frankl's work, you would take time to think about the meaning of your work. This might mean taking some time in your busy schedule for contemplation and determining the answers to the difficult questions that really matter in your career. You should ask yourself questions such as, "Why am I here? And what do I want to do with my life?" You examine the meaning in your work by asking: "Where can I make a difference? And what do I see myself doing in 5 years?" Finally, you should think about the global question of: "For what do I want to be known?"

Many HCAs find it helpful to write a personal mission statement based on this process of contemplation. They review this statement at least annually (often on their birthdays) to see if it is still true or needs revision. It also serves as a compass for making career decisions. For example, comparing your personal mission statement with that of your organization can be very insightful. Do you respect its mission? Is it reasonably compatible with your own? This assessment gives some guidance when considering a new position or thinking about a job change, because it would be difficult to support an organization that you do not respect or whose practices directly oppose your core values. You will learn more about personal mission statements and ethics in Section IV of this text.

Conducting an ethics self-assessment is also helpful to identify your true "ethics bottom line." You need to think about your own definition of integrity and not just the textbook definition. For example, you could ask yourself, "What principles or events would cause me to resign?" Or, "What principles am I willing to state publicly and act upon?" The ACHE has a self-assessment tool that many have found helpful in this process (ACHE, 2009). It helps you to examine your ethics in an organizational context. You will read more about this when you examine codes of ethics in a later chapter.

You then need to take the time to write these statements down for your personal ethics code. You can put them in a place where you can easily refer to them, such as the middle drawer of your desk. The brave HCAs state their personal ethics in a document suitable for framing and post them in their offices. This means that, not only are they willing to articulate their "ethics bottom line" but also they are willing to have staff know what it is. This lessens the temptation for hypocrisy.

After self-assessment comes the process of building and maintaining your professional competency as an HCA. When you graduate from school, you will possess certain knowledge, attitudes, and skills that make you competent to practice healthcare administration in certain settings. While you should have a positive feeling about your accomplishment, it is only the beginning. You will add many more levels of competence as you progress through your career. Much of this will come through actions and self-assessment of those actions that builds to experience. You might want to seek out a mentor to assist you in building your experience-based competence. Be careful to find a person that you can trust. This person should also be at least one or two levels above you in the organization. He or she should also be a person who is willing to take time to help you assess your strengths and areas for improvement in an honest, but not ego-crushing, manner. Mentors can also provide insight into the arcane organizational culture and its unwritten rules so that you do not step on someone's toes because of your ignorance.

Once you have identified your strengths, do not be too complacent. You cannot rely just on these areas or always assume that they will be there. Just like a muscle, if your strengths are not used and reinforced, they will diminish. You must continue to use and build those areas. You also need the humility to work on areas of improvement. When you are a new graduate or in a new position, you have a honeymoon period where you are not expected to know everything. Take advantage of that time to ask questions and listen to the answers to those questions. You will be forgiven for not knowing everything and you can learn much during this period.

You also need to consider your own continuing education opportunities. These can be met on a formal or informal basis. For example, consider taking continuing education courses through your local ACHE, MGMA, or community resources. If you are strong in a certain area, you might consider becoming a part-time teacher or workshop leader. Nothing helps to reinforce what you know or to make you learn new areas like teaching them to others. Some organizations have programs for administrators where they do the job of one of their staff (nonclinical, of course) for one day or one-half of a day. Participants in these programs report a great increase in their understanding of staff's contribution to the organization. Staff also appreciates an administrator's willingness to understand their role in the organization, so it is a win-win situation. Finally, if you are in a position to do so, become a mentor to a new HCA or an experienced one who has recently joined your organization. Your efforts will help to reinforce your own learning and assist in the career building of another.

Competent HCAs do not isolate themselves from their communities. You need to take advantage of opportunities to be involved in appropriate organizations as either a member or an officer. These organizations can include the local Rotary Club, the Kiwanis, or the Boy Scouts or Girl Scouts. You might also consider being on advisory boards for HCA programs at local colleges, public health programs, and other health-related organizations. Remember that you are always representing your organization when you do anything in the community, so you will have to pay attention to your words and actions. However, putting yourself "out there" to have a better understanding of the real issues facing your community is worth the extra effort. It also improves your image and that of your organization.

In light of your busy schedule, just how are you supposed to find time for all of this competence assurance? First, you cannot afford not to find some time for it. You are the role model and cannot expect something from staff that you are not willing to do yourself. Second, making the time investment discussed here can have a substantial return on investment. Not only can you build up your career, but you can also have a greater understanding of what you want in life. Third, you will have a better understanding of your organization, your staff, and your community. This will help you to be more effective in your daily operations as an HCA. Finally, you will be a more complete person who has a good level of self-understanding and desire to grow and adapt to the ever-changing environment that is today's healthcare administration.

Summary

In this chapter, you can see that healthcare organizations exist in an age of multiple accountability. You are expected to comply with regulations from a great many external organizations that serve to protect the public's interests. You learned that there is a need to be an advocate for your organization and profession through maintaining current knowledge and getting involved. The chapter also presented your responsibility for ensuring your own competency and that of the staff. Because you are part of a trust-based industry, competency assurance is vital to ethical organizational behavior.

Cases for Your Consideration

The Case of the Novice Nurse

As you read this case, consider the following questions. Responses and comments will follow the case.

1. How effective was the orientation process for intensive care unit (ICU) nurses at St. Dismas Hospital?

2. What could have been done to prevent this situation from occurring?

3. How do you think Lawanda's family feels? What about the client's family?

4. What action needs to be taken to address this situation and decrease the damage to St. Dismas?

Case Information

Lawanda Person was a recent graduate of a BSN program. She had only one year of experience in Medical/Surgical units when she was hired by St. Dismas Hospital to be a staff nurse in the ICU. The situation for this case occurred during the fourth week of her six-week orientation. On that particular day, she was assigned two clients who suffered an anterior myocardial infarction (MI) and were both 48 hours post event. One of the clients was still on a ventilator. Lawanda had been assigned to be the medication nurse, should a code happen during her shift. This meant that if codes were called, she would be the team member to give physician-ordered medications to the clients.

Just before her shift was to end, Lawanda's ventilated client went into code. The code team arrived and CPR was begun. The code had lasted over 20 minutes when the nurse behind her handed Lawanda a syringe. Without any further action, she injected into the IV line. Immediately, the client reacted to the medicine and his heart stopped. The client was pronounced dead at 10:30 P.M. Lawanda felt sad that the client died, but knew that she had done everything she could to save him.

After the code, the nurse supervisor completed the documentation and checked the procedures used. She discovered that the wrong medication had been injected into the client. Apparently, there was a mix-up in the medication drawer, and the syringe was drawn from the wrong bottle. The nurse manager and the physician were immediately notified, and an investigation was begun.

The next day at the beginning of her shift, Lawanda was called to the nurse supervisor's office. She was told about the medication error that was made on the code. The nurse supervisor said, "You killed that client last night. You were the one who was in charge of the meds and you did not check them. You are going to lose your license over this." She told Lawanda that she must call and report herself to the state board of nursing. In addition, she might be subject to fines and jail time for the medical error she had made. The nurse supervisor also threatened to put her on suspension. Even though Lawanda was visibly upset by this news, the supervisor told her to "get some backbone" and finish her shift.

Lawanda went back to the ICU and, at the first chance she could, called her parents to tell them what had happened. They told her that they would do whatever they could to help. However, this did not make her feel better. She could feel the cold stares of the staff who would not speak to her during the shift. She tried to be attentive to her patients, but the supervisor's words echoed in her head. She was a murderer! She might go to jail! She began to imagine what was going to happen to her during a full investigation of the event and how her mistake was going to cost her everything she had. She thought about the humiliation of being taken before board and losing her license.

Somehow, she made it to the end of her shift and then she made her decision. She went to the medication drawer, took a bottle of potassium and a syringe, and put them in her pocket. On her way out of the lobby, she entered the restroom, locked the door, and gave herself a fatal dose of potassium. Her body was found by the housekeeper later that evening and an emergency call was made, but it was too late. The CEO was called and he made the necessary notifications including the hospital's attorney. He also called Lawanda's parents. Understandably, they were shocked and angered by the news and accused St. Dismas of "killing our daughter." Soon after this conversation, they contacted their attorney and alerted the press.

Responses and Commentary on Questions

1. How effective was the orientation process for ICU nurses at St. Dismas Hospital?

   On the surface, it seems that this is not an effective orientation program at all. After all, a client died as the result of a medication error that could have been prevented. However, the program itself perhaps was not completely responsible.

First, you need to consider the hiring practices that preceded the orientation process. It could be argued that St. Dismas, like many other hospitals, was facing a nursing shortage and, therefore, had to take a chance on a nurse with limited experience, and none of it in the ICU. However, the overall costs of this decision were great. A client and a nurse lost their lives, and the hospital faced the potential for tremendous negative publicity. In fact, it took several years before it regained public trust completely. In addition, Lawanda was assigned full care for two clients even though she had not finished the entire orientation program. Perhaps this was just too much responsibility for her at this stage of her orientation process.

Comment: This case makes a good argument for having a well-designed orientation program to be completed by your staff. You need to consider not just an orientation to the routine practices for your institution, but also prevention strategies. It is a good idea to have your organization's legal support personnel evaluate your program to see if it contains the most significant information. In terms of prevention of medication errors, some organizations have begun using **poka-yoke** or error prevention practices, including bar coding for medications. If such practices are active in your organization, they certainly need to be featured in your orientation program. You also need to evaluate the program frequently and actually review these data and use them to make appropriate updates. An out-of-date or inaccurate orientation program will not help the staff or the organization.

2. What could have been done to prevent this situation from occurring, other than instructions given in the orientation program?

You must begin at the beginning. During a code, there is a great deal of stress, even though protocols have been clearly defined. However, in the haste to save a life, sometimes these procedures are overlooked or omitted. Clearly, Lawanda was not the only person to make an error here. The nurse who was responsible for obtaining the drug failed to check and recheck to make sure she had the correct medication as ordered by the physician. When Lawanda received the medication, she should have verified that it was the correct one before injecting it. Failure to follow the protocols was the cause for making and not catching the medication error.

What about the actions after the code? The correct procedure for documentation and verification of the process was done by the nurse supervisor. When she did find a problem, she followed the correct procedure for notifications. It was also correct that an investigation needed to be conducted and the individuals involved needed to be made aware of the seriousness of what occurred.

However, the way she dealt with Lawanda was very inappropriate. First, the supervisor assumed a tone of accusation and blame even before the full investigation was completed. She also threatened Lawanda with jail and loss of license rather than finding the underlying cause of the situation. In her anger over what happened, she failed to consider the effects her words would have on this novice nurse. Rather than deal with the situation fairly and apprise Lawanda of what could happen and why, she chose to present the worst-case scenario without complete knowledge of the situation. Then, to add to the problem, she told Lawanda to complete her shift, thereby potentially endangering clients.

The nurse manager should have been given proper instruction on how to handle situations where bad news must be given. Lawanda had a right to know what had occurred and what was being done about it. She also had a right to be told in a professional manner. In addition, there should have been a policy concerning her status while things were being investigated. Minimally, she should not have been working with clients on the day that she learned of the incident and the investigation. The potential for causing unintended harm to clients was too great.

You should also look at the behavior of Lawanda's coworkers. By ignoring her and, even worse, talking about her when her back was turned, they demonstrated a presumption of guilt. Perhaps some compassion or support was too much to expect, but they should have treated her in a professional manner. In addition, no one seemed to be watching the medication drawers, which made it very easy for Lawanda to obtain her fatal dose. Do her coworkers have any ethical burden here? Perhaps they should have been educated about appropriate behavior in such circumstances.

3.   How do you think Lawanda's family feels? What about the client's family?

Can you even imagine how Lawanda's parents felt? They were only aware of the situation at St. Dismas on a surface level. They had one quick phone call from their daughter, who seemed terribly upset by what the supervisor had said. However, she was going to finish her shift, so they had no real indication of how severe those feelings were. Perhaps, they were feeling some guilt for not going to the hospital and insisting that Lawanda come home. However, she was an adult, and they did not want to interfere. They were also angry with the facility staff for their treatment of their daughter and felt that the way Lawanda was told about her situation caused her suicide.

As for the client's family, they certainly were upset. While an MI is a serious problem where death can occur, they lost their loved one through an error made by people that they trusted. Besides the grief from the loss, they are probably feeling confused and angry. It would not be at all surprising if St. Dismas received a telephone call from their attorney.

4. What action needs to be taken to address this situation and decrease the damage to St. Dismas?

Because this situation now involved the law and the media, there was a need to be in contact with whoever provides legal counsel for the hospital. This person would have provided St. Dismas administrators with information on how to deal with any action that is taken against them and how best to handle the press to protect the hospital's interests. In addition, an internal investigation needs to be conducted so that all of the facts are known. Any appropriate actions would need to be taken and documented.

In dealing with the press, the hospital would be best served to have a designated spokesperson who would be forthcoming with the appropriate level of information. The spokesperson should be cautioned to avoid the use of "no comment" (it only makes the person appear to be guilty) and instead to direct the inquiry to the appropriate contact person. Staff members who were involved should be instructed not to speculate in the press so that the situation does not become even worse. Regaining the public's trust in St. Dismas Hospital after such a situation would take much additional effort and time.

The Case of Patient Safety and BFOQs

As you read this case, consider the following questions. Responses and comments will follow the case.

1. What motivated Sara and Emma to report their supervisor?

2. What should Stan do in this case?

3. What needs to be done to prevent future situations of impairment?

Case Information

Stan Delouse was the assistant director of HR at Seraphina Compassionate Care Center (SCCC), a specialty hospital for the treatment of cancer. On Monday morning, he was greeted at his door by two of the RNs from the Evergreen Floor. After introducing themselves as Sara Katz and Emma Smith, they informed him of the reason for their visit.

It seemed that Linda Chard, their nurse supervisor, was no longer able to do her duties. She was, they said, "so fat that she does not even leave the desk anymore unless it is to take a smoke break." They described her as being only five feet four inches tall but weighing at least 250 pounds. While her weight was not a new issue, her latest incident caused them to be concerned enough to report it to HR.

On Sunday night, one of the patients on Evergreen had a code. Ms. Chard was the first one in the room but she could not even begin to provide basic CPR. She was too heavy to reach across the bed and assist the patient. Further, she appeared to be having symptoms of shortness of breath herself. Fortunately, Sara and Emma were there almost immediately and began the correct procedures. The two nurses did not want to be seen as "tattletales" but they were very concerned that Ms. Chard's health condition was putting patients in jeopardy. In addition, they felt it was unfair that they had to cover the supervisor's duties because her weight and shortness of breath interfered with her ability and desire to do them. They both wanted Stan to address this issue, but they also had some fears of retaliation.

Responses and Commentary on Questions

1. What motivated Sara and Emma to report their supervisor?

   First, you can consider an ethics-based motivation for their actions. They work in a facility that is dedicated to meeting the needs of patients who are in varying stages of pain and suffering. Consider what it took to report on someone who has power and authority over them. They might genuinely be concerned that Linda's health could compromise that care and jeopardize the healing of patients. They also might be somewhat concerned with the injustice, as they view it, of having to do Linda's work as well as their own. They are asking for an investigation into the matter.

   On the other hand, they might be angry with Linda for something totally unrelated to the situation. Their motivation might be less than ethical and include a desire to cause difficulty for their supervisor. Perhaps, they are prejudiced against people who are overweight or obese and or who are health professionals who smoke. Stan needs to investigate this information about Linda without making a prejudgment of fault.

2. What should Stan do in this case?

   First, Stan should review the job description related to Linda's current position. Were there specific BFOQs that related to the physical ability to do the job? If yes, it makes his job a little easier because Linda would have been hired under these conditions. If physical abilities were not spelled out, he might have to contact the legal team to get advice before taking any direct action.

Next, he needs to consider the source of his information and its motivation. He should be sure that other issues are not present here and that the information presented is accurate. He might contact the director of nursing (DON) and ask her to stop by his office. Then, he could have a confidential conversation about the situation that was just presented to him. He could verify the information given and ask for further information. Do Linda's health issues truly have an impact on her ability to meet the needs of SCCC's patients?

Assuming the answer is yes, Stan needs to handle the situation with a concern for the ethical treatment of staff. First, he needs to prepare himself for a meeting with Linda. Remembering the cost of termination, recruiting, and rehiring, he must develop a plan to solve the problem without having to fire Linda. The DON should be consulted about this plan and invited to come to the meeting. Asking Linda to come to the HR office could create anxiety, but he cannot afford to ignore the problem. Therefore, he starts by holding the meeting in his office. He begins by telling her the reason for the meeting and stating the facts as he knows them, including the BFOQs for her position. Then, he should take time for compassionate listening.

Because this situation potentially threatens her livelihood, Linda might be angry and defensive. Stan should allow her to react and to give her version of the case. After she completes her comments, Stan should make note of them and ask for her ideas about how to resolve the situation. This will help her be a part of the solution and not the victim of it. Perhaps she really has the answers to her own problems. Stan should also introduce his plan for solving the problem, which might include support for Linda to enter smoking cessation programs and referrals to weight management services. There should be a reasonable time line with checkpoints so progress can be monitored. If the DON is present, she can assure Linda that she supports the plan. Before Linda leaves the office, she should sign off on the plan and receive a copy. Another copy should be placed in her HR file.

This meeting might have been stressful for all concerned, but it does not solve the problem. Stan still has the responsibility to follow up on the actions and time lines. He should be in frequent contact with the DON to verify that Linda has taken the agreed-upon actions and is making progress toward solving her health problems. He should inquire about her job performance and check to see if it is now meeting standards. It is hoped that there will be progress at each of the checkpoints and the problem will be solved. However, if there is no resolution, Stan must be willing to take appropriate action up to and including dismissal. The patient must always come first in any healthcare organization.

3. What needs to be done to prevent future situations of impairment?

As you read earlier in the chapter, employment of competent personnel begins with the job analysis stage. Therefore, this incident might trigger a re-evaluation of the nurse manager position and its job requirements. If additional requirements are needed, the job description and BFOQs should be changed appropriately. Stan should also review the policies and procedures for handling situations where impairment occurs, regardless of its source, to be sure that they support appropriate action. Of course, staff education might be needed in the future on the subject of impairment. Stan should always keep in mind that he needs to balance safety and quality care for the patients with compassion and respect for the humanity of the staff. This is no easy task, but one that is essential to an ethics-based healthcare facility.

Web Resources

American College of Healthcare Executives (ACHE)
http://www.ache.org/hap.cfm

American Hospital Association (AHA)
http://www.aha.org

Health Insurance Portability and Accountability Act (HIPAA)
http://www.hhs.gov/ocr/privacy

Joint Commission on Accreditation of Healthcare Organizations (JCAHO)
http://www.jcaho.org/

Medical Group Management Association (MGMA)
http://www.mgma.com/

National Committee for Quality Assurance (NCQA)
http://www.ncqa.org/

References

American College of Healthcare Executives. (2009). *ACHE healthcare executive competency assessment tool 2009*. Chicago: Author.
American Hospital Association. (2003). *The patient care partnership: Understanding expectations, rights, and responsibilities* [Brochure]. Chicago: Author.

Annison, M. H., & Wilford, D. S. (1998). *Trust matters: New directions for health care leadership.* San Francisco: Jossey-Bass.

Covey, S. R. (1989). *The 7 habits of highly effective people.* New York: Simon & Schuster.

Dye, C. F. (2000). *Leadership in healthcare: Values at the top.* Chicago: Health Administration Press.

Fottler, M. D., Hernandez, S. R., & Joiner, C. L. (1997). *Strategic management of human resources in health services organizations* (2nd ed.). Albany, NY: Delmar.

Joint Commission on Accreditation of Health Care Organizations. (2008). *History tracking report: 2008 to 2009 requirements accreditation program: Hospital chapter: Ethics, right, and responsibilities.* Available at: http://jointcommission.org/NR/rdonlyres/8C588. Accessed November 3, 2008.

National Committee for Quality Assurance. (2008). *About NCQA.* Available at: http://www.ncqa.org/tabid/675/Default.aspx. Accessed November 3, 2008.

Shortell, S. M., Gillies, R. R., Anderson, D. A., Erickson, K. M., & Mitchell, J. B. (2000). *Remaking health care in America: The evolution of organized delivery systems* (2nd ed.). San Francisco: Jossey-Bass.

Worthley, J. A. (1997). *The ethics of the ordinary in healthcare: Concepts and cases.* Chicago: Health Administration Press.

CHAPTER 6

Market Forces and Ethics

Markets change, tastes change, so the companies and the individuals who choose to compete in those markets must change.

—An Wang

Points to Ponder

1. What is the relationship between market forces and ethics?
2. What were the ethical roots of managed care?
3. Why should a healthcare administrator (HCA) be concerned about ethics and managed care?
4. What ethical issues have been introduced since the advent of alternative/complementary medicine?

Words to Remember

The following is a list of key words for this chapter. You will find them in bold in the text. Stop and check your understanding of them.

case management	disease management
gatekeeper	HEDIS®
integrated medicine	managed care
practice profiling	utilization review

■ INTRODUCTION AND DEFINITIONS

What forces in the marketplace affect the business of health care? To answer this question, first consider who is a potential user of the healthcare market. The most encompassing answer is everyone! Because everyone may need our services, we must be aware of what happens in the communities that we serve. Changes in the economy and market forces that affect our community also affect the business of health care. For example, think about what happens to your market when a new research discovery hits the news. Even if the results are not definitive, there is often an almost immediate public response. Physicians' offices are inundated with telephone calls for the procedure or product. On a more serious scale, think about what happens when there is a major scandal in a healthcare facility somewhere in the United States. When reported on the national news, the public's mindset can paintbrush the entire industry with the sins of the few. Trust is questioned and your telephone begins to ring with questions.

In this chapter, you will explore examples of economic issues and general market forces with emphasis on they affect the business of health care. Because managed care is such a powerful market force, a separate section is devoted to it. You will learn about its history and status. This information can assist you in thinking about ethics principles and how to apply them when dealing with managed care. Because the increased role of the consumer is also a major market force, you will explore an example of a consumer-driven phenomenon—the rise in **integrated medicine** (IM). There will be a summary to suggest some key concepts to remember in dealing with market forces in an ethics-based way.

■ GENERAL MARKET FORCES

In thinking about how the market influences the business of health care, it makes sense to start with the general economy. Recent events, such as the rising price of gasoline, the housing market crisis, and the banking bailouts, make Americans realize that economics is more than a course people study in college. It affects individual and businesses; health care is no exception. For example, when there is an economic recession, people lose their jobs. A loss of healthcare coverage often accompanies this job loss. While COBRA benefits can assist with maintaining coverage, many cannot afford the coverage or do not have the financial resources to purchase private insurance. Without insurance, they may put off procedures that are needed and risk conditions that are more serious in the future. This decision adds to healthcare costs for the individual and the system as a whole. If care cannot be delayed, the unemployed person may face serious debt or even bankruptcy.

Another example of how economic changes can affect the business of health care happens when gasoline prices rise quickly. Let us look at the how this occurs. The healthcare industry uses a wide variety of materials, which are manufactured all over the United States and abroad. Therefore, no matter the source, materials must be transported to the healthcare site where they are used. When gasoline prices rise beyond normal fluctuations, vendors have to pay more to purchase and transport healthcare supplies. This cost is passed on to the customer. Therefore, healthcare institutions have to pay more for the materials that they need to do business and charge the patient a higher rate. These are just two examples of the effect of economic change, but they demonstrate why we must pay attention to the larger economy as well as the market forces that are part of our communities.

What are the ethics ramifications of changes in the economy? Ethics thinking and decision-making becomes more challenging when there is an increase in the emphasis on fiscal responsibility. For example, if your costs increase without a matching increase in revenue, you may have greater difficulty meeting payroll, purchasing needed materials, and maintaining your business. It is easier to forget ethics when survival thinking overcomes patient thinking.

In an economic downturn, ethics issues concerning providing care for the uninsured are even more troubling. If the system struggles to provide care in good economic times, how can it manage when there is an increase in the uninsured? How do you provide just care and still stay afloat financially? In addition, the issue of justice may also surface as patient complaints about the fairness of increased charges for the same services. It is easy to see that difficulties with the economy can strain ethics resources as well as fiscal ones.

In addition to the overall economy, several market forces influence the business of health care. You have only to enter a healthcare facility to experience a major one of them—technology. The strides that have been made in this arena and its potential for the future pose serious business and ethics issues. In fact, technology has had such a profound effect on your business that an entire chapter is devoted to it (see Chapter 8).

Another market influence that cannot be ignored is the aging of the American population and the role of baby boomers in that phenomenon. Shi and Singh (2008) state that in 2030, when most of the boomers are in retirement, they will represent 20% of the U.S. population. Even today, they make up over 12%. What is the impact of the aging of this "bolus of boomers"? History gives you a clue. When the boomers hit first grade, the schools changed to accommodate their large numbers. When they hit college age, the colleges expanded. When they began to buy homes, the real estate market changed. Now, they are aging. What do you think will happen to the healthcare market?

Because chronic disease is more prevalent with the onset of aging, you have to anticipate a different kind of healthcare service. This will require a major change in thinking and system design, as health care today is still in the acute care model. However, you can also see this as a stellar business opportunity to increase your revenue stream by providing services that this population wants and needs. What might be included in these services?

Remember that aging boomers tend to be educated, affluent, and quality-seeking. They are willing to spend their resources to prevent the onset of chronic disease or to lessen its severity if it already exists. They want high quality of life right up until the end of life—and are willing to pay for it. What does this mean for your business? Prevention, once thought to be the purview of "health nuts," will be a business opportunity. Goods and service related to the quality of life among the elderly will increase. The boomers will expect their healthcare system to provide geriatric services at a reasonable price (Coddington, Fischer, Moore, & Clark, 2000). Community- and institution-based care will have to be evaluated and expanded to meet this new market demand.

Not only will this market force bring change to the type and delivery of health care, it will also bring its own ethics issues. For example, how will the healthcare business maintain its profit margin if demand for care exceeds its resources? The boomers represent a powerful voter block. Will their power allow them to take more than their fair share of the health resources at the expense of younger generations? What about the human resources issues here? Will your business experience a "wisdom drain" as boomers retire and positions need to be filled? Is there a way for you to use this new "leisure class" of boomer retirees to benefit your organization and its efforts for community health? These are just a few of the ethics issues that this market force will generate in the immediate future. You might not have the answers now, but you will need to seek them in the future.

You can see by these examples of market forces that prudent HCAs need to maintain a current knowledge of cultural and community trends in order to stay ahead of them and keep their organizations' competitive edge. Tunnel vision will only cause you to miss market opportunities for your business or face unnecessary ethical challenges. In light of these challenges, there is a need for each facility to carefully define or refine its mission and make it address market force concerns.

■ MANAGED CARE AND ETHICS

Managed care has been part of healthcare delivery in one form or another for over 50 years (Morrison, 2000) and has become a major influence on how you do business. It contributed to moving the foundation of health care from a social justice or care model to an emphasis on business practices. As a response to the limitations of fee-for-service and healthcare inflation, managed care was designed to control costs and increase appropriate access. Managed care coverage now appears to drive the provision of care, because facilities are reluctant to offer what is not funded. The result has been a corporate system that might not meet the needs of the individual consumer or the community at large.

Health care is now a highly competitive business where profit margins are tight and a struggle to meet your mission exists. You must deal with multiple regulations imposed by government and managed care contracts to control costs, prevent abuse, and regulate practice patterns.

The response to managed care from the greater community is not always favorable. The public, while generally liking their individual practitioners, tends to have negative feelings about managed care in general. It finds the limitations of choice and coverage, **gatekeeper** referrals, and other features to be annoying at best. In addition, this system of delivery has been the target of the media that looks for prime time issues to cover. Entertainment venues also reinforce a negative image for managed care. For example, think of the portrayal of insurance coverage—or lack thereof—in such films as *As Good as It Gets* and *John Q*. Politicians also find it a convenient target and strive to protect voters from its abuses through an increasing amount of regulation (Pearson, Sabin, & Emanuel, 2003).

A market force with this much impact also brings significant ethical issues. For example, what happens when managed care no longer can control costs and access? If you fail to negotiate contracts to cover your expenses and profit, how do you still provide services when you cannot make enough money to keep your doors open? What happens to patient autonomy when third-party payment directs available care? How will you provide care for those not under a contract? In addition, what is your role as an ethics-based HCA in negotiating contracts and maintaining standards? These are just a few of the potential ethics questions that managed care raises.

The first step in answering them is knowledge. In the case of managed care and ethics, the idea that knowledge is power is not a cliché. The more that you are informed about these organizations, their missions, and their past and future, the more you can be successful forming business relationships and making sound ethical decisions. The next few sections of this text will provide you with an overview of history, current status, and future concerns in managed care. You must remember that there are whole courses and textbooks on managed care, so these sections will not make you an expert on the subject. In order to keep up with current trends in this business, you must, to paraphrase Dory in *Finding Nemo*, "Keep reading, reading, reading."

Historical Foundations

Why begin with history? Organizations do not exist in a vacuum: they have a foundation and a philosophy. Understanding their history will help you to understand the traditions that govern their thinking and actions. Therefore, history does matter in your ability to make educated business and ethical decisions. Even though some think that ethical managed care is an oxymoron, this delivery system was actually founded because of an ethics concern. The health maintenance organization (HMO) (earliest form of managed care) movement actually began in 1938 when the Kaiser Company was trying to find a way to provide health care for its workers. The company made an agreement with its partners to contract with local facilities to prepay for worker health care coverage. Kaiser Company paid for any expenses associated with accidents, and employees paid seven cents per day for other healthcare needs. By addressing both preventive and acute care, Kaiser was better able to maintain a healthy work force and gained a reputation as a benevolent and ethical company.

However, managed care did not remain a social movement for long. In 1971, President Nixon, in reaction to rising healthcare costs, pushed for the creation of HMOs. He hoped that this delivery system would correct the abuses of fee-for-service and eventually provide health care for all Americans. His interests led to the HMO Act of 1973 with its certification program. From that point, despite protests from the American Medical Association and others, managed care began to grow with promises of decreased healthcare costs, increased healthcare benefits, quality control, and patient satisfaction.

Current Situation

Managed care evolved from its roots as a social experiment to its present state through a series of incremental changes in coverage and delivery options. Managed care has penetrated the healthcare market in ways that could never have been imagined by the Kaisers in 1938. Almost all employer-financed healthcare options include a managed care plan. In fact, many people think of managed care as a synonym for health insurance. Even federal and state governments have used this model for delivery to dependents either through contracting or through their own versions. So managed care has evolved into a complex system with many options. Today, you might be dealing with an HMO, IPA, PPO, POS, EPO, TriCare—or all of these options at once. This alphabet soup of delivery systems came into being when managed care was opened to the for-profit sector (Morrison, 2000).

The managed care industry has been successful in using business practices to control access to services and cost of delivery. For example, the use of the primary physician as a gatekeeper for access to hospitals and specialists has reduced unnecessary hospital stays and treatments. Consumers do not have unlimited choices in treatment or physicians unless they are willing to pay more for this option. **Case management** and **utilization review** were instituted to coordinate patient care and oversee the appropriateness of that care. While this has not met with great favor from practitioner or patient, it has helped to control healthcare costs. Finally, **practice profiling**, the bane of many physicians, allows managed care organizations to compare practice patterns between physicians, in similar practices, for evidence of practice excesses or even fraud and abuse (Shi & Singh, 2008).

Despite these efforts, managed care has not lived up to all of its economic promises. For example, although President Nixon saw managed care as a way to insure all Americans, the rate of uninsured has increased substantially. Healthcare costs and medical inflation continue to rise despite the efforts of the managed care industry. The dominant business model for managed care organizations has become a for-profit model. This means that earning from profits and savings are given to stockholders instead of being used to reduce rates for employers or patients (Moore, 2009).

Managed care organizations have attempted to influence the quality of patient care through various utilization reviews and practice profiles. Benefits of managed care include a greater emphasis on patient satisfaction and standardization of some medical practices that has led to better patient outcomes. Some procedures have been moved from hospital to same-day surgery settings and hospital stays have been reduced. In its effort to control costs, managed care has emphasized preventive care and the control of chronic disease (Moore, 2009). In addition, the National Committee for Quality Assurance accredits managed care organizations through a detailed process involving self-study and site visits. This organization has worked to monitor quality through a set of standardized measurements called Healthcare Effectiveness Data and Information Set (**HEDIS®**). These efforts have benefitted both the individual and the community.

Despite all of this good news, managed care may have done all it can to control costs and produce quality care. Even with its evolution to adapt to consumer demands, costs to provide care continue to rise and managed care contracts may not cover these costs. If physician groups, hospitals, and other providers cannot do business based on managed care contracts, there is a temptation to save money by withholding needed services or to under treating managed care covered patients. In addition, with the increased access and use of the Internet, consumers are becoming much more perceptive with respect to their benefits under their managed care plans. They are demanding even more choice about how their healthcare dollar is used and the kind of services that are covered. In addition, information technology (IT), fraud, abuse, and other concerns have led to more scrutiny of managed care companies and increased legislation including the Health Insurance Portability and Accountability Act (HIPAA). These and other factors mean that managed care may need to make serious changes for its future survival.

Future Concerns

The Institute for the Future (2003) predicts that managed care must reinvent itself if it is to be profitable in the future. Key to these changes is addressing the issues of choice, **disease management** and IT. The system may need to create tiered options that offer a choice of benefits and costs so that consumers can be more directly involved in their healthcare options. To remain viable and profitable, managed care will have to determine how best to care for chronically ill patients who need high-cost treatment. This can be accomplished through better use of disease management practices. It is hoped that as knowledge of this area expands, best practices will be identified and adopted. These approaches should provide appropriate care and reduce overall costs.

IT is already a force in the managed care industry, but it is predicted to become even greater. It can be hoped that its use will help to control healthcare cost inflation (Institute for the Future, 2003). Managed care should be better able to identify practice patterns that yield cost-effective care and adopt them more systematically. Through use of IT systems, improved data collection, and effective indicators, quality should be improved throughout the industry. In addition, it is predicted that the use of IT will improve the accuracy of diagnosis and help consumers make better prevention and treatment decisions.

The future for managed care looks to be one of change and more change. Certainly, its demise is not imminent. Rather, through mergers and acquisitions, it appears that it will become dominated by a few, highly successful companies. The trend toward for-profit managed care organization has already begun and promises to continue the emphasis on marketplace model. To grow as an industry, managed care's path will be filled with the business and financial challenges mentioned here and perhaps many others to be identified. As you can imagine, ethics concerns will also be a part of the future of managed care.

Where Is the Ethics?

The interaction between managed care and the healthcare system introduces ethics issues that stem from conflicts between patient autonomy, the overall benefit for managed care members, and profit margins. For example, a conflict occurs when patients need for expensive services that are not covered by the contract. Denying such care could cause unnecessary suffering or even premature death, but providing uncovered services to everyone could have a negative impact on the facility's profit margin and viability. Incentive programs, gatekeeping, inclusions, or exclusions in plans, marketing, and disclosure of information are also examples of potential ethical problems related to managed care.

Perry (2002), Darr (2004), and Anderlik (2001) discuss incentive programs and the ethics issues surrounding them. Typically, incentives are incremental or lump sum payments designed to reward desirable practice patterns. An ethics concern is that these incentives unduly influence physician practices to the detriment of the patient. For example, a primary care physician might choose to treat the patient rather than refer that patient to a specialist, in order for the physician to meet an end-of-year bonus. However, if a patient's needs are beyond the scope of this physician's practice, the patient might not receive appropriate care. The decision also leaves the physician open to possible malpractice litigation.

As an HCA, you can take several actions to address the ethics of incentive programs. First, consider the scope of the program. If incentives are too broad, they can prove too tempting and produce a negative long-term effect on patient care. If they are too narrow, patient variability can make them impossible to meet. You also need to consider the incentive's effect on overall income. If the percentage is too high (for example, 25%), then it might inappropriately influence patient care decisions. If it is too low (for example, 5%), then it can fail to control costs. Remember that when incentives are linked to improvements in quality and effective practice innovation, they can be used for positive change. Maintaining patient trust and benefit should always be considered when deciding on accepting or implementing an incentive plan.

The gatekeeping function used in managed care can also bring ethical concerns. On the one hand, it serves to coordinate care and provide the best possible outcomes for the patient. It fosters cooperation between providers so the best practices can be identified and customized for the individual patient with consideration of level of acuity and comorbidity. On the negative side, the gatekeeper can function as a barrier to care. The physician is put in the middle between the patient and the payer. He or she becomes the agent for rationing care based on cost-effectiveness. In some cases, the physician's background does not prepare him or her to make decisions about providing or denying access to specialty care. For example, physicians are not well educated in the areas of mental health, yet they can deny these referrals. Some ethicists see the gatekeeper role as inappropriate for physicians because they should be an advocate for patient care. Others feel that this role is highly ethical because it serves to hold down healthcare costs for the whole community.

What should you do about the ethics of gatekeeping? Anderlik (2001) suggests that there is no solid research evidence to support strict rationing principles and stringent adherence to clinical protocols. Physicians' clinical judgment should be considered, as it is also a viable part of a patient. To support their judgment, physicians should be given information about costs and benefits of treatments. They should be encouraged not to recommend treatments that can only minimally benefit the patient. In addition, they should make greater efforts to educate patients about treatment decisions. Of course, policies that clearly define covered and noncovered treatment and the rational for the exclusion need to be in place. Such policies will assist physicians to make more appropriate gatekeeper decisions.

Several community-level ethics issues have been associated with managed care including its impact on the least advantaged in society. Managed care works as a business and not a force for social justice. Therefore, its policies are designed to improve its profit margin and not necessarily the overall health of the community. Providing care for those who cannot afford copays, who require numerous visits, or who have complex physical and social health problems, is simply not good for their business.

Despite this business position, competition has led managed care to expand to the Medicare and Medicaid market. Some studies show that HMOs have been effective in caring for elderly patients and kept them from expensive nursing home care. However, these results are not universal. Because healthy seniors need fewer services, there is an ethics concern that managed care will market to and attract these individuals (this is called "creaming"). While this makes sense in the short-term, it does not make good long-term business sense. As they age, even these healthy seniors will need more and more services that will affect profitability. What happens to those seniors who have chronic diseases and require frequent visits? Some managed care companies have tried to serve this population and have discontinued their service because of the negative impact on their profits. For an even bigger picture, think about what happens when the bolus of boomers becomes part of the Medicare system. Their numbers and increasing chronic disease experience will be a challenge for the entire managed care system.

The Medicaid population has also become more attractive to the managed care market. However, this population tends to have greater healthcare issues and poorer overall outcomes. Yet, some success has been reported by managed care in reducing inappropriate use of the emergency department and providing increased access. However, issues such as lower reimbursement rates, providing too little service, and patient skimming have also been reported. Practitioners might not want to contract for these patients because the lower rates and service restrictions prevent them from covering the cost of their service. In addition, as you saw in Medicare, if managed care begins to lose too much money on the Medicaid venture, it may discontinue service, which increases the ranks of the uninsured (Anderlik, 2001).

What is the impact of managed care on the already uninsured? First, when managed care organizations treat the healthiest of the poor, it means that the others must rely on community hospitals and public health facilities for their care. This means an additional strain on an already taxed public health budget. In addition, for-profit and not-for-profit healthcare organizations are faced with the financial impact of providing uncompensated care when managed care discontinues services or physicians will not serve this population. This whole issue of managed care's impact on social justice is an issue that may become large enough for the nation to take action. In the meantime, it continues to cause concern at many levels.

In your role as an HCA, you can be faced with the ethics issues posed by marketing managed care. Darr (2004) points out that if you are too successful in marketing the quality of your specialty care, you can adversely affect your bottom line. Too many high-risk patients could choose plans that access your services, causing you to lose money. Does this mean that you should have high standards of quality for your services, meet those standards, but keep it quiet? Darr advocates just stressing the quality of your general services. Again, you are seeing the conflict between the individual patient's needs and right to information and the collective good of members and the organization in general.

Anderlik (2001) also suggests that marketing can be an ethics problem when promises are made that cannot be delivered. In the highly competitive managed care business, salespeople might be tempted to inflate benefits and choice options to close the sale. This can also occur when contracts are discussed and negotiated. In negotiations, your role includes doing your homework, questioning all claims and presentations, and asking about the sources for information. You should negotiate in good faith, but not give away too much information. Remember the managed care company is there to close the deal, but you are trying to get the best possible contract to benefit your organization.

If you are in a position to work for a managed care organization in marketing and advertising, be sure that you give appropriate information (Anderlik, 2001). Check the accuracy of all materials (print, media, or Internet) before they become public so that they present a positive but accurate picture. Make sure that your sales representatives are well trained on your existing products. One training session might not be enough. Certainly, when you introduce a new product or service, you must make sure that your staff is sufficiently trained to provide accurate information. While such extensive training can seem like a high cost decision, it is easily justified if you consider the cost of legal action or negative press about your managed care organization. You will also want to evaluate how your sales force presents your organization and its products. This can be accomplished through follow-up telephone interviews with employers or other data collection methods. Should you find a problem, be sure to counsel appropriately so that actions are not repeated.

Finally, the issue of informed consent and disclosure of information in managed care should be considered. When a person enrolls in a managed care plan, he or she consents to having his or her care rationed. Therefore, no ethics issues should arise when information about options that are not covered are withheld. However, this assumes that the decision to enroll was an informed one, which might not be the case. Another argument on this issue is that the patient/physician relationship should be the best source of what to disclose and to whom.

What you have been learning about ethics should offer some assistance with the issue of consent and disclosure. The patient should come first. While the plan may offer a certain range of services, the patient has the right to know if other effective options are available. However, such information must include a balanced view of options including cost (to be borne by the patient), benefits, and success rates, among other things. You should also make every attempt to provide user-friendly information about treatment options. For some patients, this can mean updated information on your Web site. Others might not have computer access or the desire to use this communication tool. For them, you will need well-designed, accurate, and understandable booklets or pamphlets. Remember that the patient might be receiving news that evokes an emotional reaction. Whenever possible, allow time for information processing before asking for consent.

Moore (2009) suggests that it is possible to have a managed care organization that practices on an ethics model. Her vision of this HMO includes a large group of salaried physicians and a non-profit business model. In addition, the clinical practice would be controlled by the physicians because they would have input into quality management efforts and practice reviews. Members of the HMO would also be included in operations through membership on ethics committees, reviews of benefit coverage, and participation in education programs. This model should decrease the potential for conflicts of interest and the temptation of under treating patients.

So far, in this chapter, you have seen how managed care grew from its roots in social justice to its current state as business. This growth has brought with it many ethical issues that must be considered by both the managed care organization and its business partners. Perry (2002) gives you some general guidelines that should prove useful in dealing in managed care situations.

1. Be careful to use accurate marketing and advertising so the choice is truly informed.
2. Protect patients' rights to confidentiality. HIPAA rules go along way here, but they do not address everything.
3. Remember your responsibility to hire competent healthcare staff and ensure their competence.
4. Establish practice guidelines based on evidence and supported by your physicians.
5. Have appropriate appeal policies in place that do not punish the person who asks for the appeal.
6. Remember your community and maintain a commitment to education, research, and uncompensated care.

In addition, you will need to rely on the organization's mission and values for your decisions. Asking the question "Does this fit with our mission and values?" frequently should help you discern the correct decisions. As you will see in Chapter 10, the use of organizational ethics committees is also helpful in dealing with difficult managed care-related ethics issues. The latter half of the chapter discusses the ethics attached to IM, also known as complementary/alternative medicine (CAM).

■ INTEGRATED MEDICINE (IM) AND ETHICS

Why IM and Why Now?

In 1993, David Eisenberg and his group at Harvard Medical School stunned the medical community with a report in *The New England Journal of Medicine*. They estimated that there were over 425 million visits to complementary/alternative medicine (CAM) providers in the United States every year, which exceeded the number of primary care provider visits. The cost was 13.6 billion dollars, most of which was paid directly by the consumers. Although this study was criticized for its methods, it became one of the most widely cited research efforts of its type and demonstrated a much wider use of these practices than suspected (Eisenberg, et al., 1993). It began a major re-examination of what was once thought to be only quackery or fad.

Eisenberg and colleagues (1998) repeated this study in 1997 with even more startling results. The increase in users of CAM services was found to be 629 million, which was an increase of 47% from the previous study. CAM has become a multi-billion dollar business in the United States. In addition, most of the subjects combined CAM practices with conventional medical care. However, they did not often inform their physicians about their CAM use.

The initial terminology for this consumer-driven movement was alternative medicine, meaning that was used in place of conventional medicine. Then, it was called complementary medicine because it was used to support conventional medicine. Currently, the term "integrated medicine" is used because most people use it in conjunction with convention medicine. Just what is it? It is actually an eclectic collection of philosophies and practices. This collection is centered on a holistic view of the client, the healing properties of the body, and prevention as well as treatment of disease. IM does not see humans as being reduced to cells and diseases to be treated, but rather as unique individuals who are part of the environment in which they live. IM in the United States encompasses well over 200 different types of practices, many of which have their roots in healing systems that are thousands of years old (Micozzi, 2005).

The consumers who have directed this movement tend to be edu-cated, affluent, and female, but its use is not limited to just this group. Clients of IM desire to be partners in their health care and seek infor-mation on their own. They also are aware of the need for prevention and view IM as a way to decrease the likelihood of serious illness or to prolong the quality of their lives. Evidence of their belief in this system of health care is demonstrated by their willingness to pay billions of dollars in out-of-pocket expense to use IM services.

A major market for IM services seems to exist among people suffer-ing from chronic disease. They seek relief and/or control over their symptoms and are often disappointed by what traditional medicine has to offer. They have a need to have control over their problems and find that IM offers a greater sense of control. They need to be a partner in their care. Traditional medicine's lack of definitive treatments for chronic diseases helps to explain the growing appeal of IM.

A visit to the National Center for Complementary and Alterative Medicine Web site (NCCAM) reveals that IM users also include tradi-tional medicine in their treatment. Even though consumers use both systems, they often are not entirely pleased with the traditional system. Their experience is that conventional medicine is often too impersonal, expensive, and rushed. In addition, they find the side effects of conven-tional medicines to be undesirable. IM practitioners, in contrast, spend far more time with each client, including him or her in treatment plans, and use more personal modalities. In addition, practitioners stress pre-ventive practices and areas that complement traditional medicine's approach. According to NCCAM (2008), the IM/CAM practices used most commonly include chiropractic care, massage, herbal medicine and other natural products, and yoga. Clients seek relief from back, neck, joint, and arthritis pain through these practices. They also seek assistance with anxiety, depression, and insomnia. This list is not sur-prising when you consider that 60% to 90% of all traditional medicine visits are for stress-related problems.

Even with its increased popularity, traditional medicine's reaction to this consumer-driven movement has been mixed at best. Despite clini-cal studies by the NCCAM, many still find this form of healing to be total quackery and even ridicule patients who use it. Criticisms include that it is not grounded in scientific theory, does not have demonstrated long-term studies on safety and efficacy, and that practitioners are not qualified to treat based on medical school criteria. Even practices with thousands of years of documented effectiveness, such as acupuncture, are branded as fads or just the result of the placebo effect. Herbal med-icine, despite extensive research in Germany and other countries, con-tinues to be touted as a waste of money. In addition, negative findings associated with CAM or IM seem to garner high levels of attention in the mass media.

However, traditional medicine's response is not all negative. Since the National Institutes of Health began supporting serious research in CAM/IM, physicians have slowly begun to be more interested in the area. Most of the U.S. medical schools now offer courses in this area. There is even a Physicians' Desk Reference for Herbal Medicine available to provide updates for busy practitioners. Pharmacy and nursing schools are expanding their coverage to include herbal medicine and other areas. The NCCAM sponsors in research on these modalities and supports training programs.

In addition, a NCCAM study revealed that 26% of conventional medicine practitioners referred patients to IM practitioners. Hospitals and specialty centers including cancer centers have capitalized on the holistic care concept by adding IM practices to their existing offerings. Some of these facilities include music therapy, massage, guided imagery, and acupuncture as a way to provide patient-centered services. In addition, long-term care facilities have added IM to their services to improve the quality of life for their residents. Examples of this service expansion include music therapy and pet therapy.

Insurance companies are becoming more willing to include IM as a covered benefit because it has the potential for preventing more costly treatments. Managed care organizations are particularly interested and provide supplements that cover services of IM providers in their networks. These providers are credentialed to offer the best possible service to the consumer. In addition, credentialing for IM practitioners has become more standardized. Licensure and/or certification are required for major professional groups such as acupuncturists, massage therapists, and naturopathic physicians. The trend toward the use of IM practices appears to be growing, and the number and duration of clinical studies has increased.

Where Is the Ethics?

The integration of two systems of health care with very different views of patients and their needs has the potential for many ethical problems. If future predictions are correct, IM will be a part of your healthcare business on some level. It will be important to consider these potential ethics issues and do what you can to prevent them. First as clinical or hospital director, you must have an informed practice in order to correctly diagnose and treat patients who also use IM. While your professional staff might not agree with what your patients do, they will still expect you to honor their autonomy and to make accurate diagnosis of their condition.

Failure to have a basic knowledge of IM practices will prevent your staff from providing the most informed care and can have drastic results. For example, some herbs affect the blood's ability to clot. If they are taken with prescribed blood thinning agents, the results can even be fatal. A well-informed practice is able to prevent such problems by gaining patient information about herb use and by knowing the action and drug interactions of what the patients are using. Physicians and nurses could also answer questions about IM practices in a fair and evidence-based way. Continuing education programs and resource materials might be needed to do this, but the expenditure of money and time will be worth it.

Informed consent is another ethics issue related to IM. Some have argued that healthcare practitioners should discuss IM options as well as traditional medicine with their patients. This is supported by the AHA's *Patient Care Partnership* document, which stresses the need for patients to be given information on benefits and risks of healthcare decisions. To assist with patient decision-making, physicians and other practitioners should be aware of all treatment options and be able to answer questions. Your staff will also be expected to provide objective and accurate advice about these modalities so that patient consent is truly informed. As clinical studies reveal more and more evidence about which IM practices are effective and which are not, practitioners should feel more comfortable discussing these options with patients. The policy of "don't ask; don't tell" with respect to IM will not work for the future. In fact, many practices have already added questions about IM uses and herbs to their medical history forms.

If you are considering adding IM modalities as a revenue stream, there are some areas for you to consider. First, you will want to analyze what services are readily available in your area and which of them are frequently used. You will also want to investigate which of these services are covered by insurance. This information can be obtained through Web searches and telephone surveys. Because patient safety is an ethics concern, you will always want to consider the efficacy and quality of any services. You could research Web sites such as the National Center for Complementary and Alternative Medicine, which will give you information about modalities, what they are supposed to do, and what they actually do. You would then have to take all of the appropriate steps, including gaining all the appropriate approvals, for adding IM services. Do not forget to consult the physicians and have a champion or two on your side. It is wise to start small and build. For example, add a massage therapist or music therapist after evaluating patient satisfaction and profitability of such an addition. Fortunately, Faass (2001) has written a detailed book on how best to integrate IM services into traditional practices.

As part of your ethical duty to protect patient safety, you must contract with or hire IM practitioners who are prepared in their area of service. Several of the over 200 areas of IM are now certified or licensed. For example, the American Massage Therapy Association has accredited programs throughout the United States. Many states also require a license to practice massage therapy. Likewise, there is a program for school accreditation and individual certification/licensure for acupuncture and naturopathy practice. To make this even easier, firms have been created to verify practitioner certification and to make the selection of who to hire much easier. Remember though that, while certification and licensure is increasing for many of these areas, not all practitioners have formal credentialing or are even required to have it to practice. You will have to use discernment based on your mission, research, and consumer information in those cases.

Summary

In this chapter, you have begun to explore the impact of market forces on healthcare systems and the potential ethical problems that they can create. It concentrated on two major trends, managed care and IM, but this is not the whole picture. As a practicing HCA, you will have to keep your finger on the pulse of what is happening in your healthcare market. Additional issues can arise that must be addressed. Your responsibility will be to address them in an ethics-based manner. Remember that you are trusted to provide safe, quality care for patients. In addition, your image in the community is critical to your success as a healthcare business. In dealing appropriately with market forces, organizational and personal ethics matter.

Cases for Your Consideration

The Case of the Concerned Managed Care Administrator

1. What ethical principles did this administrator use in dealing with Mr. Michigan?

2. What was the cost of her practicing ethical behavior and what were the benefits?

Case Information

Mary Ledfedder was one of the claims managers for St. Dismas Health Plan (SDHP). On Monday, she received a case from one of her assistants for review. The case involved a man named Shamus Michigan who had visited his acupuncturist. This professional found a problem in the kidney meridian. Mr. Michigan then had a full body scan at a local clinic and the scan picked up a mass in the kidney area. A follow-up was suggested. Mr. Michigan had another scan and a follow-up MRI. He was diagnosed with cancer of the kidney. Fortunately, the tumor was encapsulated and he was treated by a laparoscopic nephrectomy. He filed a claim for reimbursement for his scans, and his claim was denied.

Mr. Michigan became quite upset when he received this news. He told the claims representative that he thought SDHP discriminated against people who used IM practitioners. After all, if it were not for his acupuncturist, he might be dead instead of just losing one kidney. He could not understand why coverage was denied and after consulting with an attorney, he asked for an appeal.

Usually, Ms. Ledfedder would do a quick review of such cases and issue a form letter to the appellant. However, she felt that this case might be different and wanted more information. She contacted Mr. Michigan and asked for more details. At first, he was upset about the denial of his claim, but he listened to Ms. Ledfedder as she explained their policy. They could only pay for procedures that were ordered by a physician, not ones that were chosen just by the patient. She asked Mr. Michigan if he had a physician order for any of the tests. As it turned out, he did. The second and third tests were done based on a referral from his physician and he had a copy of his letter.

Ms. Ledfedder put Mr. Michigan on hold and checked her policy book. While such a referral was not specifically mentioned, it certainly seemed appropriate. She told Mr. Michigan to send her a copy of the information that he had so she could review it. When it arrived by fax, she found that Mr. Michigan was correct; he did have proof of a physician order. When she called him back, she was able to give him good news. SDHP would pay for the last two tests, which would lessen his financial burden considerably.

Mr. Michigan was not pleased that not all of the tests could be covered but, after talking with Ms. Ledfedder, he understood why. He thanked her for putting in the effort to help him with his situation and said he looked forward to receiving his check in a reasonable period. After their conversation, he called his lawyer and told him not to go forward with the lawsuit.

Responses and Commentary on Questions

1. What ethical principles did this administrator use in dealing with Mr. Michigan?

   At this point in your study, you should be able to identify many ethics principles for this case. Ms. Ledfedder acted with beneficence when she chose to take the extra time to review the case instead of just issuing a form letter. Her follow-up phone call and decision to assist Mr. Michigan were also acts of beneficence. In addition, she supported the principle of nonmaleficence by making sure that his claim was handled fairly and he was paid what was appropriate.

Certainly, Ms. Ledfedder acted to respect Mr. Michigan's autonomy by giving him complete information about why his claim was denied. She even went further to inquire if he had proof of a physician's order. This inquiry helped her to arrive at a successful resolution of the problem because additional information could be provided. In addition, she treated Mr. Michigan with respect even though he was angry at the plan. She was not condescending or rude in her conversation, and that kept things on a more rational basis. Finally, she practiced justice because, while she did not order payment for a claim she could not support with a policy, she did make sure that Mr. Michigan received the reimbursement for which he was entitled.

2. What was the cost of her practicing ethical behavior and what were the benefits?

    Basically, the cost of Ms. Ledfedder's use of ethical behavior was minimal compared with the cost of having to deal with a lawsuit. Even if such a suit did not reach the courts, the negative publicity potential would be great. In addition, she kept an SDHP member satisfied, so he did not wish to change health plans. If asked, he could attest to the fairness of his treatment. This was worth a great deal in positive word-of-mouth publicity for the plan. In all, practicing ethical behavior was good business practice in this case.

The Case of the Confused Abuela (Grandmother)

As you read this case, consider the following questions. Responses and comments will follow the case.

1. What principles of ethics are involved in this case?

2. What were the ethics issues for Porter Sanders?

3. How important was knowledge of IM practices to the successful resolution of this case?

Case Information

Porter Sanders was the assistant administrator of St. Dismas Home Health (SDHH) program. On Monday morning, one of his best home health nurses, Emma Ray, stopped by his office to discuss a concern. Here was the case she presented.

Ms. Ray received a physician order for a home visit assessment of Mrs. Viola Romero, an 80-year-old woman with hypertension, who was also on thyroid medication. Mrs. Romero was living independently in her own home, but the family was concerned. Her behavior seemed to be deteriorating. She often appeared confused, exhibited some unusual aggressive behavior, and cried without provocation. They were worried that she had Alzheimer's disease and contacted her physician who then ordered the visit.

During her assessment, Ms. Ray questioned Mrs. Romero about her health history and activities of daily living. She was supposed to be taking medication for her hypertension. Because she had a thyroidectomy, she was also supposed to be taking daily thyroid pills. However, Mrs. Romero also consulted with the local curandero who conducted several rituals including sahumerio (incensing) and prayer. This healer advised Mrs. Romero to stop taking all of her medicines because they were poisoning her system. Instead, she suggested drinking a mint herb tea made with olive oil added to the tea. She also sold Mrs. Romero a magnetic bracelet to wear every day to balance her energies.

Mrs. Romero believed in the powers of this healer, who had a good reputation in the community and wanted to follow her advice. Ms. Ray tried to talk to her about the problems associated with not taking her medications, which could explain her change in behavior and other symptoms. She tried to explain that Mrs. Romero was endangering her safety and her life by not taking these medications. Mrs. Romero accused Ms. Ray of not respecting her beliefs and being on the side of the physician and her family. At the end of the visit, she remained adamant that she did not want to visit the physician or get back on her medications.

After she filed her report to the physician, Ms. Ray asked for Mr. Sanders's advice on the next steps to take. While she wished to respect Mrs. Romero's autonomy and right to choose or refuse treatment, she was concerned that Mrs. Romero was threatening her life. Mr. Sanders agreed and expressed concern about the effect on SDHH if no action is taken. After a lengthy discussion, Ms. Ray decided to discuss her findings with the physician and the family.

Once the physician had a full picture of the situation, he told Ms. Ray to advise the family to bring Mrs. Romero in immediately. In his opinion, this curandero was jeopardizing her life. He needed to evaluate her status and get her on the appropriate medication immediately. Ms. Ray then visited the family and explained what happened. They were shocked and greatly concerned. The family said that they would get Mrs. Romero to the physician "if they have to drag her there."

Two weeks later, Ms. Ray received a call from the family. Mrs. Romero consented to be taken to the physician's office but cried the whole way there. Fortunately, her physician was aware of the practices of curanderos and was able to convince her that her medications were not poisons. She could still use prayer and the bracelet for balance as long as she continued to take her pills. Mrs. Romero did not want to make the physician angry, so she decided to take the pills. Her symptoms disappeared.

Responses and Commentary on Questions

1. What principles of ethics are involved in this case?

   From your study of ethics, you can see that many principles are involved in this case. One of the most obvious is the conflict between patient autonomy and paternalism. Who knew what was best for this patient? Ms. Ray wanted to honor Mrs. Romero's autonomy and treat her with respect. Mrs. Romero had the right to control her own body and accept or reject treatment, but her actions put her life at risk. However, these actions also compromised her ability to make informed decisions. Therefore, her family had to intervene in this situation. Additionally, as part of autonomy, she also had the right to truth-telling. Ms. Ray carefully provided truthful information to convince Mrs. Romero that the curandero's practices were not in her best interests. Because the belief in the power of curanderos is a part of Mrs. Romero's core culture, this was difficult.

   You can also see the dual principles of beneficence and nonmaleficence in this case. First, Ms. Ray had a moral obligation to respect Mrs. Romero's beliefs and not demean them. Even though she disagreed with these practices, she had to treat Mrs. Romero with respect and kindness. However, she also had a moral duty to do no harm. Allowing Mrs. Romero to continue this practice without any intervention could cause her great harm and contribute to her premature death. Mrs. Romero's physician told Ms. Ray to contact the family immediately, and she supported this decision.

   The principle of autonomy was also an issue for the family. They dearly loved their Abuela Viola and wanted to respect her rights. However, they were concerned that her latest actions made her too confused to make appropriate health decisions. On the advice of Ms. Ray and the physician, they took action on the situation and coerced Mrs. Romero into visiting her physician.

2. What were the ethics issues for Porter Sanders?

   Porter Sanders had a different view of the ethics in this situation. While the mission of SDHH stressed that he must respect the cultural practices of his clients, he also needed to consider the impact of Mrs. Romero's actions on his business. If Mrs. Romero was not convinced to see her physician and died as a result, it could pose real problems for SDHH. The family could choose to blame Ms. Ray and SDHH for her death and contact an attorney, the press, or both. Certainly, the publicity of such actions, even though unfounded, could be harmful to the organization.

Mr. Sanders was also concerned with providing the best advice to Ms. Ray. He needed to listen to and consider her viewpoint in this situation. Of course, since the organization functions under physician order, he had to remind her that she needed to provide detailed information to him. To protect patient confidentiality, he had to make sure that Mrs. Romero's records were complete and protected. He also needed to be sure that Ms. Ray did not discuss this interesting case with her colleagues over coffee. Mr. Sanders relied on Ms. Ray's professionalism and the policies of SDHH to maintain this ethics obligation.

3. How important was knowledge of IM practices to the successful resolution of this case?

Knowledge of IM practices, specifically the practices of curanderos, was critical to the ability to resolve this case. First, Ms. Ray needed to be fully aware of the belief system of her Hispanic client, Mrs. Romero. This knowledge allowed her to communicate more completely and honor her autonomy. She also had to understand the philosophy and practices of curanderos. Many of these healers use practices that support traditional medicine and can actually be helpful. In Mrs. Romero's case, however, the curandero was in fact giving harmful advice. Ms. Ray needed to be able to explain why it was harmful while respecting Mrs. Romero's culture.

Most assuredly, the fact that Mrs. Romero's physician operated an informed practice helped him understand her culture and explain what she needed to do. Without such knowledge, he might have ignored her beliefs (at best) or even ridiculed them. Either of those responses would not have ensured patient compliance with treatment and might have caused unnecessary harm. However, his knowledge and patience with Mrs. Romero led to a positive outcome in this case.

Web Resources

National Institute on Complementary and Alternative Medicine
http://nccam.nih.gov/

American Massage Therapy Association
http://www.amtamassage.org/

References

Anderlik, M. R. (2001). *The ethics of managed care: A pragmatic approach*. Bloomington, IN: Indiana University Press.

Coddington, D. C., Fischer, E. A., Moore, K. D., & Clarke, R. L. (2000). *Beyond managed care: How consumers and technology are changing the future of health care*. San Francisco: Jossey-Bass.

Darr, K. (2005). *Ethics in health services management* (4th ed.). Baltimore: Health Professions Press.

Eisenberg, D. M., Kessler, R. C., Foster, F. C., Norlock, F. E., Calkins, D. R., & Delbanco, T. L. (1993). Unconventional medicine in the United States. *New England Journal of Medicine*, 328, 246–252.

Eisenberg, D. M., Davis, R. B., Ettnes, S. L., Appel, S., Wilkey, S., Van Rompay, M. V., & Kessler, R. C. (1998). Trends in alternative medicine use in the United States, 1990–1997. *JAMA*, 280, 1569–1575.

Faass, N. (2001). *Integrating complementary medicine into health systems*. Gaithersburg, MD: Aspen.

Institute for the Future. (2003). *Health & health care 2010: The forecast, the challenge* (2nd ed.). San Francisco: Jossey-Bass.

Micozzi, M. S. (2005). *Fundamentals of complementary and alternative medicine* (3rd ed.). New York: Churchill Livingstone.

Moore, J. (2009). Ethically important distinctions among managed care organizations. In Morrison, E. E. (Ed.). *Health care ethics: Critical issues for the 21st century*. Sudbury, MA: Jones and Bartlett, pp. 267–282.

Morrison, I. (2000). *Health care in the new millennium: Vision, values, and leadership*. San Francisco: Jossey-Bass.

National Center for Complementary and Alternative Medicine. (2008). *Health information*. Available at: http://nccam.nih.gov/. Accessed November 16, 2008.

Pearson, S. D., Sabin, J. E., & Emanuel, E. J. (2003). *No margin, no mission: Healthcare organizations and the guest for ethical excellence*. New York: Oxford University Press.

Perry, F. (2002). *The tracks we leave: Ethics in healthcare management*. Chicago: Health Administration Press.

Shi, L., & Singh, D. A. (2008). *Delivering health care in America: A systems approach* (4th ed.). Sudbury, MA: Jones and Bartlett.

CHAPTER 7

Social Responsibility and Ethics

A community is democratic only when the humblest and weakest person can enjoy the highest civil, economic, and social rights that the biggest and most powerful possess.

—A. Philip Randolph

Points to Ponder

1. Can health care be socially responsible and still meet its business goals?
2. How do prevention services fit into health care's social responsibility?
3. What should your relationship be with public health?
4. How is quality assurance part of social responsibility?

Words to Remember

The following is a list of key words for this chapter. You will find them in bold in the text. Stop and check your understanding of them.

epidemiology
Institute of Medicine
morbidity
social marketing

infant mortality
Leapfrog Group
public health administrator (PHA)
social responsibility

■ WHAT IS SOCIAL RESPONSIBILITY IN THE HEALTHCARE BUSINESS?

To stay fiscally sound, health care must operate on business principles. However, its roots and mission are unlike any other business. Health care's foundations are centered in the idea of social justice, which, as you learned in Chapter 4, is also called distributive justice. For example, in the early days, hospitals were established either to protect the community against contagious disease or to care for those who did not have the funds or the family to provide their care. Religious orders or communities were primary providers of such care. Admittedly, by today's standards, these early efforts were abysmal, but their motivation was one of service, not profit (Shi & Singh, 2008).

The change in orientation to business-like model happened for many reasons. After World War II, the healthcare system was not adequate to meet the nation's needs and needed assistance in upgrading facilities and building new ones. The federal government passed the Hill Burton Act, which assisted in these endeavors. The use of these funds required documentation, accountability, and demonstration of the provision of charity care. Business functions to meet these requirements became more important. The rise in the use of employer-sponsored health insurance also made a strong contribution to the change to a business orientation. The advent of for-profit healthcare facilities and managed care are more recent and formidable influences on the change to a profit-centered orientation.

Despite the current business orientation, the public does not have business expectations for health care. Purchasing health care is not like purchasing a refrigerator, car, or a home. The ability to choose is limited because health care is a monopoly. Although it has been regulated and controlled to some extent, it still wields great power and influence. Because of their knowledge and diagnostic ability, physicians control what procedures are used and when they are used. The public really does not have complete freedom of choice in its health care as it does in other businesses. In addition, there is a third-party payment system, which removes the consumer from the direct costs of service. Many have no idea about the real costs of their service and are shocked when they learn how it is priced.

Because service in the business of health care is not a direct choice, the public must trust health care's ethics and hold this business to a higher standard than other businesses. They expect that the principles of ethics you read about earlier in this book will be honored. They also expect to be treated with dignity and be given care that benefits their highest good. With this level of expectation, you can see why the reaction is so strong when even a few violate this trust.

Just how are you to be socially responsible and keep your profit margin high enough to stay in business? Chapter 4 gives a beginning discussion of this problem. Darr (2004) also provides some assistance with potential solutions. He stresses that ethical practice in this case involves making well-informed choices about strategic planning, availability of services, and setting priorities. You many need to perform environment scans to understand your community's needs and resources. While economics is a factor in these choices, questions about how each decision can positively affect service to all patients, including those who are disadvantaged, should also be considered. Profits can be used to care for those who cannot afford care. In other words, profit, used appropriately, can have a positive impact on your ability to be socially responsible.

Serving as good stewards of your resources by controlling costs, improving efficiency, and reducing waste are also part of social responsibility. If you can keep costs at an appropriate level, it can mean that more people will have access to care because it is more affordable. It also sends an important message that you are not just interested in your profit margin or in a million dollar annual income, but respect your obligation to provide for the community's health. This is especially important in managed care organizations where members can "vote with their feet" when they think that you are not putting them first. Perhaps your guiding question should be, "Who or what comes first in this organization?" If you can answer "the patient" and guide all of your decisions by this response, you can make decisions that exhibit social responsibility.

Social responsibility is also displayed in the daily interaction between patients and those who care for them. In healthcare facilities, we often categorize patients who care economically disadvantaged. Those categories could be described as those we regard as deserving and those we regard as not deserving. The deserving poor can be people who have suffered from a natural disaster or some event that was not under their control. While they may be unemployed, homeless, and without healthcare coverage, somehow we feel that they deserve compassion and available treatment.

The undeserving poor are those who have made lifestyle choices with which we do not agree. They are addicted to alcohol and drugs, practice risky sexual behaviors, or fail to comply with prescribed healthcare practices. These individuals are often viewed as annoyances or drains on the profit margin. They are subtly (or not so subtly) told that they must take whatever we give them and be grateful for whatever that is. Because healthcare professionals are human, it is easy to understand that constant exposure to people who make self-harming choices could lead to such cynicism. However, society judges our facilities by how they treat the poor regardless of the reason for their condition.

Those who provide service to the economically challenged in your organization should have the benefit of education and support. It is necessary to observe how care is delivered not just in terms of numbers of procedures. You might also have to evaluate the interpersonal communication between patient and care provider to see if basic ethical principles are being applied. In-service programs in areas like patient relations, applied ethics, meaning in work, and living your mission should help to assist daily patient interaction. In addition, you should do whatever you can to reinforce ethical treatment of all patients. This might include reward programs, scheduling that includes sufficient time breaks, and recognition of service.

Social responsibility in the healthcare system is not only about fiscal policy or direct patient treatment. It can be seen in your commitment to providing prevention services and understanding and supporting public health efforts. In addition, ongoing efforts to improve the quality of healthcare services are also a form of social responsibility. In the next sections of this chapter, you will learn more about your role in each of these areas.

■ PREVENTION AS SOCIAL RESPONSIBILITY

An individual's health is not determined by access to medical care alone. In fact, medical care is only credited with a 10% contribution to overall health (Shi & Singh, 2008). The remaining 90% comes from genetics, lifestyle, and environment. This means that many of the determinants of health fall into areas where prevention can make a positive contribution. For example, research supports the influence of nurturing on early childhood health and future development. Therefore, prevention and treatment of obesity in children can decrease diabetes, heart disease, and other chronic disease rates for adults. Active prevention and treatment for substance abuse and dependency has also been shown to have a positive impact on many health-related areas including decreasing domestic violence, auto accident fatalities, divorce, and chronic disease. Prevention services have the potential to positively affect the health and quality of life for communities, regardless of individual income or status.

It would seem logical that a system that is called "health care" would be actively engaged in providing prevention services at every opportunity. Unfortunately, this is often not the case. To understand why prevention is not a priority or, in some cases, not even a consideration, you have to remember the system's origins. For many years, the limited resources of health care were directed toward the treatment of acute diseases; they were a priority for the community. An acute care system was developed to meet this demand and capitalize on available funding. Today, the U.S. healthcare system is one of the best in the world for treating acute health conditions.

In addition, in the early stages of this system, evidence of the effectiveness of prevention was limited and little or no reimbursement was provided for these services. In a fee-for-service system, what did not receive reimbursement was ignored or given minimal attention. With the advent of managed care, some prevention services were increased such as well baby checkups and certain screenings, but an all-out effort at prevention did not materialize. Cynics say that prevention is not part of the healthcare system because the system makes more money on the sick than on keeping people well. To follow that logic, it is a good business decision not to waste resources on screenings, education, and other prevention efforts but wait until illness is present.

Despite this cynical view, there has been some change in the attitude toward prevention services. Evidence has demonstrated that effective prevention practices can save money through less abuse of the emergency department, fewer preventable office visits, and disease management. More and more facilities are beginning to engage in community-based education efforts, for example, providing car safety education and infant seats to new mothers, engaging in parish nursing, and working in elementary schools in support of healthy lifestyle choices. These efforts help to demonstrate social responsibility and improve the facility's image in the community. On the business side, they provide marketing for the facility at minimal cost and can positively influence the bottom line.

What is your role in providing preventive services? As an individual, you can support prevention efforts by becoming involved. You can also contact the major charitable agencies in your community and become a volunteer. This can mean becoming a board member, being trained to provide service (such as disaster services), or supporting ongoing efforts. Remember that you always represent your organization in the community when you serve in these organizations.

In terms of your organization, you can begin by conducting an informal survey to determine what prevention services are already being provided and by whom. This information might not be known for the total organization, as this work is often done by individual departments. Then, based on data about your own patients and the community (public health data), you could begin to assess how to better meet your organization's mission and provide appropriate prevention services. A team approach would be valuable to decide what you can do and how you can do it. Your plan should include supporting existing services from public health and voluntary agencies and finding ways to fund efforts within your budget. While this can be challenging, you get a return on your investment through the potential reduction of unnecessary care, increased patient satisfaction, and improved community image.

Organizations that provide health care should also consider their own employee's health as both an ethics and a business decision. Since your ability to make a profit can be affected by the costs of providing health care to your employees, efforts to reduce healthcare costs through improving their health status make good business sense. Health Enhancement Systems (2007) explains how providing prevention programs for your employees can decrease these costs. When most of your employees are at a low risk for health problems, they contribute to an organization's fiscal health. However, if these employees' health risks increase, so does your cost to provide treatment.

Since costs relates to healthcare risk, it makes business sense to assess the level of health risk among your employees and then provide programs to decrease risk. Health Enhancement Systems (2007) reports that low risk employees use less disability insurance, worker's compensation, absences, and medical costs than those of medium or high risk. The overall cost saving for avoiding even one healthcare risk is over $300 per employees. Studies cited by Health Enhancement Systems state that for every $1 you invest in prevention programs for your employees, you can save almost $6 in healthcare costs.

What are you supposed to do to maintain the health of healthy employees and improve the health of others? The literature is full of suggestions, and you can adapt the ideas to your organization's setting and budget. For example, you can set up a walking course so that employees can walk during their lunch break. You can also conduct health assessments so that employees are aware of their risks and can be educated about prevention. In addition, you can provide incentives for those employees who choose to practice prevention. Some organizations link these incentives to benefit plans. By offering prevention programs that are attractive to employees and easy to use, you are not only affecting your bottom line. You are demonstrating for ethics foundation by showing that you value each employee and want him or her to have the best possible health.

Public Health's Role

Public health has it roots in the establishment of communities and the need to protect quality of life. Written evidence of quality of life efforts goes back to 1700 B.C. and the Code of Hammurabi (Tulchinsky & Varavikova, 2000) and continues to this day. Public health has evolved into a multidisciplinary system whose mission stresses prevention of disease and injury, promotion of healthy lifestyle choices, protection of the environment, and prevention of epidemics. In addition, it is concerned with community access to quality health services. This system is parallel to the healthcare system and links the study of disease (**epidemiology**) to prevention and treatment. Its focus is on the community rather than the individual.

Public health's philosophic roots lie in social justice and community action. This orientation means that it stresses the common good, tries to find public solutions to health problems, and assumes that everyone is responsible for the community's health. It also tends to favor central planning and a government role in health care when it is necessary. Public health tends to view health care as different from other goods and services and focuses on access to care regardless of the ability to pay. It tends to take the utilitarian view of the greatest good for the greatest number (Shi & Singh, 2008). However, according to Holland (2007), both Kantian and virtue ethics play a role in the ethics foundation of public health.

Improvements in public health have been credited with the over 30-year extension in life expectancy that occurred between 1900 and the present. These improvements included protection policies that decreased the impact of infectious diseases through immunizations and early treatment. Improvements in water quality, food processing, and waste management also had major impacts on individual health. In addition, health promotion campaigns have increased awareness about sexually transmitted diseases, nutrition, exercise, and seatbelt usage. While these efforts might not seem as dramatic as acute care, they have reaped benefits for society. Opinion polls (Turnock, 2004) have found that public health is highly respected in the United States, with most respondents stating that it was "very important" to their health. One study even found that almost half of its respondents found public health to be more important than medicine.

Despite the recognition of its contributions, public health only receives approximately 5% of the healthcare budget. If these services are so important, why are they funded at such a low level? Part of the explanation is that the public just expects public health to be there. When it is doing its job, it is ignored unless something goes wrong. The public expects that whatever funds are available will be enough to handle any emergency. Major events occur, such as the tragedy of September 11 and the aftermath of hurricanes Katrina and Ike, that emphasize the importance of public health and its role in healing communities. These events also show the need to assure future funding that is adequate for its work.

In addition, there has been a long-standing conflict between the public health system and medical system (Turnock, 2004). As public health began to develop, physicians became concerned that it would infringe on their practice. In the area of clinical services, there was a fear that they would lose paying patients to public health programs. Agreements were made and public health services were limited to those who could not pay. This relationship exists on many levels even today.

The systems also have two different orientations that can often conflict. Public health wants to use its limited resources to minimize the harm to the population. Within these resources, it tries to distribute tests, immunizations, screenings, inspections, and so on, for prevention of possible negative outcomes. Medicine, in contrast, wants to provide the maximum benefit for the individual through customized treatment. The differences in views can lead to conflict or collaboration.

Today there is a greater need for collaboration between these two divergent systems because of the need to engage in prevention as well as treatment of disease (Turnock, 2004). One of the most common areas is in the reporting of data to various state and federal agencies for use in incidence and prevalence reports. While this might seem like a time-consuming effort, it does help to give a more accurate picture of the health concerns of the community. Increasingly, hospital and public health facilities are also working together to tackle problems of mutual interest including planning for community health needs. In fact, hospitals can even include community benefit areas in their mission statements, such as linking bonuses to community health goals, and educating staff on community as well as patient outcomes. Such efforts cannot be accomplished without cooperation between the hospitals and the various aspects of public health. In addition, the need to focus on homeland security and protection from bioterrorism has also increased collaboration between public health and the medical system. All resources would have to work in cooperation if such an event occurred.

How does public health and its efforts relate to you as a healthcare administrator? First, you can be employed by any number of community-based facilities as a **public health administrator (PHA)**. This career would afford you many opportunities to practice social justice on a daily basis. You would have to use your knowledge and experience to make the best decisions for the benefit of your community. You would be monitoring the pulse of your community to be aware of its health concerns and working to get them met. While your reward might be less financially, you would have the chance to really make a difference and engage in meaningful work.

Even if you are not working in a community-based setting, local or state public health departments should be part of your administrative resources. Practicing ethical decision-making requires that you have a complete picture of whatever situation exists. Data from national, state, and local public health agencies can give you information about incidence and prevalence of conditions in your community. This knowledge can be extremely beneficial in strategic planning efforts, including budgeting and program design. If you are employed in managed care, these data can be a significant part of your financial success because you are not making decisions in a vacuum.

As the medical system begins to add a focus on prevention and community health goals, you might find yourself working more closely with public health agencies. It is a good idea to become familiar with the roles of these agencies and their key administrators. This is especially important when you assume a new position in a community. Perhaps a telephone call, a lunch meeting, or even an agency visit is appropriate to build collaboration. In addition, your facility can support public health efforts by offering space for meetings, being a part of research, or jointly working on grants to provide community programs. Such efforts not only increase your image in the community, but they can also decrease the unnecessary use of your services and actually increase your profitability.

■ QUALITY ASSURANCE AS SOCIAL RESPONSIBILITY

CQI, NCQA, HEDIS®, IHI; what do all these initials have to do with ethics and social responsibility? The answer is that they are attempts to assess the quality of services provided by healthcare facilities. Many of them were developed by nonhealthcare businesses because they recognized that quality assurance related to profits. General business still leads the way with quality assurance efforts such as ISO 9000, Malcolm Baldrige National Quality Awards, and Kaizen. However, several of these efforts have recently been adapted to health care with mixed results.

By working to ensure the best quality service in your facility, you are fulfilling your duty of beneficence and nonmaleficence (Darr, 2004). You are also practicing social responsibility through positive stewardship of resources and protecting the community against inappropriate or even fraudulent care. Because it is tempting to put your facility in the best light, you must consciously practice ethics in the way that you collect, analyze, and present data on quality of care. When gaps between what should be and what exists are found, you can be diligent in finding the ways to improve, instead of being tempted to ignore the problem. This daily ethics requires your powers of persuasion and ability to use data effectively.

The issue of quality of care and social responsibility has come to the nation's attention through the efforts of the **Institute of Medicine (IOM)** and the **Leapfrog Group**. The IOM has published several books based on extensive research into the quality of health care in the United States. Its *Crossing the Quality Chasm* (IOM, 2001) demonstrated that although progress has been made in the American healthcare system, gaps in quality exist. These gaps include issues of patient safety, incorrect use of resources, fragmentation, lack of emphasis on chronic care, and failure to use information systems and technology appropriately. IOM has profiled what it considers goals for a new healthcare system. They include areas of safety, evidence-based care, care that is just, focus on the patient and not the procedure, and reduction of waste (IOM, 2001). IOM continues to study quality issues in health care through its hundreds of reports including studies on medication error prevention, emergency care, and evidence-based medicine.

The IOM reports and other healthcare concerns led to the development of the Leapfrog Group. It was founded by the Business Roundtable and supported by the Robert Wood Johnson Foundation (Leapfrog, 2008). This Group is a consortium of healthcare purchasers who have agreed to purchase health care based on patient safety, quality, and healthcare affordability. It has identified Four Leaps that form the basis of evaluating hospitals. These areas are the use of computer physician order entry systems (CPOE) and evidence-based hospital referral. In addition, Leapfrog considers staffing in hospital intensive care units and scores on their safe practices surveys. The organization works with hospitals to establish target dates for meeting their recommended quality standards.

Because of its efforts, the Leapfrog Group has been influential in getting hospitals to speed up implementation of these standards. These efforts are aimed at reducing medication errors and improving the overall safety of healthcare delivery. In addition, to improve overall quality, members of this group have agreed to certain concepts when dealing with healthcare providers. These include incentives for systems that provide value and improve safety, increasing accountability of health plans through comparison ratings, and providing education for employees. In addition, Leapfrog Group provides information about the safety of hospitals to the consumer through an online Web site.

The IOM reports and the Leapfrog Group are just a few of the efforts that have been created to address quality in health care. It is clear that this will be a part of your professional career no matter where you are employed in the healthcare industry. How can you demonstrate your social responsibility in the area of quality control? You will need to understand the standards under which your facility conducts its practices and patient care efforts. The standards are not always stable, so you must check appropriate Web sites and other sources to make sure that you are working with the latest information. In addition, you will be responsible for the quality of the data that is collected to demonstrate compliance with the standards. This means that your staff understand how to collect the data, how to report it, and the importance of its accuracy.

In addition, be sure that you practice the highest level of ethical behavior when you report data to your next level. The accuracy of collecting data is your responsibility, so you may want to conduct spot checks on a periodic basis. Reporting data can also be an ethical dilemma for you. While it can be tempting to present your department as being "perfect," it will not benefit you in the end. You cannot affirm your quality or make improvements if your data are inaccurate or even fraudulent.

Your responsibility for quality assurance can also be met by serving as a member of one of the evaluation organizations. Depending on your background, you can become a member of a quality review team or a policy review board. It is very beneficial to be part of the decision-making process that directly affects how you do business in health care. Remember that these organizations also need administrators; this is another career opportunity for you in the future.

Summary

Practicing social responsibility not only makes good ethical sense; it also makes good business sense. Remember that many healthcare organizations receive at least part of their funds through government or community sources. These funds are given in trust. In other words, the community expects that healthcare organizations act with social responsibility and serve as good stewards of these resources. They want them to make every effort to provide necessary and quality care, reduce waste, and control costs. In addition, care must be respectful and compassionate regardless of a person's social economic status or ability to pay. Organizations such as the IOM point out gaps in what should be and what exists and bring greater attention to the area of social responsibility. As a healthcare administrator, you should be aware of the efforts of these organizations and be proactive in addressing their quality concerns.

The public sector is not the only group concerned about social responsibility. As you have seen, employers are also increasingly aware of the quality of services you provide to their employees. Awareness of issues such as patient safety and value for funds invested is increasing. Employers are trying to change the system by using their buying power to provide incentives for improving quality care and stewardship of resources through various organizations. Surely, social responsibility is part of your business and ethics future.

Cases for Your Consideration

The Case of the Devoted Dentist

1. What principles of ethics governed Dr. Francis Loreto's business decision?

2. Why was Dr. Blaise Loreto concerned with his father's latest business decision?

3. What compromise was made?

4. What lessons can you gain from the Doctors Loreto?

Case Information

Dr. Francis Loreto practiced dentistry in Maryville for over 40 years. As a young dentist, he made a decision to practice his own version of social responsibility by providing free dental health services to all of the clergy in his town. This included priests, nuns, ministers, and the local rabbi. This beneficent act, while not increasing his bottom line, was greatly appreciated and increased Dr. Loreto's reputation in the community. Recently, a seminary was begun in the town and Dr. Loreto decided to extend his service to seminarians who needed care.

Dr. Loreto's son, Blaise, joined his father's practice five years ago and supported his father's practice decision. However, he thought that extending this benefit to seminarians was just too much. He had a vision of hundreds of students demanding free care and bankrupting the practice. He actually wondered about his father's business sense. He knew he had to talk some sense into him before he ruined the practice.

During their weekly business lunch, Dr. Loreto listened patiently to his son's concerns and suggestions to stop providing free care to clergy or at least, not extend it to the seminarians. Then, he explained that he had made a commitment to those who serve God in Maryville, and his word meant everything to him. He did not want to renege on his promise. This service was also part of the practice's image in the community; patients respected the practice because of it. To stop might actually decrease paying business because patients might see them as serving dollars and not the community. However, he did acquiesce to continuing to monitor the impact of his decision on the practice's profit margin and being open to further discussion if it became a problem.

Dr. Blaise Loreto was skeptical but also wanted to honor his father's ethical decision, so he agreed. The practice continued as before with only a minor increase in uncompensated care costs. The seminarians respected Dr. Francis Loreto's commitment and did not abuse his generosity. When he passed away after 50 years of practice, the whole community honored him as a man of ethical service. His son continued his commitment to the clergy of Maryville to honor his father.

Responses and Commentary on Questions

1. What principles of ethics governed Dr. Francis Loreto's business decision?

   The most obvious principle involved here is beneficence. In this case, Dr. Francis Loreto decided to practice this ethics principle on an individual basis by providing uncompensated care for each clergy member. He also practiced beneficence for the community by caring for its entire clergy, regardless of their faith orientation.

This practice decision was made early in his career as his way of honoring the work of these members of his community.

Dr. Loreto was also practicing social responsibility as he saw it. Even though providing the clergy free care lowered his profit margin, he was willing to take the financial risk. His practice experience told him that he could absorb these costs and that the community benefit was well worth the cost. Even though he did not intend it, his commitment to social justice was actually a practice builder. People chose his practice because they felt he had a strong moral compass and would provide them with quality care. They saw him as motivated by services and not just a need for more profit.

2. Why was Dr. Blaise Loreto concerned with his father's latest business decision?

   Dr. Blaise Loreto was a recent graduate from dental school and was oriented toward maintaining and growing the business part of the practice. He did not always understand why his father would provide care when the clergy should be able to pay for it themselves. He tolerated his father's practice because he respected him, but the idea of seminarians being given free care frightened him. He was justifiably concerned that such a practice might erode the profit margin too much and negatively affect the viability of the dental practice.

   He saw social responsibility in a different light. He was thinking about the principle of the greatest good for the greatest number. Maintaining the practice and having a solid profit margin would keep them both in business. This meant that they could provide quality dental treatment to many people in Maryville. In addition, having this economic base would enable them to provide some charity care for those who really deserved it. If his father's commitment to the clergy got out of hand, they might have to close the business. This meant that the many would suffer because of compassion for the few.

3. What compromise was made?

   Dr. Blaise Loreto wanted to honor his father and maintain his practice. He listened carefully to all of his father's ideas, and they reached a compromise. He would monitor the financials of the practice and, if his father's decision began to decrease the profit margin, they would discontinue serving the clergy. Dr. Francis Loreto agreed to this compromise because he loved his son. But his experience told him that his decision was the right one. As it turned out, the clergy did not take undo advantage of his generosity, and he was able to maintain his commitment to social justice until he retired. His son also came to see this as a good business practice and continued it.

4. What lessons can you gain from the Doctors Loreto?

Sometimes it seems like the problems in society are so great that no one can make a difference. People can be overwhelmed by it all and just do nothing. The Doctors Loreto demonstrated that everyone could make a commitment to social justice in some way. This means searching for the correct fit between a community need and your ability to meet that need. Research and collaboration with public health and other community leaders can assist in finding your niche. Once the need is identified, it requires some creativity to find ways to address it and not overwhelm your profit margin. The goal is to make a difference in the community through action from your organization or from your personal commitment.

The doctors showed that social justice can also have a positive effect on business. The practice gained a reputation in the community for its service to all clergy. Of course, the two dentists were clinically competent, but many people chose them because they were also compassionate. The practice continued to grow by word-of-mouth referrals and both partners had a healthy profit margin, even with the uncompensated care for clergy. In addition, the clergy respected what the dentists were doing and never abused their generosity.

The Case of the Proactive Public Health Administrator (PHA)

1. How does this case demonstrate the role of public health in social responsibility?

2. How important was social marketing to the success of the program?

3. How important was collaboration to the success of this program?

4. How did this program improve the visibility and image of the health department?

Case Information

Sandra Peoples was the director of a small county public health department. Frequently, she reviewed reports on the incidence of health problems in the zip codes served by her clinics. In her latest review, she noticed that her two zip codes showed the highest rates of infant injury and deaths from automobile accidents. She was startled by these numbers and contacted the chief executive officer (CEO) of the local hospital to check on its experience. He confirmed the numbers. She also contacted the local chief of police and found that tickets for noncompliance with infant car seat laws were also increasing for parents in her zip codes. When tickets were issued, the most common response was, "I can't afford a car seat."

These conversations made Sandra aware of a problem that hurt the most vulnerable in her zip code area. She knew that she had to do something. First, she made a visit to all of her clinics and talked with the staff and the clients. She soon learned that buying a car seat was not a high priority for the mothers served by the clinics. They were more concerned with feeding and clothing their children, paying rent, and keeping the electricity on. It became even clearer that car seat compliance was a problem.

Armed with this information, Sandra called a staff meeting to brainstorm solutions. It was decided to research sources for grant money, as the department's funds would never cover this new expense. The staff determined that car seats needed to be provided along with an education program to ensure that parents would use them properly. They also found that the federal Department of Health and Human Services awarded grant money for creative projects that helped to save lives.

After several sessions, a grant proposal was filed. It included a three-pronged approach to the problem. First, parents would qualify if they were in the department's service area (verified by proof of residency) and had a financial need. The program would consist of attendance at a 45-minute class on car seat usage and a demonstration of the participants' ability to use it correctly. In addition, the chief of police agreed that when all officers who serviced the zip code ticketed a noncompliant driver, they would also provide a flyer about the program. The CEO of the hospital wrote a letter in support of the grant and agreed to provide data on reduction of infant injury and death.

It was funded. Sandra received funding for 9000 car seats for the year. They would arrive in shipments of 3000 so that storage would be less of a problem. However, the grant funding turned out to be a mixed blessing and a source for creative problem solving.

First, the shipment of car seats arrived in a semi and she had no one to offload them. However, she did have an acquaintance who was a director of a residential treatment center. He sent over some of the residents who made short work of the offloading process. She also had to find places to store all of the car seats until room could be made in a central supply area. Her clinic temporarily became car seat central with all available space used to store car seat boxes.

Next, her social marketing campaign using the police department, staff of the obstetrics department at the hospital, and clinic personnel was almost too effective. The first class day she had over 150 people lined up to take the class. She had to think quickly to schedule two additional class sessions that day and ask some of the clients to return on the next day. She learned to plan for the popularity of this program. She even learned to separate parents into groups to better facilitate their learning (teens, Hispanics, and others).

All of this planning paid off. Sandra checked with both police and hospital emergency department staff and found that there were fewer severe injuries and deaths reported for infants in her zip codes. She also found a decrease in the state's statistics, so she was able to demonstrate the effectiveness of her program. Anecdotal evidence also supported the impact of the program. Almost every day someone in the clinic was thanked for their efforts to improve the safety of infants in the service zip code areas.

Responses and Commentary on Questions

1. How does this case demonstrate the role of public health in social responsibility?

   Sandra Peoples was a PHA who really took an interest in the epidemiology of her service area. She routinely scanned the statistical reports about the zip codes for her service area and tried to keep up with trends. In this case, she was alarmed by what she read about **infant mortality** and **morbidity** from car accidents. Her response was based on the social justice philosophy; she looked at the impact of this problem on the community she served. This included the families involved but also the emergency department and even the police department. She wanted to take a proactive approach to solving the problem for the whole community. She also knew what her budget was for the year.

   Also in keeping with the social justice focus of public health, Ms. Peoples used a team approach to find the resources to meet her community's need. Her grant proposal had to be competitive to be awarded funding so as she wrote it, she tried to anticipate any objections. She got the support of the community for what she wanted to do, which certainly was a factor in gaining funding.

   Once the program was in place, Ms. Peoples and her staff did everything they could to ensure that whoever received a car seat knew how to use it. It would not have been socially responsible just to give away free car seats without teaching the parents how to use them correctly. Improper use of the seats would also not be effective in solving the problem. The staff actually had the participants demonstrate the correct use of the seats before they would issue them a certificate for the car seat.

2. How important was social marketing to the success of the program?

   Social marketing is used extensively in public health because budgets are usually very restrictive and do not have room for expensive marketing campaigns. In this case, Ms. Peoples used the police department (through flyers), the obstetrics department of the hospital, and her own clinical staff to make her community aware of the program. Evidently, it worked quite well because she was somewhat surprised by the number of participants in the early days of the program. She had to change her schedule of classes to accommodate. She also had to be careful not to run out of car seats between shipments. If the car seats were not available when parents came for the classes, it would have been disastrous for the program.

3. How important was collaboration to the success of this program?

   You probably have figured out that public health efforts often rely on collaboration with various members of the community. In this case, it began when Ms. Peoples contacted the police chief and the hospital CEO for information. Her efforts to build relationships with these important community members paid off. They also supported her grant proposal by writing letters and offering to inform clients about the program.

   Once the grant was funded, collaboration was also needed. Ms. Peoples's acquaintance with the director of the resident treatment center really helped when she needed some willing hands. The residents were happy to help in such a worthwhile effort. In addition, the police officers gave out flyers advertising the program when they stopped someone for an infant car seat violation. Ms. Peoples knew this was effective because her staff reported that many clients came into the clinics with the flyer in their hands. Certainly, the hospital staff contributed to the success of the program by informing those clients who might qualify. The public health department clinic staff should not be overlooked. Their support of this program really made it work.

   Finally, collaboration was important in documenting the program's success. Hospital emergency department statistics, the number of police warnings and tickets, and documentation by clinic staff helped to demonstrate the effectiveness of the program. Without this support, it would have been more difficult to show how it improved the infant mortality and morbidity rates.

4. How did this program improve the visibility and image of the health department?

   It soon became known in the community that the public health department was trying to do something to help keep infants safe while traveling in cars. The clients saw this effort as one of concern for their needs. They told others about the program, which also helped in the **social marketing** efforts. In addition, a local television program found out about the program and interviewed Ms. Peoples and two of her clinic staff. She told them how important the program was in preventing infant injury and urged others to be sure to use car seats. This program was so successful that it received funding for a second year.

Web Resources

Public Health information
http://www.apha.org/

The Leapfrog Group
http://www.leapfroggroup.org/

The Institute of Medicine
http://www.iom.edu/

References

Darr, K. (2005). *Ethics in health services management* (4th ed.). Baltimore: Health Professions Press.
Health Enhancement Systems. (2007). *Keeping healthy people healthy: A business case.* Midland, MI: Author.
Holland, S. (2007). *Public health ethics.* Malden, MA: Polity Press.
Institute of Medicine. (2001). *Crossing the quality chasm: A new health system for the 21st century.* Washington, DC: National Academy Press.
Leapfrog Group. (2008). *Fact sheet.* Available at: http://www.leapfroggroup.org. Accessed November 26, 2008.
Shi, L., & Singh, D. A. (2008). *Delivering health care in America: A systems approach* (4th ed.). Sudbury, MA: Jones and Bartlett.
Tulchinshky, T. H., & Varavikova, E. A. (2000). *The new public health: An introduction for the 21st century.* San Diego, CA: Academic Press.
Turnock, B. J. (2004). *Public health* (2nd ed.). Sudbury, MA: Jones and Bartlett.

CHAPTER 8

Technology and Ethics

It is only by the rational use of technology; to control and guide what technology is doing; that we can keep any hopes of a social life more desirable than our own: or fact of a social life which is not appalling to imagine.

—C. P. Snow

Points to Ponder

1. What is the relationship between technology and health care?
2. Why is information technology so important in healthcare administration?
3. What are the issues surrounding future technology development?
4. What is the relationship between technology and ethics?
5. What is your role as an ethics-based healthcare administrator?

Words to Remember

The following is a list of key words for this chapter. You will find them in bold in the text. Stop and check your understanding of them.

assisted reproductive
   technologies (ART)
decision support systems
health information
   technology (HIT)
neuroenhancements
radio frequency
   identification (RFID)

collaborative technology
electronic medical record (EMR)
neuroengineering
neuroethics
telemedicine

■ TECHNOLOGY AND ITS IMPACT ON HEALTH CARE

Medicine has embraced technology, making it a driving force in the U.S. healthcare system from both a treatment and economic standpoint. Shi and Singh (2008) use the term "technology diffusion" to describe technology's influence on values and culture. In the United States, this diffusion is so extensive that many Americans equate "good medicine" with the amount of technology that is used, even if it is not appropriate. Diffusion also influences the education of practitioners, who increasingly rely on technology regardless of cost.

Technology has become an integral part of clinical practice. For example, where would diagnosis be without a fetal monitor or a CAT scanner? Can you imagine health care without intensive care units, pacemakers, or bone marrow transplants? Telemedicine has already made long distance consultation a reality. Will it change how medicine is practiced? As you read the next section of the text, you will see an example of one form of technology has affected the business of health care. Information technology is now part of how the healthcare system's billing, materials management, budgeting, and quality control processes.

Technology cost is an issue for the business side of health care. Although practitioners and patients enjoy the advantages of the increasing use of technology in all its forms, these benefits affect the cost of providing care. Hospitals have been particularly affected by this increase because, to accommodate advances in technology, they have to invest large amounts of capital. Administrators need to consider more than the cost per patient in their decisions about acquiring new technology. Concerns about whether the use of technology increases or decreases the overall cost of patient care need to be addressed. In addition, information about the rapid improvements in many of these technologies and their quick obsolescence should be part of making purchase decisions. Administrators should remember that purchasing technology is not the end of the cost considerations. Technology support is often ongoing and is a cost factor. A thorough cost-benefit analysis is necessary when making purchase decisions about technology.

The diffusion of technology also poses problems beyond cost. Its benefits are extensive, but the apparatus might not be readily available in certain geographic areas or to certain populations. For example, rural Americans have just as much need for an MRI as their urban counterparts. However, access is not available because the technology can be just too expensive to purchase and maintain. Health problems can go undetected. Technology access is creating two healthcare systems: one for urban dwellers and one for rural.

When you add low-income populations to the picture, the divergence becomes even greater. For example, the insulin pump as a treatment for diabetes has been shown to provide health benefits. However, the cost of the pump and supplies for one year averages many thousands of dollars. This means that benefit is limited to those who are well insured or wealthy. Given the additional costs, should technology should be limited to only those who can afford it? Does technology create a two-tiered healthcare system: one for the insured and one for the uninsured? You will explore more of these and other ethics issues created by the diffusion of technology in a later section of this chapter.

Information Technology (IT)

Inexpensive computer systems and increased availability of the Internet has caused profound changes in the amount of available information and the speed of access to it. American businesses have increasingly embraced this technology and used it to great advantage. In fact, IT is a large part of the American way of life, from how our cars operate to how we pay our bills. It means that we can converse instantly with friends all over the world and access information that only experts knew in the past. Health care, while slower to make the required capital investment in IT, is beginning to catch up. Information is becoming a critical part of its potential for success.

There has certainly been an explosion of health information. For example, if you type the word "health" into your search engine today, you will get 1,210,000,000 hits in 0.16 seconds (Google search)! This small example gives you an idea of the expansion of access to knowledge. However, there is a drawback. Although there are some Web sites with reliable information, currently there is no system for quality assurance of Internet information. The lack of information filters can cause problems for consumers and providers alike because it is difficult to discern its quality.

Despite the gaps in quality, you cannot afford to ignore the impact of information technology on health care. Every aspect of the system from patient encounters to waste management has seen its influence. It has even spawned its own industry of health information management, or health informatics, administrative positions (e.g., Chief Information Officer), and degree programs. In order to appreciate technology's influence, you need to consider its relationship to clinical care, business practices, and the consumer. These relationships also create significant ethics issues.

Clinical Applications   In the area of clinical care, technology is predicted to change dramatically the way that medicine is practiced. Patients use the Internet to research their diagnoses and come to office visits armed with information. Since the information presented may be incorrect or misleading, its use may be viewed as a nuisance because it adds to visit time. However, it also can open doors to communication about the patients' concerns and save time in the end. Patient use of the Internet may also contribute to physician use of this technology. If the source of information is reputable, the Internet can add to his or her currency of knowledge.

Telemedicine is another example of the application of IT in clinical practice. It combines computers, videoconferencing, and digitized medical records that can be transported via satellite or high-speed telephone lines (Coddington, Fischer, Moore, & Clark, 2000). Consultation can even include remote reading of MRIs or radiographs. Telemedicine is used for consultation in military installations, correctional facilities, and some rural healthcare facilities. It also helps in physician education through live remotes and interactive sessions. Because telemedicine is new and not reimbursed by insurance, it currently does not add to the profit margin of hospitals that have incorporated it. However, it holds the potential to serve populations where access to specialists is limited.

The use of e-mails is increasing as a vehicle for communication between physicians and patients. Brooks and Menachemi (2007) found, in a study of over 4000 physicians, that 16% used e-mail as a way to communicate with patients. In addition, 63% found it useful for communicating with other physicians, business contacts, hospitals, and pharmacies. Reaction to the use of e-mail for patient communication has been mixed. Some practices find this a highly effective tool for patient triage and a time saver. Others resent the intrusion e-mails make on their already busy schedules. However, as it becomes more and more common, consumers' demand might increase its use in clinical practice.

One of the most visible examples of IT in clinical practice is the **electronic medical record (EMR)**. This innovation not only has an impact on clinical practice, but it also affects healthcare business practice and law. The idea of the EMR is not particularly new. The Institute of Medicine (2001) called for a standardized electronic record as early as 1991 and stressed its importance again in 1997. However, even though evidence is building that the EMR can decrease medical errors and lower costs, progress toward automation has been slow.

Patient privacy and securing personal information are concerns with respect to EMR adaptation. The concern about patient privacy led to the enactment of the Health Insurance Portability and Accountability Act of 1996 (HIPAA), which has become a part of the operation of healthcare facilities. Since IT makes medical information more easily accessible, questions about the ownership of medical information and who can have access to it are becoming increasingly important. The issue of one's civil rights and the need for patient consent must be considered when making decisions about disclosure of patient information (Budinger & Budinger, 2006).

There remain concerns about financing an extensive change to the EMR. Capital investments for purchasing new equipment, locating and installing new software, upgrading the legacy systems, and providing appropriate training are significant. In addition, such capital investments can be very difficult for physician groups, rural healthcare facilities, and public health settings. In addition to funding issues related to the EMR, healthcare administrators (HCAs) must be concerned with the work force that has varying degrees of knowledge and acceptance for the change to electronic rather than paper records. Previous negative experiences with IT, frustration with necessary standardization, and the loss of income from disruptions have contributed to slow adoption by clinicians. Consumers also have concerns with this technology. While some find it to be an exciting innovation, many are distrustful of automation, or do not have access to it. This, coupled with a response from physicians, can cause the healthcare system to operate parallel record keeping systems (paper-based and paperless). Imagine the expense, confusion, and error potential that dueling systems can cause.

The American Medical Association (AMA) has taken the lead in providing physicians and other practices with information about how to make the transition to the EMR. In fact, it has an entire section on its Web site devoted to many areas of **health information technology** (**HIT**). This section includes information on the risks and benefits of HIT, practices options, and implementation strategies. It also includes information on assessing software and vendor needs (AMA, 2008). In addition, the Institute of Medicine and the Leapfrog Group continue their efforts to make EMR and HIT part of the healthcare practice throughout the United States.

These brief examples illustrate some of the changes that IT has made in clinical practice. In the section on emergent technologies, you will encounter the change projections for the future. All of these changes will challenge your thinking on the ethical practice of healthcare delivery.

Business Practice Applications   IT now provides a foundation for many of the business practices used to operate the healthcare system. It holds the promise of providing accurate data to assist with critical areas such as strategic planning, financial analysis, quality improvement, and performance assessment. IT facilitates necessary reporting to external agencies, including accrediting bodies and government entities. It can also support daily operations of a healthcare facility.

In the financial aspects of health care, for example, IT can make payroll, accounts payable, cost accounting, and budgeting more accurate and timely. It can simplify claims processing by making it an electronic exchange of information rather than a paper one. This ability has greatly decreased the amount of time needed for reimbursement and could increase its accuracy.

In the area of human resources, IT can assist in maintaining employee records, as well as charting turnover and absenteeism, and increases labor cost assessment. IT programs are available for conducting background checks on applicants, which reduces the cost of this preventive action. In addition, technology has already decreased employee-training costs by using an online format rather than a classroom one. IT also assists with providing continuing education programs and maintaining records of continuing education units.

IT makes strategic planning more efficient by using **decision support systems.** These systems include software that allows the HCA to create databases for efficient retrieval of information, to design decision models, and to create reports. In addition, programs are available to assist with disaster planning to increase your readiness. To use these systems appropriately, you must be able to discern the quality of information and be sure that it was collected appropriately. To be useful, information needs to be timely, collected using a standard protocol, unbiased (as much as possible), and in sufficient quantity to allow for accurate decision-making (Glandon, Smaltz, & Slovensky, 2008).

IT is a major tool for the business aspects of health care. However, there are costs associated with this tool, especially when inappropriate purchasing decisions are made. To avoid such decisions, the HCA must keep informed about technological advances without becoming overwhelmed by "techno-hype." Gathering information from users as well as vendors will enhance the ability make the best decisions for the organization. Even though the HCAs are not computer experts, they will be active in scheduling, training, recruiting and hiring, maintaining systems, and ensuring security.

Consumer Applications   The Internet is the most obvious consumer use of IT. The increased emphasis on prevention and patient responsibility has contributed to the patient's need for accurate and understandable health information. The Internet is perceived to be a low-cost delivery system for providing this information to large numbers of consumers. Web sites have been created to address everything from diagnosis to prevention. The most common consumer uses of the Internet include researching diagnoses, seeking information about drugs and their side effects, and looking for a physician. On the prevention side, consumers want information on nutrition, fitness, and the location of support groups. Even mental health interventions are included through sites called e-therapy, cyber therapy, or life coaching.

Just like the physician, the consumer can be overwhelmed by the amount of information on the Internet. Vehicles for filtering and credentialing Web sites are just beginning to be created. Until they are more available, consumers are cautioned to choose Web sites that are designated by reputable organizations, reviewed by experts, and clearly identify their sponsorship. In addition, consumers need to be aware that their use of Web sites can be monitored without their knowledge.

This can occur at their workplace to prevent inappropriate use of the Web or it can be used by an online vendor to track preferences in books, magazines, or clothing. Consumers should always be cautious about how they use IT and its affect on their privacy.

You can see that IT holds great promise for increased efficiency and patient safety. Of course, it also introduces ethics issues that will challenge both the system and the individual. HIPAA and other laws are attempting to address autonomy and privacy of records, but they will not be enough. As IT becomes more sophisticated, problems will surface that need to be addressed. Policies and procedures must be developed and staff must be trained in them. Ethics should be a part of both the development of these procedures and the training process.

■ EMERGENT TECHNOLOGIES AND FUTURE ISSUES

Clinical Applications

Technology is advancing at such a rapid pace that today's fiction is becoming tomorrow's reality. Books like Michael Crichton's (2006) *Next*, where genetic research and gene manipulation are used to create completely new species, are becoming closer to reality. Concerns about the rapid progress of technology and its side effects continue to surface. The ethics debate often centers on the progress of emerging technology versus its ethical ramifications. Ethicists ask, "Why on earth should it be the case that 'what we ought to do,' should follow from what we can do?" (Gastmans, 2002, p. 18). This concern will certainly be a challenge for the future as technology continues its rapid expansion.

Budinger and Budinger (2006) list **neuroenhancements** and **neuroengineering** as two of the many emergent technologies that can have profound ethical consequences. The technology used in these fields allows an interface between the human brain and machines. The authors include "deep brain stimulation, brain-computer interfacing, regenerative neurology, brain imaging, and psychopharmacology" as part of the technology involved in neuroenhancement and neuroengineering (p. 448). These areas are so challenging that a separate field of ethics, **neuroethics**, was created to address them.

Why are these advantages in technology so ethically challenging? A brief examination of each should assist in answering this question. First, deep brain stimulation uses electrodes in areas of the brain for the treatment of neurological problems such as pain, obsessive-compulsive disorder, depression, and strokes. While this technology appears to be promising, ethics issues of weighing harm over benefit exist. At present, there is not sufficient information to determine if a patient who receives deep brain stimulation would have a greater quality of life or suffer side effects or yet unknown consequences. Researchers in the field of deep brain stimulation are studying ethics-related issues such as protocols for who should receive such treatment, the training needed for providing treatment, and the strengths and limitations of the technology (Budinger & Budinger, 2006).

Brain-computer interfacing also uses electrodes to affect how the brain works with the body. In this case, electrodes are implanted in the brain so that they can signal sensorimotor pathways of paralyzed patients. The patients can then use robotic prosthesis or even computer cursors through their thoughts. Regenerative and rehabilitative neurology includes implementation of stem cells, gene therapy that could replace diseased tissue or increase brain function, and treatment of spinal cord injuries.

New developments in brain imaging have been proposed as the ultimate lie detector in criminal cases and as way to profile people who may become violent. Finally, psychopharmacology could be used to develop personalized drugs that assist with self-confidence, phobias, or alertness (Budinger & Budinger, 2006).

The emergent technologies associated with neuroenhancement and neuroengineering, on their surface, promise great patient benefit. However, they also could lead to an ethical slippery slope where misuse could become common use. For example, technology that could potentially improve the lives of spinal cord injury patients, amputees, and others could also be used for enhancing athletic performance, creating greater intelligence, or profiling to identify a potential criminal. The potential for violating the principle of autonomy is strong unless controls are carefully placed on their use. In addition, justice with respect to who should get these treatments will be an ongoing debate. Patients, physicians, and family members will have to balance beneficence with nonmaleficence to determine if the risk is worth the benefit. Most assuredly, study and debate will be needed before these technologies and others become a common part of the medical treatment arsenal.

Another area of emergent technology is concerned with assisting human reproduction (Budinger & Budinger, 2006). These technologies are collectively called **assisted reproductive technologies (ART)** and continue to be developed to assist infertile couples in their quest for parenthood. ART includes procedures such as in vitro fertilization, gamete intrafallopian transfer (GIFT), and intracytoplasmic sperm injection (ICSI). In addition, diagnostic techniques are available to identify potential abnormalities before fertilization and implantation including embryo biopsy. Success rates of ART and the number of infertility clinics are increasing as is the sophistication of this group of technologies. Graber (2009) considers 40 ways to create a child in his discussion of the ethics issues surrounding ART! They include several incidents where the father of the child is listed as a technician and a child has two different sets of parents (germ-cell parents and social parents). The future of this technology promises to challenge health-care ethics on many levels.

Business Applications

The business of health care will also be affected by emergent technologies that challenge us to do the same work with less people through its use. These technologies promise to make our jobs as administrators more efficient and effective. Two technologies that are currently being perfected and can be adapted to healthcare settings are **collaboration technology** and **radio frequency identification (RFID)**.

The idea of instant collaboration between groups whether they are in the same building or in different countries has captured the imagination of computer innovators. Systems are being perfected that would allow healthcare administrators to design strategic plans and conduct business transactions through online meetings and sophisticated audio and video conferencing. The systems, currently under development, capitalize on social networks and offer advanced technology without having to replace the existing systems. In addition, these collaboration or human networking systems promise security features and policy management to control use and prevent abuse. Cisco WebEx Connect® is an example of this type of business technology (Cisco Systems, Inc., 2008). With the increase in mergers and integrated systems in health care, collaboration systems will be more common because they can increase ability to hold virtual meetings while reducing travel costs. In addition, systems can expand the use of their human capital by accessing talent without the limitations of distance and time.

Radio frequency identification (RFID) uses specialized radio frequencies to identify and track property or people. The system includes a microchip and antenna, called a tag, which can transmit information to a reader. The reader can transfer radio frequencies to digital data for computer analysis (Roberti, 2008). As an addition to bar coding, RFID shows promise for tracking expensive healthcare equipment and supplies and reducing theft and shrinkage. Widespread application is currently limited by the lack of transparency between systems and the cost of implementation. However, these issues may soon be resolved as technology advances.

The pharmacy industry is beginning to explore RFID for making supply chains more efficient and preventing the development of counterfeit drugs. Several large hospital systems are also exploring RFID as an inventory management system. In addition, veterinary medicine uses this technology for tracking pets. The system also shows promise in patient-related applications. One example was its use during the evacuation of the elderly and disabled during hurricanes Gustav and Ike. Evacuees were issued wristbands containing RFID tags to facilitate identification and tracking (Roberti, 2008).

These are just a few examples of emergent technologies that will have impact on the healthcare system in the immediate future. The rapidity with which they become readily available and cost effective for use depends on several factors. First, there must be a willingness to make the capital investment in technology. Such a substantial investment of funds can be a major business concern for the facility, especially if it does not have a substantial budget. However, there may be no choice: physicians and consumers will demand availability of technology's "latest and greatest." The decision to invest in emergent technologies can result in the need to limit other services, causing ethical dilemmas for the administrator.

■ TECHNOLOGY AND ETHICS

Because of its cost and scarcity, technology has always posed challenges concerning the balance of money and mission. For example, when dialysis was a new technology, hospitals had to create committees to decide who would receive this expensive treatment and who would not. Imagine how painful those ethics committee decisions were. As technology diffusion increases, the entire system including insurance companies will struggle to decide who and what to cover. So, as technology dependence increases, so will the need for ethics-based decision making to balance economic and human concerns. The next two sections examine some of ethics issues that emergent technologies can create.

Technology, Ethics, and Society

Profound does not adequately describe the potential impact of emergent technologies on society and ethics. Progress, while highly valued, comes with a price. Many ethicists believe that such progress could create issues that will change how Americans value each other. "Ethics has to do with the question how we ought to live or act; technology with new ways and means to do (new) things" (Gastmans, 2002, p. 18). American society will have to decide on the acceptable balance between technology's new ways to live and the ethics of using these options. Justice requires that it also address who should benefit from technology, those who can afford it, and those who need it.

Another major ethics issue for society is that, for the first time, technology will be able to do more than just improve life. It has the potential to alter the nature of being human. ART will soon make it possible to create designer babies, cloned organs, and other medical wonders. Will this progress change how humans value each other? Could technology help to create two different species of humans (one genetically superior to the other)? Thinking ethically, does technology have the right to alter what has taken millions of years to create?

Some of the concerns about technology's progress and its ethical ramifications are rooted in the fear that human dignity and autonomy will be lost. For example, what would happen to those who are not genetically superior? Will they still have rights in the society? Should clones that are not perfect or embryos that are implanted become stem cell incubators? Rawls might suggest that in a just society, self-interest would dictate that consideration be given to how technology is used or not used. Decisions to purchase and use emergent technologies should be made through ethics decision-making as well as fiscal management.

The loss of autonomy is another major societal concern. First, we know that technology gives great convenience. For example, we can buy almost everything we need, pay our bills, and do our banking online. We can be billed for our toll road use through a photograph of our license plate. When we call in our pizza order, they already know our name and address. Technology makes our lives more efficient and saves us time and money.

This convenience seems wonderful, but it is not without cost to autonomy. For example, online companies are profiling customers using massive databases of information. This allows them to suggest products to you as you surf the Internet. However, have you given permission for your personal information to be collected and used? Additionally, when personal computers are lost or stolen, especially from government or healthcare agencies, the risk of compromising personal information is increased. Talented hackers also add to this risk. The result is that the business and the consumer must be aware and do everything possible to protect personal autonomy. We also need to consider what limits should be placed on technology to preserve personal autonomy.

Technology, Ethics, and the Business of Health Care

Hospitals, both urban and rural, already feel the need to supply the "latest and greatest" technology to meet the demands of their physicians and consumers. This capital investment can strain an already tight budget and cause some administrative headaches. As technology advances and more choices for enhancing and prolonging life emerge, decisions about who will get technology and who will pay for it will become even more intense.

One ethicist discusses the need to apply utilitarian principles to making these decisions (Gastmans, 2002). If economics principles are used, the benefits of technology could be maximized to provide the greatest good for the greatest number of patients. Tough financial decisions based on scarcity of resources should be used to provide the best quality of life. Treating the worst off, while compassionate, might not make the best sense when it prohibits treatment for those who have a greater chance for quality life. While such issues have been debated before, emergent technology creates a greater need for serious consideration.

Because the goal of health care is supposed to be improving health, policies will have to be developed that considered factors like quality of life years remaining, severity of disease, and cost/benefit of treatment. Of course, such policies can be challenged by physicians who see their role as advocates for their patients and by consumers themselves. Denial of treatment, no matter how futile, will never be a popular solution. However, emergent technologies will increase the need to find an acceptable balance between economics and ethics.

In addition to financial concerns, emergent technologies will mean a change in the way business is conducted. Technology assessment skills of both clinical and business applications will be essential for administrative effectiveness. Cost-effectiveness analysis, including the expense of hiring tech support staff, maintenance, frequency of obsolescence, as well as the cost of the technology, will have to be a routine function. Policies and procedures will also have to be developed for appropriate use for all of the technologic innovations. In addition, facilities will have to assess the level of risk they are willing to take if the technology does not turn out to be profitable. Ethical healthcare business practice involves balancing mission and margin. Technology can help or hinder this balancing act, depending on how decisions are made.

The healthcare insurance business will also face challenges from emergent technologies. It will have to decide what to cover and at what level. For example, many experimental treatments are not covered, so the financial risk for such treatments rests with the consumer. However, as technology increases the speed of innovations, more and more procedures will move from "experimental" to "routine." Consumer demand will force companies to increase what they cover in their policies, which will most assuredly increase the rates. In light of this potential increase and the difficult economic situation, employers are taking a hard look at the value of providing employee health coverage versus loss of profit. Imagine what might happen to business if insurance rates triple or quadruple.

On the positive side, emergent technologies promise to create new business opportunities. While these new businesses will provide job opportunities and revenue sources, they will also have an ethical obligation to provide value through quality services using appropriately credentialed providers. In addition, ethics will mandate that educational institutions adequately prepare professionals for service in these new entities. To avoid educational fraud, they will have to evaluate their curricula to be sure that graduates are ready for the ever-changing healthcare market.

■ TECHNOLOGY AND THE ROLE OF THE HEALTHCARE ADMINISTRATOR

Technology also changes your role as an ethics-based HCA. First, you have an ethical duty to make intelligent decisions about the purchase of technology. This means that you must rely on more than the information presented by vendors. You will need to seek out unbiased information from several sources and read it. This, on the surface, sounds simple but much of what you have to read can be saturated in techno-jargon. You can only make the best decision for your organization when you truly understand what you are purchasing, how much it costs to maintain, how quickly it will need to be replaced, and how easy it is to use. Making the best decision not only demonstrates your stewardship of resources, it also makes financial sense by limiting excessive spending and waste.

Technology can also force your organization to make tough decisions about rationing of care. Because trust matters in health care, it should not be ignored when considering the impact of your economic policies on your patients and their families. If such policies are created based solely on economics and not on your articulated mission and ethical principles, you can become vulnerable to potential lawsuits and/or negative community image. In short, you cannot make these policies in a vacuum; ethics committees, ethicists, and others will have to assist. You might have to assume what ethicists call a paternalistic position when deciding about technology's role in your organization (Gastmans, 2002). This means that you will have to consider potential harm and threats to patient dignity.

Summary

The information is this chapter is just a beginning for understanding the impact of technology on ethics and ethical decision-making. Each healthcare organization will continue to struggling with this issue. As a HCA, you will be faced with the challenge of balancing a lucrative revenue stream with the ethics base of your organization. The only way to be prepared to assist in this process is to stay vigilant. Read, surf the Internet, and conference to keep your knowledge at the cutting edge. Consider reading more than the healthcare literature to understand what is happening with IT in the business community. You will also have to consider "what if" situations before your organization is faced with a "must do" decision. Dialogue among practitioners, ethics committee members, and community representatives will also enhance your level of preparedness when decisions must be made.

Cases for Your Consideration

The Case of the Techno Ankle

As you read this case, consider the following questions. Responses and comments will follow the case.

1. Why did Dr. Aidan set up a multi-staff conference?
2. What ethics theory and principles apply to this case?
3. Will this conference change Dr. Aidan's decisions about technology?

Case Information

Dr. Shane Aidan was frustrated! He was a well-respected orthopedic surgeon, but this case was becoming more and more perplexing. Fiona Ecne, a 40-year-old woman, broke both bones in her ankle in a home accident. The repair required two surgeries and was successful. However, the wound in her ankle would not heal. Consequently, Dr. Aidan ordered a negative pressure machine to assist in healing. While he was not an expert in the use of this machine, past experience led him to believe that it would speed healing.

However, something was clearly different about this case. Although Ms. Ecne had technology and home care through wound specialist nurses, very little healing was happening. In addition, Dr. Aidan received a complaint about the quality of care provided by the wound care specialists. He wondered if they were contributing to the lack of progress. He was concerned about the loss of credibility to his practice and even considered the potential of a lawsuit. Consequently, he decided to take control of the technology dilemma.

He called a meeting during Ms. Ecne's next appointment. Attendees were representatives from the company that created the technology, wound care specialists from the home health agency, his office staff nurse, and Dr. Aidan. Using Ms. Ecne's ankle as a prop, the representatives discussed the purpose of the machine and how to change the dressings correctly. They also observed the wound care specialist as she applied the dressing and offered suggestions. Both Dr. Aidan and his staff nurse asked questions about how the technology applied to Ms. Ecne's particular wound, and how to enhance future healing. After serving as the prop, Ms. Ecne was finally allowed to ask her questions. In the end, all those who attended felt more knowledgeable about the application of this technology to Ms. Ecne's case.

Responses and Comments on Questions

1. Why did Dr. Aidan set up a multi-staff conference?

   Consider Dr. Aidan's dilemma. He was relying on technology to assist healing in a difficult case. However, he was not completely familiar with all of the aspects of the latest version of this technology. Therefore, he could not answer all of the patient's questions or assure her that she would be healed in a timely manner. His staff nurse also could not provide such assurance. In addition, he had concerns about the competence of the home health wound care specialists and their contribution to the slow healing. He was considering changing agencies. The logical course of action was to get all parties together and do some technology calibration. This might assure that all parties involved in Ms. Ecne's care were working together from common knowledge.

Dr. Aidan might also be concerned about a potential lawsuit and its affect on his practice. The ability to bring all the participants in Ms. Ecne's care together would allow them to communicate and create better understanding. This understanding could mediate any future harm in her care. Dr. Aidan hoped that she would view this meeting as quality assurance on her behalf. This perception might prevent her from consulting an attorney. In addition, he could verify that the wound care specialists had the most current information on the technology. This knowledge could give Ms. Ecne assurance that her home care would contribute to her healing rather than cause further harm.

2. What ethics theory and principles apply to this case?

    In this case, you can see the principle of deontology at work. Even though the bones had healed, Dr. Aidan still had a duty to the patient. He needed to make sure that she could resume her normal life. This duty included the complete healing of her surgical wounds. Calling a meeting of the professionals who contributed to her care and making sure that they had correct information on the technology was one way to demonstrate active deontology. He continued to practice his duty to the patient by making sure that her wound care specialists were also properly trained on the latest technology.

    While deontology is the most obvious theory at play here, you can also consider utilitarianism. Dr. Aidan was concerned about making the best decision for his practice. Having a meeting at his office during a patient's appointment meant that he incurred costs. For example, he did not see other patients during the meeting, and that was a loss of income. However, if he used a cost/benefit analysis based on utilitarian in principles, he could determine that the cost of holding a meeting was well worth the benefit of preventing future problems with this technology. In addition, this meeting might prevent thousands of dollars in lost revenue if a lawsuit could be prevented.

    With respect to principles, beneficence and nonmaleficence were evident. Dr. Aidan wanted to prevent future harm to Ms. Ecne by making sure that technology was used correctly. He also needed to understand its features better so that he could use it correctly in the future. Before he prescribed this technology, he wished to be sure that it functioned to prevent harm by increasing healing time. In terms of beneficence, Dr. Aidan made the decision to take time out of this practice and have a meeting. While this action was not required, it demonstrated his concern for the patient and her healing. He also hoped that Ms. Ecne would view his actions as taking extra steps to benefit her care.

Another principle to consider in this case is autonomy. The autonomy of the care providers was respected because they were allowed time to ask questions and gain knowledge necessary for the correct use of the technology. However, Ms. Ecne's autonomy was not completely respected. During the appointment, she acted more as a prop than as a person. However, at the end of the conference, she was allowed to ask questions which demonstrated some level of respect for her as a person.

3. Will this conference change Dr. Aidan's decisions about technology?

Dr. Aidan will need to consider his future decisions about the use of technology based on ethics and economics. From an ethics view, he will consider the benefit to the patient compared to the potential harm. As he learned in this case, technology used improperly can add to a patient's problems rather than promote healing. He will have to be very well informed about all aspects of each type of technology before he prescribes it. To be able to keep up to date with the advances in technology related to his practice, he will have to engage in continuous learning.

From an economics view, Dr. Aidan must be careful not to succumb to the "lure of the latest." That means he will have to weigh the cost of immediately obtaining the newest technology versus the benefit of this technology for his patients. Perhaps, it will be more economical to wait until the price declines before purchasing the newest models. He will also have to remember that newer is not always better. Again, his decisions must be based on research rather than on the influence of a well-spoken sales representative.

The Case of the Lemon Baby

As you read this case, consider the following questions. Responses and comments will follow the case.

1. What principles of ethics should be considered in this case?
2. How does this technology affect the business of health care?
3. How does this technology affect the nature of families?

Case Information

Introduction

This case is based on a scenario that was used in the author's ethics classes for several years, and it is always popular. When it was first introduced, students thought it was so bizarre that it would never happen. They thought that it was just an academic exercise and that they would never have to deal with such a situation. Now, the case is much closer to reality; some clinicians are even providing this service at a basic level. The case illustrates the need to balance the business potential of technology with the ethics issues it creates. It goes back to Gastmans's (2002) question of, just because you can do something, should you?

The Case

The Center for Reproductive Technology has made great strides in clinical applications of genetic engineering for reproductive services. For a fee of $150,000, it can provide a "baby to specs." The potential parents fill out an extensive questionnaire that gives their preference for gender, eye color, hair color and type, potential height and weight, intelligence potential, athletic potential, and other variables. They also complete three interviews including a psychologic evaluation and a marriage stability profile. Standard consent forms are also a part of the client acceptance process.

The procedure uses the egg and sperm of the parents, or donor if necessary, and genes are engineered to meet the parents' specifications. The improved embryos are then implanted in the mother or surrogate mother for delivery. All efforts are made to ensure the quality of the product delivered. Customer satisfaction rates have been reported as 95%, and the Center has turned a very high profit share to its investors.

The Doctors Smalley took advantage of the services offered through the Center. They had long wanted a male child to carry on the Smalley name. Dr. Herbert Smalley wanted a male baby who had the ability to be a star athlete. Dr. Matilda Smalley wanted a child with high intelligence potential so he could maintain the family tradition of graduating from Harvard. The procedures went well and their surrogate mother gave birth successfully. The problem was that the child had the wrong eye and hair color, and was female.

The Center's chief executive officer, Kit Ptolemy, received a call from Dr. Herbert Smalley, who was enraged at the lack of product quality. He had paid $150,000 for a male child with certain genetic traits and potentials. What he got was a female child who did not meet any of the stated characteristics. He demanded an explanation. Mr. Ptolemy calmed him down and told him that he would investigate immediately.

After checking into the situation, Mr. Ptolemy found that there had been a mix-up in the computer system. The surrogate mother was implanted with improved embryos from another order, which was for a red-haired, blue-eyed, Caucasian female with high beauty and intelligence potential. There was no data concerning who received the actual Smalley implant so it could not be traced. Because the Smalleys were African American, Mr. Ptolemy could see how they could be angry about this error.

Mr. Ptolemy called the Doctors Smalley back and explained what happened. He offered to reimburse them for their fees. That is when Dr. Herbert Smalley exploded. He told Mr. Ptolemy that he would not raise a white female child in his home even if she were free. He wanted his full refund and, tomorrow morning, he would be bringing the baby back to the Center. She would be their problem, not his.

Responses and Comments on Questions

1. What principles of ethics should be considered in this case?

First, look at the business aspects of this case. The Center for Reproductive Technology made a risky financial decision that paid off. They invested huge amounts of capital in technology and staff to be able to provide a service that many wanted and could afford. In fact, Mr. Ptolemy thought that the fee of $150,000 was a bargain in light of the Center's capital investment.

The administration of the Center felt it was meeting their business obligation to provide a quality product as promised. They tried to prevent any unsatisfactory consequences by insisting on extensive interviews with potential parents of this product, including an assessment of their psychological and marital stability. In addition, as part of a capital-based society, they felt that they had an obligation to make a profit and provide a dividend to investors. To fail in this effort would be bad for business and violate corporate ethics. Up until the time of the Smalley error, the Center was meeting these obligations and saw itself as a thriving business with great growth potential.

From a purely capitalistic view, the Center was an ethics-based business. However, when you look beyond the business aspects, you can see some serious ethics issues. First, the Center regarded human embryos and full-term babies as "products," not humans. This is a violation of the principle of autonomy, because their view did not value and respect human life. Buber's idea of moral relationships also applies here. When humans become "its" instead of valued individuals, it can change the way they are treated in society. The Center, through its designer baby technology, is actually contributing to a negative valuing of individuals.

How do other ethics principles apply to this case? Although it can be seen as providing a societal benefit, the Center's policies do not comply with utilitarian ethics. The ability to design children is limited only to those who are wealthy enough to afford such technology. Therefore, the greatest good is not provided to the greatest number; it is limited to a few. Rawls's principle of differences could be used to argue that these parents are helping to contribute to the future. They are creating genetically superior children. Therefore, they felt that they should they be given the special treatment. However, is this true? Kantians would reject this idea and say that the Center has an ethical duty to obey the categorical imperative. Apparently, they do not feel that providing designer children should apply to all in society—only to those who can pay for it. The Center's action could not be defended by this ethical test. Finally, the principles presented by Mills also question the ethics of this business, because it does not seem reasonable to create a different type of human being without first considering the impact of such a decision on society as a whole.

2. How does this technology affect the business of health care?

This case goes to the root of how technology will be implemented in health care and the impact it can have. The potential for profit will make many technology-based businesses very attractive especially if traditional healthcare services begin to be less profitable. They hold the potential for changing how administrators think about healthcare delivery. So many questions need to be answered. For example, is health care going to continue to be centered on the service of increasing or maintaining health, or is it to be a products-based industry? How do you invest capital in technology and still have enough resources to provide quality services? What about paying for technology applications? Will those who are uninsured or medically indigent be denied life-saving or life-enhancing benefits? What if the technology's products are not needed, but are profitable? How do you make appropriate decisions?

Technology's potential seems almost limitless in terms of what it can do for and to the human body. This potential can greatly benefit business and society as well. However, difficult decisions will have to be made to determine just how far technology should go. From an ethics standpoint, each organization will have to determine a balance between demand for new technology, investment versus profit potential, and ethical considerations.

3. How does this technology affect the nature of families?

Certainly, the Smalleys have a different view of the family than most. They wanted to have the perfect child who would grow up to meet their expectations. Their view of the ideal family was supported by their access to technology that could provide them with the kind of child that they wanted. They were able to pay for this technology, and it was legal. Frankly, they felt that it was nobody's business what they did in their own home. Their only problem with this was that the Center did not deliver. Their error produced a very unacceptable product—a redheaded, white, female child. They had no desire to spend their time and money raising a child who was not the correct gender or even the correct race. Full refund and a return of the defective product seemed fair. After all, if their Lexus child was really a lemon, it could be returned.

You can see from this response that the designer baby business can introduce completely new issues about the nature of what it means to be a family. Will there be issues about designer children versus "natural" children so that one will be valued over the other? Can you imagine the issues this change might create for social workers, psychologists, and counselors who have to deal with the psychologic impact on the family and individuals? What should happen in schools? Are they prepared to educate a group of super children? How will the nonengineered children fare in school and in society in general?

In the author's classes, several groups tried to grapple with what to do with the "rejected products" or children who were born, but did not measure up to the specifications. They acknowledged that the Center might have to take these children back, much like adoption agencies do today. Therefore, they decided that they could create a spinoff business by running a discounted adoption center that would place these babies in the homes of those who wanted designer babies but could not afford them. This suggestion, while made facetiously, sparked a class debate about what would happen to the children who did not measure up and the impact on the family and society in general.

Web Resources

American Health Information Management Association
http://www.ahima.org/

Joint Healthcare Information Technology Alliance
http://rodp.ridne.net/node-53318.html

Radio Frequency Identification Journal
http://www.rfidjournal.com/

References

American Medical Association. (2008). *Health information technology*. Available at: http://www.ama-assn.org/ama/pub/category/16195.html. Accessed November 28, 2008.

Brooks, R. G., & Menachemi, N. (2006). Physicians' use of email with patients: Factors influencing electronic communication and adherence to best practices. *Journal of Medical Internet Research*, 8(1), e2. Available at: http://www.jmir.org/2006/1/e2/. Accessed May 19, 2009.

Budinger, T. F., & Budinger, M. D. (2006). *Ethics of emerging technologies: Scientific facts and moral challenges*. Hoboken, NJ: John Wiley & Sons, Inc.

Cisco Systems, Inc. (2008). *Collaberation*. Available at: http://www.cisco.com/en/US/netsol/ns870/index.html. Accessed November 30, 2008.

Coddington, D. C., Fischer, E. A., Moore, K. D., & Clarke, R. L. (2000). *Beyond managed care: How consumers and technology are changing the future of health care*. San Francisco: Jossey-Bass.

Crichton, M. (2006). *Next*. New York: HarperCollins.

Gastmans, C. (Ed.). (2002). *Between technology and humanity: The impact of technology on health care ethics*. Belgium: Leuven University Press.

Glandon, G. L., Smaltz, D. H., & Slovensky, D. J. (2008). *Austin and Boxerman's information systems for healthcare management* (7th ed.). Chicago: Health Administration Press/AUPHA.

Graber, G. C. (2009). The moral status of gametes and embryos: Storage and surrogacy. In E. E. Morrison (Ed.). *Health care ethics: Critical issues for the 21st century*. Sudbury, MA: Jones and Bartlett, pp. 61–70.

Institute of Medicine. (2001). *Crossing the quality chasm: A new health system for the 21st century*. Washington, DC: National Academy Press.

Roberti, R. (2008). Frequently asked questions. *Radio Frequency Identification Journal*. Available at: http://www.rfidjournal.com/faq. Accessed November 30, 2008.

Shi, L., & Singh, D. A. (2008). *Delivering health care in America: A systems approach* (4th ed.). Sudbury, MA: Jones and Bartlett.

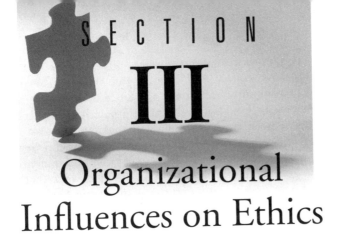

SECTION III

Organizational
Influences on Ethics

■ INTRODUCTION

Ethics is not just theory or words for discussion. It must be practiced daily in health care organizations. In fact, organizational culture can greatly influence the application of ethics. In turn, your ethics decisions can have an impact on your organization's culture. Your understanding of your organization's mission, espoused values, structure, and financial status can enhance this symbiotic relationship. In order to be an agent for ethical change, you need to understand how your organization works and responds to ethical issues. In addition, you must be aware of your power and its use for influencing ethics-based decisions. The chapters in this section will assist you with this responsibility. They explore various organizational areas including finance, culture, compliance to the law, and view of the customer as they relate to ethics practices for health administrators.

In Chapter 9, *No Mission, No Margin: Fiscal Responsibility*, you will examine how health care receives its funding. The complexity of health care finance adds to its ethics issues. However, like other industries, health care must maintain a solid bottom line so that it can keep its doors open, pay its employees competitively, and maintain quality service. Unlike other industries, its mission is supposed to be based in service to the individual and the community and not on profit building. In this chapter, you will examine some of the ethical issues that occur when mission and margin compete. You will also study the concept of fiscal stewardship that should be prevalent in all aspects of health care delivery.

In Chapter 10, *Organization Culture, and Ethics*, you will learn about the different cultures that exist in health care and how they present ethics concerns. You will also examine management culture and its influence on ethics and what can happen when administration is not controlled. Adams and Balfour discuss this in their 1998 book, *Unmasking Administrative Evil*. The chapter also discusses the functions of ethics committees and their assistance in ethics decisions and policy formulation. In addition, several ethics decision-making models are presented to assist you in working with these committees.

Chapter 11, *The Ethics of Quality*, begins with a brief review of how organization's view compliance to externally imposed standards. Then the chapter goes beyond compliance to examine ways that external agencies are working toward improving quality in health care. The chapter discusses these organizations' efforts and how they affect health care facilities. In addition, the features of Kaizen activities and the Lean Thinking model are presented. As the chapter title suggests, the ethical implications of quality assurance are featured in this chapter.

In Chapter 12, *Patient Issues and Ethics*, you will look at the ethical issues affecting the patient from the organization's view. In an era of health care accountability, the communities you serve hold you to certain standards of patient satisfaction. This chapter examines the struggle between paternalism and patient autonomy. It also explores the ethics of measuring patient satisfaction and its affect on you as a health administrator. Finally, the chapter introduces the concept of patient-focused care and explains how organizations are trying to implement it for both ethical and business reasons.

CHAPTER 9

No Mission No Margin: Fiscal Responsibility

Can anybody remember when the times were not hard, and money not scarce?

—Ralph Waldo Emerson

Points to Ponder

1. How are the financial aspects of health care different from those of other businesses?
2. Why does the way profit is made affect community trust?
3. How can mission and profit margin be balanced?
4. What other key ethics issues exist in the financial side of health care?
5. What can you do to increase stewardship and balance financial decision in your organization?

Words to Remember

The following is a list of key words for this chapter. You will find them in bold in the text. Stop and check your understanding of them.

medically necessary   O Team   stewardship

■ SHOW ME THE MONEY

The quote by Ralph Waldo Emerson, the 19th century philosopher, that begins this chapter could easily have been written about today's healthcare financial situation. Even though health care is relatively recession proof, the system can still feel the effects of tight economic times. Even the best of times, the demand for health care exceeds its resources, especially in the case of the uninsured or underinsured. Despite government and private sector efforts, the system still has difficulties providing needed care and finding the funds to pay for it. Financing creates numerous problems for organizations that want to be true to their mission and yet stay fiscally sound. A quick review of how health care is financed should assist you to understand health care's unique monetary problems and the associated ethics.

First, you need to recognize that health care is a business, but that its funding is like no other business. Suppose you have decided to buy yourself a Ferrari. Your budget can handle it, and you have even selected the color. You go to the dealer, choose your car, and obtain appropriate financing. Your dealer is paid and you have a tangible product—your new car. In this situation, you are in charge of the purchase. If you cannot afford a Ferrari and/or cannot obtain financing, you have other options, like driving a lower cost vehicle or even using public transportation. The Ferrari dealer is not responsible if you cannot finance this purchase, but he or she does not make a sale.

In the case of most businesses then, customers have power because they decide to purchase items based on factors like need, perceived value, available finances, and even location of the services. The supplier does have certain obligations that can influence sales and profit, such as delivering a quality product at a competitive price. There are sometimes safety regulations to be met depending on the product for sale, but compliance can be used in product marketing.

What happens in the healthcare business? Shi and Singh (2008) discuss the maze-like complexity of healthcare financing, which includes a myriad of public and private sources. From the private sector, health care is funded through third-party organizations called health insurance companies. Access to these entities is most commonly provided by employer benefits, and options vary from Blue Cross Blue/Shield types of payers to various forms of managed care (i.e., health maintenance organizations, preferred provider organizations [PPOs], and independent practice associations). Employees usually pay part of the cost of such insurance through premiums, deductibles, and copays, but employers pay the majority of it. In difficult economic times, employer funding of health care can be increasingly difficult.

The public sector also funds health care, and this funding varies by population. Active duty military persons and their dependents, military retirees, and veterans have funding systems. State and federal government employees and retirees have a different system. Retirees and certain other qualified members have another system. Qualified poor persons, children, and those with disabilities have a system. Native Americans and other qualified populations also have a financing system. Each of these systems has regulations, policies, and procedures for including or excluding people and services. Cost reimbursement schemes can be different in each system, which adds to confusion, time, and staffing needed for reimbursement.

How do those who are not employed or in a covered population pay for their health care? These groups of patients fall into categories of the uninsured. If they are wealthy, they simply write a check for services rendered. However, many of the uninsured are not so fortunate. They often lack necessary coverage because their employer does not or cannot provide it. They may not be able to afford private healthcare premiums. These population groups can also be unemployed, children, or unqualified for public sector programs. Sometimes, they are given uncompensated care from hospitals, clinics, or charity from nongovernment agencies. They can also make financial arrangements with the facility (e.g., payment plans) or charge services to their credit cards.

While the complexity of payment seems obvious, it should also be noted that not all health care is covered, even for the insured. For example, dental and eye care are not universally covered and often require separate insurance policies. Prevention services such as nutrition counseling, exercise programs, and integrated medicine services are just beginning to be included in health insurance plans even though their potential for lowering cost is proven. Mental health services, which could be of benefit to millions of Americans, also have limited coverage. Out-of-pocket payment is often the funding source for these types of services.

Because health care is so expensive, insurance serves to protect consumers from bearing too heavy a financial burden. However, it also removes them from having an accurate understanding of the cost of care. Many do not even look at the costs incurred and only pay attention to their deductibles or their out-of-pocket costs. Some healthcare reformers think that this financial distance is part of the difficulty in reforming the cost structure of health care.

In addition to the complexity of the payer system, you also need to consider what happens with the demand side of the healthcare market. In other businesses, the consumer, often influenced by marketing, creates a demand. However, in health care, it is the provider or the payer who influences the demand. For instance, you cannot decide that you would like to have an MRI. It must be ordered by a referring physician and authorized by your insurance carrier. If you did not go to medical school and do not have the knowledge of a physician, you must trust the professional's decisions about what is best for you. In addition, the drug industry contributes to demand through their extensive advertising campaigns. These advertisements are often so convincing that consumers are sure that they have a particular disease and need a particular drug even before they see a physician!

In addition, the payer and the provider of care make the decisions about what is considered **medically necessary**. Physicians and other healthcare professionals are certainly well prepared to assist patients in making decisions about their health. However, many view the inclusion of the payer in deciding medical necessity with great distrust. They resent all of the rules and regulations that seem to question their professional opinion, increase the complexity of practice, and restrict their practice decisions. Physicians and the public often question whether or not a for-profit company can make equitable decisions about who should be given care and when they should receive it (Pearson, Sabin, & Emanuel, 2003).

What does all of this complexity mean for the system? First, it adds to the overall cost of providing care. In order to receive payment for services rendered, a myriad of knowledgeable personnel must be employed. These individuals need to know ways to navigate through the complex rules and regulations and obtain optimum funding for the organization. Does the need for these personnel take away funds that could be spent on providing care? Can this complexity be a source of employment for those who are on the business side of health care?

Second, the complexity can lead to many ethics challenges. The lure of profit over service can lead to both ethics and even legal problems. For example, while the most appropriate reimbursement code should be used for maximum return; there can be a temptation to code for the dollar and not for the diagnosis. This practice is called coding creep, which can become a legal issue if the organization is audited. In addition, since certain services can be better funded, reimbursement, rather than community need, can become the driving force for treatment. While this might be helpful for the bottom line initially, when the market is saturated, organizations are forced to compete for "insured hearts" and "well-covered cancers."

You are beginning to see that the financial complexity of the healthcare system poses difficulties for the organization in both the clinical and administrative areas. Reform efforts have attempted to simplify the system, but these efforts have not resulted in simplifying its financing. While there is much that could be done to improve the overall funding process, any reform must fit within the uniquely American position of trying to balance market-driven business with social responsibility.

■ MARGIN VERSUS MISSION: A DELICATE BALANCE

Simply put, healthcare organizations need to make money. When an organization shuts down due to lack of funds, the community is angry and feels betrayed. Yet, being solely motivated by profit seems beneath the higher mission of caring for the sick and injured. Profit-driven organizations can even be perceived as crass or unethical. Since no healthcare organization wants to advertise itself as putting profit over patients, a true dilemma exits. How do you maintain an adequate profit margin and remain true to social justice for your community?

As you just reviewed, care is provided in a uniquely American financial environment where the market is determined by the professionals and by the confusing array of payers. The ethical struggle for healthcare administrators (HCAs) is to find the balance of the yin of quality care and the yang of profit and market survival. To achieve this balance and maintain an ethics-based organization, you must realistically assess both aspects and make decisions that are appropriate for the organization and the community it serves.

No doubt, you have heard about the power of mission when it truly drives the functions and decisions of the organization. This can happen only when it is clearly and operationally defined, well understood by all, and used consistently at all levels of decision-making. Mission, in an ethics-based organization, needs to include the elements of delivery of quality services within the framework of community needs and mandates (Boyle, DuBose, Ellingson, Guinn, & McCurdy, 2001). To function, it must also be founded in appropriate and adequate resources including personnel, equipment, supplies, and funds. While these recommendations make perfect sense, they are often difficult to achieve. Remember that unlike other businesses, health care must also comply with complex and conflicting standards from many external agencies. While these standards are intended to protect the public's interests, they add to healthcare costs and must be included in financial planning.

In ensuring a balance between mission and profit margin, ethics-based organizations first must demonstrate congruence with their mission through their actions. For example, they cannot have two standards for the treatment of patients: one for those who are well funded and one for those who are not. Giving one group respect and the other minimal service does not demonstrate mission. Similarly, treating employees differently based on their ability to create revenue streams not only fails to demonstrate mission, but can also threaten quality of care and organizational image. In keeping with Frankl's (1971) concepts, an environment should exist where employees are given the opportunity for meaningful work. Valuing employees as people and acknowledging their service is just one action toward creating such a climate.

In addition, mission needs to be lived beyond organizational doors (Boyle, DuBose, Ellingson, Guinn, & McCurdy, 2001). This means that it needs to be lived in the community. Employees are also part of the community and need to provide quality service within the organization and be examples of ethical citizens outside of the organization. In fact, because of their place of work and responsibilities, they are held to a standard of behavior. They are often seen as a reflection of their organization and even health care itself.

Healthcare organizations also have a responsibility to model ethical citizenship by acting in accordance with community standards, being fair in their treatment of vendors, and paying their bills on time. When it is appropriate, organizations should act as community advocates. They can also encourage individual employees to provide service to the community through their volunteer efforts. Encouraging this commitment to community might include recognition of community service in newsletters and sponsorship of community events.

How does profitability fit in with mission? Boyle and colleagues (2001) and Pearson and colleagues (2003) present different aspects of mission and margin. First, ethics-based organizations need to take a big picture view of balancing patient care and profitability. This starts with the **O Team** (chief executive officer [CEO], chief financial officer [CFO], chief operating officer [COO], and chief information officer [CIO]) and the board of trustees. The budget must be seen as both a financial document and an ethics statement. It should be thoroughly assessed with attention to quality care, community needs, and adequate staff compensation. It should also be a statement about the organization's ethics. If profit is the sole motivation for budget decisions, the organization can face problems with community image and marketability. In the end, profit-only organizations can actually lose revenue. As Annison and Wilford (1998) suggest, trust is lost because there is a perception that your organization's goal is solely to make a profit. Confidence in your facility can also be lost. Because this confidence is at the core of your business, you run the risk of even more severe financial problems. Your internal customers (e.g., physicians) and your patients will find other venues to meet their healthcare needs. Given these examples, you can see that the O Team and the trustees must maintain trust and confidence by considering both the fiscal and ethical aspects of any financial decision.

The O Team is not the only group responsible for making the budget a statement of ethics. Orlikoff and Totten (2007) suggest that members of the board of trustees should also act as stewards of their organization's resources. This responsibility is based on the idea that, particularly in nonprofit facilities, trustees represent their communities and are the guardians of these resources. Trustees need to understand the issues that their facilities face and still oversee the ethical use of resources.

Trustees are also not alone in their **stewardship** role. In fact, all administrators should act as stewards of resources including money, equipment, and personnel. Steward-type administrators will protect resources as if they were their own. They are also trusted to ensure the quality, availability, and best use of these resources. Peter Block (1996), in his book called *Stewardship: Choosing Service over Self-Interest*, discusses health care's need to spend its money responsibly. This means taking ownership and accountability for what happens in the organization. It also means paying attention to fit—fit between the organization and the community and between staff and the organization. Block suggests that good stewards also hold their employees accountable. This means treating staff with real respect, trusting them with decisions, and avoiding excessive micromanagement.

Boyle and colleagues (2001) offer some specific ideas to address stewardship and working toward balancing mission and profit margins. These include paying careful attention to your patient mix. While it can be tempting to exclude uninsured or low-payment Medicaid patients, it might not play well in your community image. In order to maintain a good profit margin, organizations should also work toward efficient use of all services and cut down on inappropriate use. This could mean programs like "Dial a Nurse" and community education efforts. Pearson and colleagues (2003) suggest that loss of income from low- or nonpaying patients can be lessened by assessing needs, using outreach efforts, and working with community agencies.

Waste reduction represents another area of stewardship. For example, when you authorize spending, be sure it is used for essential functions as defined in your mission. In addition, model behavior that you expect from your staff concerning the use of resources. Hoarding materials and over ordering might seem like a good idea but can lead to waste. Resources are finite and need to be used appropriately whether they are for clinical or business practice. Remember that you are always an example and your personal actions to reduce waste carry a strong message.

Boyle and colleagues (2001) also caution that care should be taken in capital expenditure decisions. While growth is needed for organizational survival and maintenance, these decisions should be carefully considered in light of mission and outcome. Technology can be helpful here by providing software to assist with projections on maintenance costs, projected obsolescence, and other data. Of course, conducting product research, using competitive bids and astute questioning of selected vendors should help in making appropriate decisions.

Balancing profit and mission might force you to consider decisions that are more drastic. These actions might include staff and salary reductions and program elimination. In some cases, these options have become necessary for an organization's survival. They should not be taken lightly because, while they can help short-term financial problems, they have a steep cost in diminished employee and community trust. It can take many years (if ever) to rebuild this trust, so drastic decisions should be made only after careful data analysis and with a plan for dealing with their impact. When they are made, attention must be given to communication, including providing an explanation for the action and treating those affected with dignity and beneficence.

Health care is a unique business that is conducted in unique organizations. Therefore, there is no one formula for balancing mission and profit margin. The issue is not that health care has to make money. In fact, the community feels betrayed if an organization closes its doors. This issue more about how the money is spent. It is also about congruence between what you say is your mission and how you act fiscally on that mission. When profit appears to be a stronger motivation than patient care, trust can be lost. If Annison and Wilford (1998) are correct, a loss of trust means a loss of the essential element for the existence of a healthcare organization. Decisions about ethics-based financial policies need to begin with the O Team and trustees. They also need to be consistently implemented throughout the organization.

Beyond Mission/Margin Balance: Other Concerns of Finance and Ethics

Nowicki (2007) also finds decisions about finances and resource allocation to be one of the top ethics issues in healthcare finance. However, he adds conflicts of interest and billing as potential areas of concern. Billing can include issues of fraud and abuse, which can move the organization into legal problems.

Conflicts of interest can exist for the individual (discussed in the next section of this chapter) or for entire organizations. Conflicts can also exist within the external community and the internal communities of the facilities. Employees worry that "pink slips will fall like rain," and often the most talented people bail out before the unpleasantness begins. Additionally, fiduciary boundaries become confused and trustees feel conflicting loyalties. Conflict of interest situations are further enhanced when mergers are between religious or civic-based organization and a for-profit one. These types of merger raises concerns are about mission, values, public image, and even service offerings.

Darr (2005) stresses that reducing these situations requires awareness that interests between parties can be in conflict. Epstein (2007) suggests that you determine the definition of a conflict of interest for your organization. After you are clear about the potential conflicts, then you can decide what to do to control them. It is also important to know whether or not the conflict is supported by law. If a conflict has legal support on either side, then the law must prevail. However, many conflicts of interest are not backed by law. In such instances, mission and values, fiscal impact, employee considerations, and other factors must be considered.

Examples of potential conflict-of-interest situations where there might not be legal support include employment outside of the organization and behavior during personal time. An organization has the right to expect its employees to provide adequate time on task for salary paid to these employees. Moonlighting can affect the employee's ability to provide satisfactory performance. However, there might be circumstances in which outside employment does not adversely affect the organization and can even enhance its image. Therefore, each situation should be examined carefully for potential conflicts of interest and resolved in favor of the organization.

Another example of conflict of interest that is not backed by law could be personal time behavior. While the organization cannot and should not have policies to control all of its employees' behaviors outside of the employment setting, certain behaviors negatively affect the organization's image and should be addressed. For example, many organizations used to offer alcoholic beverages at social functions. This became a problem when employees did not limit their consumption and were involved in traffic accidents or other serious problems. Employees' actions produced a negative image in the community when it became known that the organization provided the alcohol. Currently, most organizations either refrain from any alcohol at functions or restrict its use through cash bars and limited access. In addition, healthcare organizations have policies and procedures regarding the recreational use of alcohol and other drugs and support prehire and random screenings. Because this personal behavior has a direct impact on patient care and the facility's image, action is taken to rehabilitate or remove employees who violate policy. The interests of the organization must take precedence in this situation.

In his classic work, Worthley (1999) discusses conflicts of interest for healthcare organizations. First, he states that the five "hallmarks of conflict of interest" are "competing obligations, appearance, myopia, fairness, [and] power" (p. 153). You need to identify the interests involved and determine if they, as obligations, compete with each other. The second, appearance, is most critical in healthcare organizations. If the situation is perceived as a conflict of interest by the board of trustees or the community, then it is in fact a conflict of interest. Such situations need to be avoided if possible or resolved if necessary. He also notes that people engaged in conflicts of interest might not see them as a problem (what he calls myopia). They might be motivated by what seems to be good "business sense" and fail to perceive the potential impact. Fairness is also an element to be considered in conflicts of interest. Actions should be fair to all groups and not give one group an unfair advantage. Finally, Worthley says that power is usually a part of a conflict of interest. Organizations and people in these potential situations need to think about the limits and impact of their authority.

Worthley (1999) suggests that conflicts of interest need to be addressed in both formal and informal infrastructures of an organization. On the formal side, policies and procedures should be designed to prevent potential problems and deal with them as they arise. For example, is it a conflict of interest when a pharmaceutical company pays for a continuing education unit (CEU) course and lunch for all of your nurses? Should your physicians and residents get free cruises masked as CEU opportunities? What should you do about vendor gifts to your purchasing department? On the surface, this might look like business as usual and have little influence on decisions, but Worthley found that such practices do influence practice decisions. Because patients have a right to expect that prescribing or purchasing products for their care is based on their needs, many healthcare organizations have created policies to limit gifts, for example, from vendors. A dollar limit or a no-gift policy can be established and published for all staff and vendors. In addition, some organizations audit their purchasing departments to be sure they use fair practices in making vendor decisions. HCAs are expected to be role models for these policies and to enforce them when necessary.

The informal policies of an organization also need to address the gray areas surrounding conflicts of interest. This is done through the organization's attitude toward these behaviors. For example, does anyone question the appropriateness of eating all those free lunches or using all those free supplies? Do individuals honor the policy of outside employment? Are they aware that they represent the organization in the community by what they do or what they fail to do? Consistent policy application and reinforcement help to maintain a culture where conflicts of interest are reduced.

Finally, another classic work by Worthley (1997) reminds us that conflicts of interest can be reduced when you take time to define your responsibilities and values as an organization. This might not be an easy task, because all healthcare organizations have multiple responsibilities and often-conflicting values. To reconcile conflicts, he recommends using awareness, creativity, discussion, and reflection to move toward a common understanding and good policies. Professional organization statements like that of the American College of Healthcare Executives and of the American Hospital Association can provide guidance for working on this goal.

Billing and Finance Ethics

Nowicki (2007) includes billing practices as both an ethical and legal issue for healthcare finance. Some of these practices, while remaining within the letter of the law, violate basic ethics principles. For example, if an organization delays as long as possible in refunding overpayments from insurance companies or is slow to pay its vendors, it can help its bottom line. However, it risks a negative impact on its level of trust in the community and possibly its future contracts. More than just legality should be considered in billing practices.

May (2004) discusses ways to improve revenue cycles, as well as billing practices and financial outcomes. When the revenue cycle is handled appropriately, there is less temptation to violate the ethics of finance. She suggests that you include billing data in making decisions, model a processing cycle instead of a fixed stream, and increase ownership and accountability among employees. Efficient work processes coupled with staff training can decrease the time between charge filing, billing, and payment. Performance measures in several areas are provided including registration, coding, charge capture, and patient payment. Finally, May encourages you to discuss billing with patients to foster a clear understanding of deductibles, charges, and payment. She even suggests the use of a financial counselor in the emergency department to assist with patient needs.

On the negative side, billing practices can become so unethical that they lead to fraud and abuse. Shi and Singh (2008), among others, have claimed that at least 10% of healthcare spending might be the result of these problems. Fraud and abuse have been a well-known secret in the industry and until recently were largely ignored. It was difficult to detect fraud and abuse, and prosecutions were rare. In addition, the complexity of the regulations and changing interpretations made it easy to defraud unintentionally. This leads to a "Do it if we don't get caught" attitude among some healthcare facilities.

How does fraud happen? It can occur if you intentionally falsify codes or costs or provide services that are not needed. You also defraud when you bill for services that were never provided. Examples of these practices include billing for dental restorations when the patient is edentulous, recording a higher code when the service was actually a lower code, and having a pattern of the same error without any effort toward correction. In addition, if you provide referrals for patients and receive kickback payments for those referrals, you are committing fraud. Shi and Singh (2008) cite fraud and abuse as a major concern for Medicare and Medicaid.

In an effort to better control fraud and abuse, the federal government has attempted several reform actions through the Department of Health and Human Services and the Office of the Inspector General, including Operation Restore Trust. Initially, this program investigated home health, skilled nursing homes, and medical supply companies for Medicaid/Medicare fraud. However, it has expanded to other areas. The Health Insurance Portability and Accountability Act enacted in 1996 also has provisions for dealing with Medicare and Medicaid fraud. They include encouraging reporting of fraudulent practices, database construction, and increased conditions where penalties and sanctions occur (Nowicki, 2007).

While these and other efforts have increased attention on fraud and abuse prevention, they have also added to the expense of providing health care. Time spent (e.g., for completing reports), personnel, and money are being used to ensure compliance, track violations, and resolve any issues. As the system becomes even more complex in the future, it is likely there will be additional regulations from both the public and private sectors to try to control fraud and abuse.

Summary

What should you do to balance profits and mission? No matter what your position is within the healthcare system, money matters. You will be dealing with financial matters whether it is monitoring the budget, requesting funds, or planning for future needs. There are several things that you can do to make ethics-based decisions on financial issues. For example, high levels of accountability and public scrutiny require sound ethics-based decisions and are especially needed when it comes to finance. You should consider the organization's mission as you participate in the various aspects of the budget cycle and be careful to monitor expenses against budget codes. Remember that knowledge is power. You must read financial documents related to your area and understand them. Be sure to question codes that are not appropriate for your area and amounts that appear to be in error. Have correct documentation of expenses to support any questions that you have. Remember that to say nothing means you agree with the report. Your annual evaluations might well be based on your financial stewardship as well as your productivity.

Greenspan (2004) recommends that all healthcare organizations consider certifying their financial statements to avoid the perception of manipulation, deception, or even fraud. He suggests that you review your payments. He also stresses that in a time of financial constraint and staff shortages, there must be a balance between mission and cost accountability. Your stakeholders in the community must believe that you are truthful in your financial statements during such challenging times. Further, it is critical to educate all of your staff about how you do business so that they report information accurately and represent your organization well. Finally, he encourages all CEOs to authenticate financial statements even if the law does not require it. Making this extra effort can provide assurance that all is well in your financial house.

Remember that you are the role model for stewardship. Even though you have written policies in place, your actions create the real policy for your department. If you create unnecessary waste and abuse resources, you send a loud message that the policy does not matter. While it is not necessary to become the finance police, be aware that you are accountable. Be willing to ask for details about requests for funding whether it is to pay for CEUs, travel, or new equipment. Whatever you authorize should support the mission of your organization. If it cannot be justified, be prepared to say "No." The ethics of finance is not just for the O Team; you are a large part of making it the norm for your organization.

Cases for Your Consideration

The Case of the Lost Chapel

As you read this case, consider the following questions. Responses and comments will follow the case.

1. What organizational ethics issues are illustrated by this case?

2. What could have been done differently?

3. What was the true bottom line in this case?

Case Information

St. Basil the Great Hospital was founded by the Sisters of Mary in 1894 with a mission of caring for those who had the greatest need. One of the first buildings in the hospital complex was a chapel dedicated to St. Basil, the patron saint of hospital administrators. This chapel became a spiritual center for the facility and the community and served as a site for many weddings and funerals.

In recent years, the hospital was part of a merger with a for-profit hospital chain but, because of community recognition, it was able to retain its name. The merged hospital placed great emphasis on fiscal stability and its commitment to shareholders for profitability. To that end, the O Team (e.g., CEO, CIO, COO, and CFO) conducted a facilities review on utilization and cost benefit. The chapel did not make the cut for effectiveness because it was not used on a daily basis to meet patient needs and required funds for maintenance and upkeep. However, the land on which it stood was very valuable and could be used as a site for a high-rise parking lot. Because parking was a real need at St. Basil's and a profit could be made from fees, it was decided to tear down the chapel and put up a parking lot.

After some discussion, the Board of Trustees approved the proposal. A request for bids for demolition was to proceed immediately. However, when the news hit the community, a problem occurred. Local churches and community organizations had not been consulted about the potential demolition, and they demanded a meeting to discuss what, in their view, was a tragedy. The request was denied and they were told that the decision was a "done deal." Next, they offered to fund its upkeep and save the chapel from demolition. They were told that St. Basil's had an obligation to shareholders, and a parking lot more positively affected the bottom line. Finally, they tried to save the site by having it declared a historical landmark, but their request was denied.

Frustrated, the group, now called "Save Our Sanctuary," went to media outlets for help. The local television featured several pieces on the issue including coverage of a candlelight vigil to mourn the death of the chapel. The local newspaper ran two feature-length articles telling the story of couples who had been married in the chapel, and the potential loss of a piece of the community's history.

Members of the O Team, while not happy about the community response, felt that it was well within their rights to make business decisions that would have a positive impact on their bottom line. They thought all this "sound and fury" would soon blow over, so the bulldozers and other equipment did their work, and the 115–year-old chapel was destroyed. However, there was an additional cost for their actions. The positive relationship that St. Basil had with the community was severely affected. Because of its new image of profit over decency, many of its physicians and well-insured families chose to use other hospitals for their care needs. Contributions to the hospital were severely reduced. Census numbers were also reduced in both inpatient and outpatient facilities, and the parking lot soon became a liability and not an asset.

Responses and Commentary on Questions

1. What organizational ethics issues are illustrated by this case?

   First, you can see that this is a case about balancing mission with profit margin. The O Team was trying to make sound fiscal decisions based on their definition of contribution to mission and revenue generation. Certainly, a chapel could not produce the revenue of a parking lot. Besides, it was actually costing the organization money through the costs of upkeep.

   What the O Team did not consider was the impact of destroying the chapel on St. Basil's image and ultimate financial situation. It did not see that destroying a chapel to put up a parking lot would cause great anger in the community. They did not think about the community's response, which turned out to be extremely negative. Once they learned of their concerns, the O Team simply dismissed them. After all, the community would get over it and profit had to be made.

   This case also points out some of the difficulties in mergers between for-profit organizations and religion-based facilities. In the view of the O Team members, they were being fiscally responsible to their shareholders to decrease waste (the chapel) and increase profitability (the parking lot). Those from the religious-based organization saw the destruction of part of their history as a great loss. Despite their objections, they were outvoted in every way and money prevailed.

   This case also is an example of utilitarianism ethics without consideration for Kantian ideas. The O Team based this decision on trying to do the greatest good for the greatest number. By removing a building that was not frequently used and replacing it with something that would provide convenience, they were able to provide a benefit for more customers. In addition, the funds generated by parking fees could be added to the operational budget and help defray costs for areas like uncompensated care. In addition, they were practicing ethics by being true to their shareholders by increasing their return on investment potential.

By treating the chapel and the people who used it as a means to an end, they violated a basic concept of Kantian ethics. The community was not even consulted. When they asked to be heard, they were given only marginal attention. Buber would say that they were treated like "Its" and their protests, feelings, and recommendations were ignored. The O Team believed that, in the end, these people did not matter and the parking lot would be seen as an asset to the community. However, the community felt otherwise.

2. What could have been done differently?

First, the O Team was correct in assessing St. Basil's assets and utilization or resources. They wanted to be able to assure the shareholders that property was being used to its best advantage for patient care and profitability. In addition, they certainly had an ethical responsibility to be good stewards of the hospital's resources and to make business decisions.

However, what they failed to assess was the priorities of the internal and external community. They were acting with a one-sided view of the situation (tunnel vision) and lacked an understanding of the bigger picture. To begin with, they were now partners with a religion-founded facility. It should have been obvious that a 115-year-old chapel would have some meaning for those who chose to work at St. Basil's and for the community it served. Conducting some form of information gathering to determine the importance of the chapel and the impact of tearing it down would have added to their understanding of the situation. However, they chose to disregard their own employees and the community they served.

They also failed to anticipate the long-term impact of their actions on the community. Although they might have realized that some protest would occur, they truly believed that the purpose of their business decision would provide a positive impact on their bottom line. Despite queries from the community and offers of alternative solutions, they chose the parking lot over the chapel. This decision, right or wrong, painted them as Scrooge-like administrators who cared little for the community and its history.

There could have been other solutions to this case. First, the O Team, armed with data about the use of the chapel, could have presented the problem to its board of trustees. Instead of using politics and power to overrule any protests, it could have asked the board to develop a solution to meet the parking needs and the needs for preservation of the chapel. Perhaps the internal and external community could have been involved in a positive way to raise funds to move the chapel to a different site or find another way to provide parking and revenue. This solution would, admittedly, take more time, but decreasing the negative effort might have been worth the effort.

Even if the chapel could not be saved, the O Team could have done a much better job with informing the community of its decision. Providing community members and media with the rationale for the decision might have helped. In addition, the O Team could have planned some type of ceremony honoring the chapel and its meaning to the community. These actions might have been much better received than just going forward with plans. The message to the community was, "You do not matter—this is business."

3. What was the true bottom line in this case?

The bottom line in this case was a loss of profit. Because census figures were even lower in the aftermath of the chapel incident, St. Basil did not receive a solid return on investment for the parking lot. In addition, it lost a more critical asset: the goodwill of the community. For many years, the community remembered how the chapel incident was handled and declined to support the hospital at the level it did in the past. As Annison and Wilford (1998) say, health care is based on the trust of the community; once lost, trust is difficult to regain.

The Case of the Faulty Estimates

As you read this case, consider the following questions. Responses and comments will follow the case.

1. What ethics principles do you think were considered in the decision to sign contracts with the PPOs?

2. What was the motivation to underestimate the revenue deductions?

3. How did these decisions impact the organization?

4. What would you have done if you were Mr. Seis?

Case Information

Mr. Para Seis was to be interviewed for the position of Senior Vice President for Operations (VPO) at Clairmont Hospital. He carefully researched and reviewed all of the financial data on this facility and found that it had a strong net worth. He also was impressed with the executive team including the CEO, CFO, and executive vice president (EVP). Of course, he was delighted when he was offered the position.

After being there only a month, Mr. Seis was called into the EVP's office for a private meeting. He learned that the EVP had signed a confidential agreement with the local PPO. If patients chose Clairmont over other area hospitals, the facility would be given bonus money. The EVP decided to make this decision without informing physicians because they were also on staff at each of the competing hospitals. He did not want to deal with their "hassle." However, once the physicians learned of the "deal," they decided to boycott Clairmont. During the last two weeks, the census had dropped by one-third and continued to fall. Mr. Seis struggled to help the organization overcome this problem.

However, Mr. Seis also did not know that the CEO, not wanting the boycott to affect the financials of the hospital, ordered the CFO to underestimate the deductions from revenue. By the end of the fiscal year, this inflated the net income and made the financial position look solid despite the income losses. All appeared to be well until an external auditor uncovered some problems with the figures and the true bottom line was revealed: it was zero. The CEO and the EVP were fired over the secret contract issue and the CFO for practicing "creative accounting." Mr. Seis was the only senior management team member left to deal with this financial disaster.

Responses and Commentary on Questions

1. What ethics principles do you think were considered in the decision to sign contracts with the PPOs?

   The EVP considered the positive impact the agreement could have on Clairmont's financial picture. If a significant number of patients chose this facility over others, there would be financial benefit through increased census and bonuses. The increased numbers might also be used in marketing the facility.

   He was aware that local physicians had staff privileges at each of the area hospitals, so he chose not to inform them of the agreement. He did not view his action as a betrayal of trust; it was just good business. However, the physicians did not see it this way and responded by conducting a boycott. Imagine their negative comments about Clairmont.

2. What was the motivation to underestimate the revenue deductions?

   Consider the position of the CEO in this situation. She sees the hospital census dropping because of the actions of her subordinate. If the shareholders and the community found out that it was "bleeding assets," there could be a panic. Surely, a bit of overestimation could bolster the financial picture until the problem could be fixed. She also knew her CFO would support this and practice his "estimation magic" on the books. She might even have seen herself as an ethical person in that she was taking this action to protect the solvency of the facility and the jobs of its employees. Apparently, the external auditor did not agree.

3. How did these decisions affect the organization?

The CEO's worst fear actually came true for Clairmont, and she was part of its creation. Although based on formulas, the estimates did not come close to reflecting the true financial picture of the hospital. In fact, after the external auditor was through, the hospital's financial position was in shambles. If this situation was not corrected, Clairmont faced bankruptcy and possible closure.

4. What should Mr. Seis have done?

Consider the unfortunate Mr. Seis. On the surface, he did all the correct things before accepting the position of VPO. He looked at the financial statements, assessed the working environment, and liked the personalities of the senior team. He had no way of knowing that he was walking into an ethics nightmare.

When he found out about the secret agreement and its aftermath, he was surprised. However, he tried to work within the situation as it existed and make sure that operations did all it could do to improve the bottom line. He instituted waste control measures, monitored staffing and overtime, and generally tried to do his part toward fixing the problem. However, the underestimation of deductions provided Mr. Seis with inaccurate information. Like the board and others, he thought that Clairmont was financially stable. He was also betrayed by the actions of the CEO and the CFO.

Perhaps he would have been better off to resign the minute he learned of the secret deal. However, he did not have the whole picture at that time and decided to give Clairmont the benefit of the doubt. Besides, he had just uprooted his family and moved them. Resignation did not look like an attractive option after only one month on the job. By working to fix the problem, he gave the impression that he supported the action. However, he wanted to do all he could to help staff keep their jobs. This situation caused him many sleepless nights and bouts of acid reflux. In the end, he was the only one not fired for unethical financial practices, but he found it difficult to secure a new position. His professional reputation was tarnished by his association with Clairmont's unscrupulous senior management team.

Web Resources

American College of Healthcare Executives
http://www.ache.org/

American Hospital Association
http://www.aha.org/aha/index.jsp

Health Care Compliance Organization
http://www.hcca-info.org/

References

Annison, M. H., & Wilford, D. S. (1998). *Trust matters: New directions in health care leadership.* San Francisco: Jossey-Bass.

Block, P. (1996). *Stewardship: Choosing service over self-interest.* San Francisco: Berrett-Koehler.

Boyle, P. J., DuBose, E. R., Ellingson, S. J., Guinn, D. E., & McCurdy, D. B. (2001). *Organizational ethics in health care: Principles, cases, and practical solutions.* San Francisco: Jossey-Bass.

Darr, K. (2005). *Ethics in health services management* (4th ed.). Baltimore: Health Professions Press.

Epstein, R. A. (2007). Conflicts of interest in health care: Who guards the guardians? *Perspectives in Biology and Medicine, 50*(1), 72–89.

Frankl, V. (1971). *Man's search for meaning: An introduction to logotherapy.* New York: Pocket Books.

Greenspan, B. J. (2004, May/June). Certifying financials. *Healthcare Executive, 19*(3), 42.

May, E. L. (2004, May/June). Managing the revenue cycle: Success factors from the field. *Healthcare Executive, 19*(3), 10–16, 18.

Nowicki, M. (2007). *The financial management of hospital and healthcare organizations* (4th ed.). Chicago: Health Administration Press.

Orlikoff, J. E., & Totten, M. K. (2007). Stewardship in action. *Healthcare Executive, 22*(5), 56–59.

Pearson, S. D., Sabin, J. E., & Emanuel, E. J. (2003). *No margin, no mission: Health-care organizations and the quest for ethical excellence.* New York: Oxford University Press.

Shi, L., & Singh, D. A. (2008). *Delivering health care in America: A systems approach* (4th ed.). Sudbury, MA: Jones and Bartlett.

Worthley, J. A. (1997). *The ethics of the ordinary in healthcare: Concepts and cases.* Chicago: Health Administration Press.

Worthley, J. A. (1999). *Organizational ethics in the compliance context.* Chicago: Health Administration Press.

CHAPTER 10

Organization Culture and Ethics

We could learn a lot from crayons. Some are sharp, some are pretty, some are dull, some have weird names, and all are different colors. But, they all fit nicely into the same box.

—Unknown

Points to Ponder

1. How does culture affect healthcare organizations?
2. How do the forces of culture influence ethical decision-making?
3. What is the function of ethics committees in healthcare organizations?
4. What can be done to increase the efficiency and effectiveness of ethics committees?

Words to Remember

The following is a list of key words for this chapter. You will find them in bold in the text. Stop and check your understanding of them.

acculturated
ethicists
Institutional Ethics Committee
professional socialization

culture clash
institutional review board (IRB)
pediatric ethics committee

■ CULTURE: A MACRO AND MICRO VIEW

Recall what you have learned about different cultures through courses in sociology, psychology, or public health, among others. You know that America is a nation of remarkable cultural diversity. This diversity adds to the country's strength but also creates special issues. Some of these issues include differing values, practices, disease experiences, and access to health care. Even though issues exist, the healthcare system has an ethical obligation to provide care for all cultural groups, and to treat them equally as members of society.

The healthcare industry employs people from a wide variety of cultural backgrounds. For example, nurses are hired who perhaps have been educated in other countries and who are not completely **acculturated** to American thinking and practices. When you consider all the patients you serve and the employees you hire, it is likely that you will encounter people whose values are different from yours. This situation can cause you difficulty, but as an ethics-based healthcare administrator (HCA), you need to make every effort to treat everyone with respect, justice, and beneficence.

In this chapter, you will learn to view culture with a macro and micro focus. First, you look at the cultural makeup of your organization and determine how it influences the organization's self-image and way of doing business. You will also examine subcultures within departments and the potential for culture clashes. Finally, you will look at the subculture of administration itself and decide its ethical practices make a difference concerning how people relate to each other.

In order to understand the impact of culture on an organization, you need to begin by defining what you mean by an organization. Daft (2006) reminds us that organizations must have goals, defined structures, and systems for organizing their activities. In addition, they are connected to the environments in which they exist. To explain the idea of organizational culture, he uses the analogy of an iceberg. The symbols and behaviors that the employees or the public sees are the tip of the iceberg. The culture in its entirety is below the surface and consists of the values, beliefs, feelings, and experiences that belong to the employees of the organization. These sub-rosa, or unseen, elements make up the practicing culture of the organization. Swayne, Duncan, and Ginter (2009) suggest the culture also includes understanding and believing in the organization's mission, vision, and goals. They agree that there may be unwritten rules about how things are done within an organization and that subjectivity exists.

It is possible to grow a community within an organization's culture when employees choose to believe and support the facility's values. In turn, culture provides a common identity that gives employees the information they need to relate to each other and meet the organization's mission. This common culture is filled with history, languages, ceremonies, stories, symbols, and traditions that help to establish a shared identity (Daft, 2006). These elements help new employees learn the way things are done, both formally and informally, and show them how to become part of the organization. Overall, this serves to represent your organization to the community.

Culture in this sense needs the capacity to adapt to the internal and external environment in order to be successful. Daft (2006) provides a greater understanding of this adaptation by subdividing organizational cultures into mission-based, clan-based, bureaucratic-based, and learning-based cultures. In a mission-based culture, the needs of populations are the focus and rapid change is not the norm. In the clan-based culture, employees' needs are the focus and rapid change is common. In the bureaucratic-based culture, things are done in a deliberate manner and the environment remains stable. In this case, change is made slowly. Finally, in a learning-based organization, emphasis is placed on adapting to change and values: caring for each other; big picture thinking and creative change are stressed. Learning-based organizations resist the temptation to be "culture bound" or to say, "We have always done it this way." and emphasize the value of change as a mechanism for success when the environment is unpredictable.

All of Daft's examples can be found in today's healthcare organizations. In fact, all four types can exist in the same organization. As an HCA, you are supposed to be driven by internal mission, but your external environment might experience rapid change. Professionals within your organization want to succeed and have a high quality of life. They expect you to provide the means to accomplish their goals. However, healthcare organizations are bureaucracies; that can make it difficult to effect change, even when it is needed. Finally, the ideal of a learning-based organization is being introduced into individual departments as a way to address the limitations of the other models. As healthcare culture tends toward being conservative, a culture shift can take time.

Ethics is now becoming a cultural issue for all organizations (Daft, 2006). Ethics violations are increasing; employees lie to employers, falsify records, and abuse drugs and alcohol at the workplace. There is an attitude that if you are not breaking the law, you are being ethical. However, organizational culture can influence day-to-day ethical conduct in positive ways through its rituals, ceremonies, and stories. If ethics is a part of the culture's traditions, it reinforces the idea that ethics matters and is not just words in a mission statement. In addition, the O Team must support and model the kind of behaviors it expects from others. As part of the administration, you too must be a role model and use ethics-based leadership. Do not just "talk" the vision; "walk" it as well. Your actions will be noticed far more often than your words. In addition, your stories, language, rituals, and ceremonies also serve to assist employees to feel a part of your organization and become loyal to it (Boyle, Dubose, Ellingson, Guinn, & McCurdy, 2001). Employees naturally wish to be part of an organization that respects them and holds the respect of the community.

How Do You Merge Subcultures?

Healthcare organizations are a gaggle of subcultures. Think of all the possibilities. Groups include the health professionals, clinical support staff, and even individual departments; each group can have multiple subcultures. Finally, you have the subculture of management and administrative services. Subcultures in these groups have their own stories, traditions, symbols, and rituals that are learned through formal and informal education and experience. The potential for **culture clash** is immense. To complicate matters further, issues also arise between loyalty to a profession and loyalty to the organization.

Subcultures hold beliefs (founded or unfounded) about the members of other subcultures in your facility. These beliefs can be destructive when assumptions are made about the motives and actions of others. Can you think of a few examples? Consider physicians. They represent the most highly educated subculture within the healthcare system. As part of their **professional socialization** in medical school, they retain attitudes and expectations regarding the behaviors of others in the system. For example, they may view a nurse, respiratory therapist, or laboratory technician as subservient and without authority to question their orders. They may also see administration as a nuisance that is designed to make their lives unhappy. Even within their own subculture, they may view certain members as being "less than" other members are. For example, a psychiatrist may be seen as less important than a neurosurgeon. These attitudes and expectations, when taken as truths, lead to behaviors that can be perceived as unethical and even cruel.

Nursing, a large subculture, has many myths and attitudes that vary by age and education. Some registered nurses (RNs) were taught to be the "handmaiden of the physician" and always to be submissive. It sounds like an exaggeration, but they were even expected to give up their seat if a physician entered the room. Other nurses were taught that they should make nursing diagnoses (a concept that is disliked by many physicians). You can see how culture clashes occur when the physician and nurse subcultures interact.

Culture clashes are also an issue between professional and support staff. Often support staff is stereotyped as not intelligent or not critical to patient care. Some report being treated as "invisible people" by the professional staff. In addition, support staff can view the professionals as self-centered and unable to communicate with the "real people." They might feel that the organization does not respect or value them. Such feelings make it easy for them to violate ethics practices. Their message is, "If they don't care about me, why should I care about them?"

You cannot leave this discussion about the power of subcultures without looking at administration. As an HCA, you have language, stories, and values that are specific to your discipline. In addition, your particular version of administration culture is a factor in how you view the organization and how you make decisions. Your position within your subculture gives you the power to influence the overall culture of the organization. For example, Lee (2004) suggests that administrators use their influence to create a culture of caring. This culture better meets the patients' need for a positive experience with the healthcare system. Caring cultures are exemplified by employees who are competent, courteous, and actively and consistently practice compassion. You can direct this caring culture through your hiring practices, policies and procedures, and example.

Although you have power to make a difference, you will face some ethical temptations because of this power. For example, Collis (1998) uses the term "managerial malpractice" as a way to describe what happens when administrators have too much freedom in decision-making and cross the ethics line. His work is based on a national study of academics, chief executive officers (CEOs), union presidents, and others and found many areas of performance weakness in terms of attitudes, knowledge, and skills. These weaknesses contribute to what he calls "fatal management sins" (p. 53). Many of the areas discussed are related to organizational culture including attitude toward employees (seen as an expense not an investment), fairness of their treatment, and creation of trust.

Adams and Balfour (1998), in their powerful book *Unmasking Administrative Evil*, use history to illustrate the negative influence administration can have over culture. This influence can lead to cultures that encourage malevolent behaviors. One example used by the authors is the civil service administration during the German Third Reich. They found that in this system, ethics was valued less than technology, and bureaucracy was valued less than people were. Therefore, it became easier to enact and implement policies that were evil, yet very efficient. The authors caution that to be an effective HCA, you need more than management theory to do your job. To be a conscientious administrator, you need to be proactively aware of the potential for evil caused by the abuse of power and consistently take action to avoid it.

You can now see that the culture of an organization greatly influences whether ethics is valued, and how it is used (or not used) in making both corporate level and daily decisions. In an environment of multiple subcultures, often with conflicting loyalties, establishing an ethics-centered culture is not an easy task. However, as an administrator, you are in a position to influence the culture's environment through rituals, stories, and ceremonies. You can articulate your own values, and most important, show your ethics by your actions. In this way, it is hoped, the employees will respect the culture they work in and follow your example.

■ THE HEALTHCARE CULTURE RESPONDS: ETHICS COMMITTEES

The healthcare system and particularly hospitals have always been faced with ethics issues requiring difficult decisions. With the advent of new technologies, more issues have come to the forefront and expanded the need to have ethics committees in place. For example, in the 1960s when kidney dialysis was a new technology, the patients who needed dialysis vastly outnumbered the availability of machines. Hospitals responded by creating ethics committees to decide which patients would receive needed treatment. These groups were often called "god squads" because of the potential for their power over life or death situations.

In the 1970s, the well-publicized case of Karen Ann Quinlan made hospitals more aware of the ethics surrounding the use of technology to prolong life. Ethics committees were charged with developing policies on the withdrawal of life support and other end-of-life issues. Although the Joint Commission on Accreditation of Healthcare Organizations (JCAHO) does not specially mandate ethics committees, today they are present in almost every hospital in some form and have far more global responsibilities. Ethics committees have even become part of other healthcare organizations, including health maintenance organizations and long-term care facilities.

Just what does an ethics committee do? To begin with, larger facilities often have three ethics committees. One is charged with general ethics responsibilities for the facility; one with issues related to pediatrics and ethics; and the last with research ethics (this one is called the **institutional review board or IRB**). These specialized committees will be discussed later in this section. The general ethics committee can be assigned different titles depending on the hospital's culture. One title is the **Institutional Ethics Committee**. The placement of the committee on the hospital's organizational chart can vary, and its position on the chart usually reflects its importance within the organization. If the administrative and clinical staff does not take the committee seriously, it becomes nothing more than window dressing. The internal organization and the external community are misled regarding the importance placed on ethics policies.

Regardless of the title, these general committees have functions in common, which include education, creation of policies, and patient case review. In the area of education, the committee can provide in-service education programs on identified or upcoming issues to staff, patients, families, and even the larger community. The educational component can also positively influence the way that ethics is valued in the organization by enhancing ethics awareness, creating an ethics dialogue, and reinforcing the vision, mission, and purpose of the facility. In addition, committee members must continually educate themselves on upcoming issues and decision-making models and orient new members (Monagle & West, 2009).

Another major function of a hospital ethics committee is policy development and review for all issues related to clinical ethics. The CEO, chief operating officer, Chief of Medical Staff, the Board of Trustees, or other key administrators can request these reviews. If policies need to be developed for recurrent issues, then an ethics committee can serve in a consultant role. Recurrent ethics issues may occur around policies on advance directives, withholding treatment, withdrawing treatment, informed consent, and organ procurement. Ethics committees can also be involved in policies relating to allocation of resources and preservation of the vision and mission of the facility. For example, they can recommend policies on community outreach, charitable contributions, and fundraising. The committee tries to make sure that policies are written in a way that will be fair to all who are affected by them (Monagle & West, 2009).

Finally, ethics committees review and provide advice on individual patient cases where there are difficult ethical concerns. The system for this review varies from facility to facility. In some cases, committee members are on call (similar to a specialist). Staff, administrators, patients, guardians, or family members all are eligible to pose a question or request an informal review from the ethics committee. Full reviews require the presence of all committee members and follow a formal procedure in making recommendations. Of course, the committee must work within the organizational structure and have a clear understanding of the articulated values and ethics position of the overall facility.

Who should be on the ethics committee? Again, the constitution of the committee will vary by institution. Generally, you find the CEO or his or her representative, clinical staff including physicians and nurses, a clergy member or a person with ethics background, and an attorney. Some facilities also include quality improvement staff, a member of the board of trustees, community members, and social workers. Members should be carefully selected. Beyond professional qualifications, a potential member should be open-minded, work well in teams, have a knowledge base in ethics, and be able to work within a framework. In addition, all members should have a sufficient commitment to ethics so that they are willing to spend the required time in meetings, training, and updating their personal knowledge.

Pediatric Ethics Committees

Pediatric ethics committees, also called infant care review committees, have the special charge of dealing with difficult ethical issues that concern the care of newborns, infants, and children. End-of-life procedures, treatment for disabilities, reporting child abuse, and disagreements between the professionals and the family require particular attention. Recommended members for such a committee include pediatricians, pediatric oncologists, neonatologists, nurses, and social workers. These members are responsible for being current on ethics issues related to infants and children, and might have to be on 24-hour call (Darr, 2005).

Institutional Review Boards

Research contributes to the understanding of disease and the improvement of health for millions of people. Unfortunately, it also has the potential for ethics violations that can cause psychological and even physical harm to participants. The roots of the IRB can be found in the Nuremburg Code of 1949, which was formulated in response to human experiments conducted by the Third Reich. It is also designed to protect people from abuses like those that occurred during the Tuskegee Syphilis Experiment in the United States.

The Tuskegee Experiment was conducted between 1932 and 1972. The Public Health Service conducted this research on 399 black men using misleading information about its purpose and procedures in order to ensure their cooperation. The real purpose was to follow the men until they died and then collect data from autopsy results. Even when information about the cure for syphilis became available, the subjects were not informed and were prevented from receiving medication. The thinking behind this human rights violation was that the benefit to society was worth the sacrifice of a few lives. It was also thought that the results would be of benefit to blacks by creating greater knowledge of how syphilis affected them. Researchers used utilitarian ethics to justify their actions, but Kantian ethics was not considered.

These and other research abuses led to the formation of IRBs in universities, hospitals, and other healthcare institutions. The functions of the IRB in a hospital are to protect research subjects and to see that protocols do everything possible to decrease risks to their well-being. This committee must also make sure that consent to participate in any research is given based on an understanding of risks and benefits, and that privacy is protected (Darr, 2005). The committee is responsible to see that informed consent procedures are stringently followed to protect potential subjects from being coerced to participate or misled in any way. Subjects vulnerable to these tactics include the mentally ill, the physically disabled, the elderly, or the economically disadvantaged.

Federal and state agencies mandate that IRBs review funding proposals before they are submitted for consideration. How a study involves human subjects defines the depth of the review, but the rights of those involved in the study are always a primary concern. Members of IRBs must have expertise in research designs and protocols. At times, they are called on to provide consultation to researchers about IRB requirements, format, or to explain the committee's decisions.

Ethicists

In addition to the committees, large healthcare facilities sometimes employ an **ethicist** as a consultant or on a full-time basis. An ethicist usually has a doctorate in ethics, bioethics, religion, or a related area and serves in both policy development and patient case review. In addition, ethicists can be a resource for the ethics committee by providing continuing education on ethics topics. He or she can guide the decision-making process of the committee using models and facilitation techniques.

■ ASSISTING THE PROCESS: CHOOSING A DECISION-MAKING MODEL

Members of ethics committees must sit on the board for more than just the "feel good" experience. To influence culture and practices effectively, committee members must view their responsibilities and status on a par with the top members of the O Team. The committee should be evaluated annually to ensure its effectiveness. By treating this committee the same as you would any other important administrative body in the facility, you send a strong message about the value the organization places on making sound ethical decisions.

As health care continues to evolve, the issues faced by ethics committees will become increasingly complicated. Committees will need to become more diverse by combining professionals with community representatives. Given these circumstances, the solutions to ethics issues will not be simple to derive. Committees will require tools to make decisions in the most effective and efficient manner. Ethics decision models can assist with this process by providing a structure to deal with situations that can be emotionally volatile. It is important to try to minimize this volatility by using a decision-making model.

Therefore, the first step is for the committee to have a selection of models from which to choose or adapt. Beginning with an agreed-on model ensures that the committee will work from a position of information and not from one of opinion alone. Knowledge of the existing models helps the committee choose the one that best meets its needs.

For example, McNamara (2008) provides a practical business-based ethics model for managing ethics in the workplace. After dispelling some of the myths about ethics in business, he provides three different models to assist in resolving ethical dilemmas. His ten-step model is based on the questions listed below.

1. What are the facts?
2. Who are the critical stakeholders and what do they value?
3. What is driving this situation?
4. What ethical principles or values should be maintained (in priority order)?
5. Who should be involved in making the decision?
6. What actions could be taken that prevent harm, maintain principles, and provide a good solution?
7. How would your best solution affect the stakeholders?
8. How can you prevent this situation in the future (check the drivers in step three)?
9. Would your chosen solution work?
10. What is the best way to build your action plan and monitor it?

This model allows the committee to identify who is affected by the decision and who should be a part of making it. It also provides a structure for evaluating possible solutions against criteria of ethics and practicality. In addition, it includes consideration of preventive ethics so that the situation is less likely to occur in the future. Evaluation and monitoring of the plan is also included as a step in the model to determine the success of implementation. The structure of this model would serve to bring a degree of rationality or practical wisdom to ethics decision-making.

Darr (2005) suggests a schematic model for decision-making that uses a decision-tree format. He suggests that the decision-making process begins with gathering information about and clarifying the problem. Then he adds a step where the committee's assumptions about the problem can be identified and discussed. After these areas are understood, alternate responses can be formulated. Responses can be evaluated based on criteria that include the reality of implementation and a cost/benefit analysis. The best response is then chosen and recommended. Darr's model also includes a comparison between what really happened during implementation and what was desired. This evaluation provides needed feedback concerning the effectiveness of the committee's decisions.

The Ethics Resource Center (2004) also created a decision- making model that contains problem analysis, alternative identification, evaluation, decision-making, implementation, and decision evaluation. This model adds another dimension called "filters" that includes ethics in the decision-making. It uses the abbreviation PLUS, which stands for policies, legal structures, universal laws, and self-standards. PLUS also includes the application of the organization's policies, any laws that apply, and the "universal principles/values" (p. 6) of the organization. Finally, each committee member considers whether he or she can support the decision as an individual apart from the committee. The model encourages the committee to consider both the ethical and legal ramifications of decisions and show how these decisions affect the organization as a whole. In addition, it allows the committee to describe the process it used to formulate its decision and to be able to explain its actions.

Several models (McNamara, 2008) that could be adapted for use by ethics committees include checklists and question-based formats. Checklists can be used to remind the committee to get the full picture of the situation before discussing the solution. This can slow down the temptation to "jump to solution" before all of the information is assessed. A number of question-type models exist that can encourage the committee to take a deeper look into the problem. For example, McNamara (2008) cites a model that features specific questions about the accuracy of problem definition, your intentions in making your decision, and who might be injured by your decision.

Models are good only when they are used and only used when they are understood. This means that the committee must be thoroughly familiar with whatever model is chosen or adapted. The committee's knowledge of the model can be continually refreshed as each new member is trained to use the model as part of his or her orientation. In addition, the model itself should be reviewed occasionally to determine if it is still meeting the needs of the organization and the committee.

Summary

Health care can be described as multicultural, which makes it a challenging work environment. It also makes this environment susceptible to culture clashes. Part of your responsibility as an ethics-based HCA is to become aware of the differences in the cultures in your organization and use your knowledge to prevent culturally based problems. In addition, you need to be cognizant of the influence you have on the overall culture of your organization. Your behaviors will be examined and speak much louder than any policy you create. Being the role model means thinking about how your actions will be perceived before you take them.

This chapter also presented some of the types of ethics committees that you will encounter in healthcare settings. While you may not be directly involved with all of them, it is important to understand their functions and how they assist your organization in meeting its ethics obligations. It is important to remember that having a decision-making model that can be easily understood and readily used increases the effectiveness of any ethics committee regardless of its emphasis.

Cases for Your Consideration

....

The Case of the White Coat Code

As you read this case, consider the following questions. Responses and comments will follow the case.

1. How does this case illustrate the impact of internal healthcare cultures on behavior?

2. How did the administration choose to handle the cultural conflict?

3. What was the result of having a policy and program that does not tolerate abuse?

Case Information

Josh O'Shaun, newly appointed CEO of Morris County Hospital (MCH), faced many problems in his 200-bed facility. One of the most pressing, in terms of patient service, was the nurse retention rate that continually caused understaffing. His root-cause strategic plan included hiring a Chief Nursing Officer (CNO) who would have equal status on the O Team. He was fortunate to hire Nicole Franz, a well-respected RN, for the position.

During the first staff meeting, Mr. O'Shaun asked for ideas on how to deal with the nurse retention issue. Ms. Franz presented research that showed that the lack of respect given to nurses contributed to this problem. With the support of their O Teams, other hospitals had instituted a policy of zero tolerance for physical, sexual, and verbal abuse. The policy was implemented through a program called Code White Coat. In this program, when a physician acted in an abusive way, the nurse could call a "code white coat" over the intercom. This action would bring available nurses to stand as witnesses to the event—and if possible, intervene in the immediate situation. Research results showed this policy led to a significant reduction of abuse incidents.

Her suggestion led to a lively discussion about the differences in perceptions of the nurse retention problem and lack of respect for nurses. The Chief of Medical Services (CMS) said that physicians were there to save lives and had a right to get angry if things were not done according to their standards. He believed that nurse abuse was not even a problem at MCH. The chief financial officer pointed out how much the current turnover rate cost the hospital but did not have an opinion about its cause. After much debate, the O Team decided to try a new policy that did not tolerate abuse in any form and then instituted the Code White Coat program at least on a trial basis. They would evaluate it after one year of its implementation to see if it made a difference in both turnover and morale. The CMS thought the program would never be used, but agreed to support it.

After the MCH staff was trained on this program, consciousness of the problem was raised and that, in and of itself, seemed to decrease the incidence of nurse abuse. However, after three months, Mr. O'Shaun heard a code white coat called. He quickly responded and found Dr. Peters, his only neurosurgeon, still screaming at a nurse. There were two other nurses present as witnesses to this action, but their presence did not stop the physician. He accused the nurse of being disrespectful, unprofessional, and not knowing her place.

Mr. O'Shaun asked Dr. Peters to come to his office immediately and contacted the CMS for a conference. He also called the CNO and asked her to have a meeting with the nurse and her witnesses. He needed Ms. Franz's report before considering final action on the situation. By the time the CMS had arrived, Dr. Peters was calmer and explained what had made him so angry. Many factors besides the nurse's behavior contributed to his outburst. However, he felt that she did not act quickly enough to his order and that he had the right to treat nurses any way he chose when lives were at stake. He was aware of the hospital's policy of zero tolerance for abuse, but he did not think he had been abusive. All he did was raise his voice.

The CMS explained that there were other ways to deal with the situation other than public outbursts. The zero tolerance policy applied to physicians as well as the staff at MCH. The CMS warned Dr. Peters that continuing such behavior could lead to sanctions, including loss of privileges if necessary. He also asked Dr. Peters if he would like to have assistance with anger management or other counseling. Seeing that the new policy was not just a joke, Dr. Peters said that he would apologize and watch his temper in the future. The CMS then said that the physician would be informed if further repercussive actions were to be imposed regarding the immediate matter.

After Dr. Peters left, Mr. O'Shaun, the CNO, and the CMS met to discuss the situation. The CMS said that he was surprised that this incident happened. He knew that physicians were demanding but never thought about the issue of nurse abuse. The CNO said that she was not at all surprised. The incident was in keeping with some of her observations of physician/nurse interaction at the facility. After much discussion, it was decided to write a letter of warning to Dr. Peters to document what was discussed in their meeting. To drive home the seriousness of the matter, the letter mandated the physician to attend an information session to refresh his knowledge of the zero tolerance policy.

Responses and Commentary on Questions

1. How does this case illustrate the impact of internal healthcare cultures on behavior?

   Recall from Chapter 3 that bullying and abuse are not considered ethical behavior, no matter who is doing it. However, because of the physician culture norms, Dr. Peters clearly did not see his behavior as unacceptable. He had been educated to believe that his status as a neurosurgeon entitled him to instant response from any nurse. His words were never to be questioned. While he was aware of the zero tolerance policy, he felt that it applied only if he physically abused a nurse; yelling was acceptable practice.

   The CMS was also part of the physician culture. Initially, he thought the whole idea of nurse abuse to be quite trivial. After all, he was not aware of any nurse being assaulted by a physician at the hospital. He thought a policy of this kind was not needed, but if the new CNO wanted to try it, he would go along. He was completely surprised when a nurse actually had the guts to call a "code." After this incident, he understood that abuse could be verbal as well as physical.

   At this point, you might well ask, "If the problem was so bad that nurses quit their jobs, how could the hospital not know about it?" You need to consider that the nursing culture is also a factor in this situation. Many nurses were taught that they were to serve as the "handmaidens of the physician." Verbal and even some levels of physical abuse were seen as just part of the burden nurses had to bear in their service to patients. They did not question it; they just learned to take it or resign. These actions resolved the problem for the individual but did not provide any information to the organization. Recent graduates of nursing schools, while still influenced by this thinking to some degree, tended to regard themselves as partners with other clinical staff. They were taught to question politely any actions that did not seem congruent with patient care. You can see how this "new nurse" paradigm could lead to a culture clash, especially if it is perceived as insubordination.

2. How did the administration choose to handle the cultural conflict?

   First, you must recognize that the action taken to address this issue was not based entirely on altruism. Mr. O'Shaun was aware that the turnover rate among nurses was causing potential problems in quality of care, morale, and costs. He was educated to seek the root cause of a problem and had the authority to work with the O Team to find solutions. Notice that he chose what might be seen as innovative, if not radical, solutions.

Mr. O'Shaun created the position of CNO, which had equal status on the O Team. This decision goes against some administrative culture norms. Nursing has not always been regarded as equal to other departments in a hospital. In fact, in the early days, nursing services were considered part of the bed charge (like linens and disposables). Creating the new position was a risk, but he knew that he needed the expertise of nurses and the support of nursing services. Putting a chief nurse on the O Team helped the necessary culture change.

Consider the courage of the O Team to create and support a policy that featured zero tolerance for all forms of abuse. While it is very easy to endorse a policy that declares it inappropriate to abuse someone physically or sexually, including verbal abuse is more controversial. The O Team had to be willing to apply sanctions for words as well as physical actions. This willingness could have had some financial risks. For example, the abuser could be someone who helped to create revenue for the facility. To remain an ethics-based facility and demonstrate justice, the O Team had to risk taking actions that might jeopardize this financial asset. In light of these and other concerns, Mr. O'Shaun had to encourage lively discussion of this innovative policy and gain support of all O Team members. In the end, even the CMS expressed support for implementation.

Consider the Code White Coat Program. Making the decision to implement it was even more courageous. O Team members were willing to counter cultural norms that might be deeply held by both the physician and the nurse groups. While they had research that showed the program worked at other hospitals, they had no way of knowing how it would be received at MCH. They risked a backlash from physicians who might resent such a program or see it as giving nurses permission to gang up on them. Physicians might even view it as an encroachment on their power and authority within the hospital. Despite the fact that the program was for the benefit of the nurses' rights and safety, the O Team had no guarantee that other nurses would respond to a code as witnesses. Perhaps the nurse who had the courage to call a code would not be supported. This could create even greater morale issues. The CMS was not convinced the program was necessary and said so. The whole team hoped that they would never hear a code called but implemented the program despite the risks.

Once a code was actually called, Mr. O'Shaun had to resolve the issue in an appropriate way. Notice that he involved the CNO and the CMS in data collection and problem solution. He needed all sides of the story to be able to make a just decision. The solution that was formulated demonstrated justice for both the physician and the nurse because it worked to change culturally ingrained behavior and was not intended to be only a form of punishment.

The CMS also showed some ethics courage here. Despite his reservations about the program, he was willing to confront Dr. Peters about his behavior and let him know that it was not acceptable. In doing so, the CMS made an ethics-based decision. He had to risk alienating his only neurosurgeon, who might resign. This would affect the revenue source of the hospital. But if he did nothing, after agreeing to support the program, he risked being a hypocrite. After weighing all the elements of the problem, he used a reasonable approach that would prevent any further incidents. His decision to take the matter seriously also sent a clear message to other physicians and to the nursing staff that the policy was more than just a piece of paper.

3. What was the result of having a policy that did not tolerate abuse?

Creation of a CNO position was a part of the solution for nurse turnover in Mr. O'Shaun's view. However, this decision required an allocation of funds for salary and benefits that came from an already frugal budget. Then, he had to respect the person whom he hired enough to hear her ideas and expend the resources to act on them. This involved an investment in policy development and training for the entire staff. From a business standpoint, Mr. O'Shaun had to be willing to make these fiscal decisions based on the potential benefits for the organization.

Although the case does not give you the results of the annual evaluation of the policy and program, you can make some assumptions based on your knowledge of ethics and the business of health care. First, in keeping with deontology, MCH sent a message to its nurses that they were valued. When a verbal abuse situation occurred, they were given the authority to call a code to stop the behavior. In addition, the program was supported by a policy that made it clear that all forms of abuse were not to be tolerated. When the first code was called, the nursing staff saw that it was taken seriously. Even though the physician involved was a major revenue contributor, his action was not covered up or glossed over. These actions created a better working environment for the nursing staff and had the potential to affect retention and patient care in a positive way.

Consider the physician culture. This new policy and program was particularly difficult for them. Even the younger physicians did not see nurses as partners and found it difficult to deal with what they perceived as a blow to their authority. However, they also learned that their Chief of Medicine took this issue seriously. After the first incident with Dr. Peters, they tended to be more careful about their verbal outbursts. The overall work environment became more pleasant for everyone and fewer and fewer code white coat calls were heard at MCH.

The Case of the Compassionate Committee

As you read this case, consider the following questions. Responses and comments will follow the case.

1. What ethics principles were included in the actions in this case?
2. How did the action of the Caneyville Hospital Ethics Committee benefit the hospital?
3. How did the action of the Caneyville Hospital Ethics Committee benefit Mrs. Smith?

Case Information

The March meeting of the Caneyville Hospital Ethics Committee in Peace City, Florida, was a particularly unusual one. The eight volunteers on the board had tackled many difficult issues in the past, but the case before them this month was notably different. A member of the Caneyville community, who was not even a patient at the hospital, had asked for a consultation. This was highly unusual, for starters. In addition, the nature of the situation and the problems that it caused for the family warranted a departure from hospital protocol.

This was the presenting situation. Mrs. Judy Smith's father (Bill Medford) suffered a closed head injury when he fell off a ladder at his home in New Mexico. His condition declined into a permanently vegetative state, and he was placed on life support. He was then transferred to a long-term care facility. Knowing that her father would not want to have such poor quality of life, Mrs. Smith did all she could to give him a death with dignity. She reviewed his Do Not Resuscitate (DNR) orders and assumed power of attorney.

Because Mrs. Smith and her three children lived in Peace City, she could not visit her father on a daily basis. Her distance from the facility was causing her grave difficulty. Each time her father coded, the staff resuscitated him and contacted her after he was stable. When she asked them why they took these actions, she was told that the administration required a family member to be present before DNR orders would be honored. She was told that the policy was designed to ensure that the true wishes of the patient were being met. The facility could be sued if someone acting on the patient's behalf had changed his or her mind at the last minute.

The situation was causing Mrs. Smith severe distress. She could not go to New Mexico and sit by her father's bedside, waiting until he coded again, and then see to it that DNR orders were followed. Her vacation days and sick leave were exhausted. Resigning from her job was not an option because she was the sole support for her children. In addition, she was her father's only next of kin. She was frustrated because it appeared that, while she had done all the right things, her wishes were not even considered at the New Mexico hospital. She came to the Caneyville Hospital ethics committee for advice.

The entire meeting was devoted to the discussion of this one case. The committee used the expertise of its members (which included a lawyer, ethicist, and physician), and its knowledge of ethics and law to discuss Mrs. Smith's case. The CEO's representative contributed some insight about the policy at the long-term facility. He said the policy had merit because it protected the facility from a potential lawsuit. He could understand why the administrators at the facility wanted a family member present.

The ethicist pointed out that, while the policy was in the best interests of the facility, it neglected to honor the wishes of the patient and his family. The facility should be true to its mission of service to patients. Perhaps it might be willing to consider the application of the policy on a case-by-case basis instead of a blanket procedure (in other words, act with utilitarianism and deontology). The committee used a decision-making model to evaluate several options and prepared a list of recommendations for Mrs. Smith. The recommendations were not binding on the part of Caneyville Hospital, but she could use them in her next discussion with the New Mexico administration.

Mrs. Smith was grateful for the time and effort the committee spent on her case. She made a trip to New Mexico to speak with the administrator she had previously dealt with and found that he was no longer employed at the facility. The new administrator met with her and reviewed the recommendations from Caneyville Hospital's ethics committee. Although he did not want to change the entire policy, he agreed to consider the circumstances of her case and make a reasonable accommodation to her circumstances. He instructed the staff not to automatically resuscitate. Instead, they were to call Mrs. Smith when a code occurred. They were to inform her of the specifics, and get her final verbal approval of the DNR order. Two weeks later, she received their call. Her father was then at peace.

Responses and Commentary on Questions

1. What ethics principles were included in the actions in this case?

   This is a complex case involving end-of-life issues and the reality of DNR orders. In order to understand all of the ethics involved here, you need to analyze the situation and the actions of the committee. First, the situation on the surface seems to be a violation of the patient's right of autonomy. Mrs. Smith was resigned to the fact that her father was not going to recover. Knowing his wishes, she made every effort to secure all of the paperwork to protect his right to a dignified death. However, because of her personal circumstances, she could not be present to be an advocate for those rights and her legal documents seemed worthless.

If you consider the viewpoint of the long-term care facility, you might have a different take on this situation. With a history of being part of one of the most heavily regulated industries in America, this long-term care facility needed to go the extra mile to protect its residents. The administrator was aware that sometimes a family wishes to hasten the death of a patient for financial gain or other unethical reason. In addition, families have been known to change their minds once the DNR order becomes a reality. The facility wanted to protect its assets and its employees by making sure that a family member was present during a patient's death so that legal problems would not ensue.

Consider the actions of the Caneyville Hospital ethics committee. It had no obligation to consider Mrs. Smith's request for a consultation. After all, she was not even a patient in the hospital. However, this committee had a reputation of compassion for the whole community and decided to provide Mrs. Smith with their well-considered recommendations. They had to base their discussion on the situation presented to them by Mrs. Smith. Notice that they tried to discuss the situation from more than just her view by listening to the input of the CEO's representative. Given more time, they could have contacted the administrator in New Mexico to get his opinion of the situation.

In deciding what recommendations to give Mrs. Smith, the ethics committee used the process that had assisted members on other occasions. It included use of a decision-making model and open discussion among all committee members. Knowledge of the ethical and legal ramifications of the situation was also part of this discussion. While this process was time consuming, the committee was able to develop a set of recommendations that could be implemented and resolve the situation.

2. How did the action of the Caneyville Hospital ethics committee benefit the hospital?

The decision of the committee to consult on the Medford case did not appear to have any direct benefit to the hospital in terms of increasing revenue or census. However, the committee's reputation of compassion reflected positively on the hospital and added to its status in the community. By deciding to volunteer their time to address a community member's needs, the committee let the community see that profit was not the only motivation for Caneyville Hospital. The community mattered.

3. How did the action of the Caneyville Hospital ethics committee benefit Mrs. Smith?

The ethics committee consultation provided several benefits for Mrs. Smith. First, she felt that her situation was important enough to be addressed by people who had ethics expertise. Being able to talk about her case to such a compassionate body gave her a voice and helped to decrease her stress level. In addition, she felt that their recommendations provided her with some tools for a meeting with the administrator in New Mexico. She could present her viewpoint in a cogent manner and feel confident about her position. Fortunately, the new administrator of the facility was more open to patients' rights than the previous one and listened to her with an open mind. A reasonable accommodation was made, and Mr. Medford was allowed to pass away with dignity.

Web Resources

Ethics Resources Center
http://www.ethics.org/

Hospital Ethics Committee Handbook Example
http://www.kumc.edu/hospital/ethics/ethics.htm

The Tuskegee Experiment
http://www.infoplease.com/ipa/A0762136.html

References

Adams, G. B., & Balfour, D. L. (1998). *Unmasking administrative evil.* Thousand Oaks, CA: Sage.

Boyle, P. J., DuBose, E. R., Ellingson, S. J., Guinn, D. E., & McCurdy, D. B. (2001). *Organizational ethics in health care: Principles, cases, and practical solutions.* San Francisco: Jossey-Bass.

Collis, J. W. (1998). *The seven fatal management sins: Understanding and avoiding managerial malpractice.* Boca Raton, FL: St. Lucia Press.

Daft, R. L. (2006). *Organizational theory and design* (9th ed.). Cincinnati, OH: South-Western.

Darr, K. (2005). *Ethics in health services management* (4th ed.). Baltimore: Health Professions Press.

Ethics Resource Center. (2004). *PLUS—A process for ethics decision making* [Electronic Version]. Washington, DC: Author.

Lee, F. (2004). *If Disney ran your hospital: 9 1/2 things you would do differently.* Bozeman, MT: Second River Healthcare Press.

McNamara, C. (2008). *Complete guide to ethics management: An ethic toolkit for managers.* Available from Authenticity Consulting Website at: http://www.managementhelp.org/ethics/ethxgde.htm. Accessed December 26, 2008.

Monagle, J. F., & West, M. P. (2009). Hospital ethics committees: Roles, memberships, structure, and difficulties. In Morrison, E. E. (Ed.). *Health care ethics: Critical issues for the 21st Century* (2nd ed.). Sudbury, MA: Jones and Bartlett, pp. 251–266.

Swayne, L. E., Duncan, J., & Ginter, P. M. (2006). *Strategic management of health care organizations* (5th ed.). Malden, MA: Blackwell.

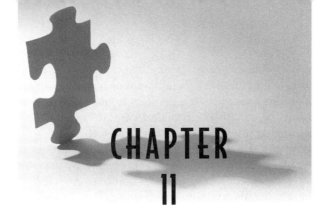

CHAPTER
11

The Ethics of Quality

Good quality is cheap; it's poor quality that is expensive.
—Joe L. Griffith

Points to Ponder

1. How do organizations view external evaluation?
2. What is quality health care?
3. What efforts are being made to assure quality?
4. How does ethics relate to the quality assurance in health care?

Words to Remember

The following is a list of key words for this chapter. You will find them in bold in the text. Stop and check your understanding of them.

Agency for Healthcare Research and Quality (AHRQ)
Centers for Medicare and Medicaid Services (CMS)
Donabedian
Institute for Healthcare Improvement (IHI)
Lean Model
Malcolm Baldrige National Quality Award
ORYX® system

■ INTRODUCTION TO THE ETHICS OF QUALITY

In Chapter 5, you studied the community's attempts to protect itself from the power of the healthcare system. Because this system literally holds the power of life or death, the community is compelled to find protection through regulations, licensures, and sanctions that are enforced by a myriad of organizations. These regulatory organizations are supposed to provide the whole community, including employers, with some assurance that these regulations are met. The community has an expectation the certain standards of care are maintained and that quality care is being provided to those who seek that care.

How do healthcare facilities view these organizations and their responsibilities? In the beginning of this chapter, you will study the idea of compliance to standards from the organization's view. You will examine the arguments for how maintaining standards serves as the foundation of quality and its limitations. You will also learn how administrators can influence compliance through their behaviors.

In the final sections of this chapter, you will learn about efforts to take healthcare organizations beyond compliance to quality. The discussion begins with the definition of quality in health care. It then provides examples of some of the many efforts that are being made to improve quality in the healthcare system. Quality assurance efforts that are adopted from other industries, such as Lean Organizations and Kaizen techniques will presented. In addition, the patient's view of quality will be discussed. The final section of this chapter will examine how the ethics theories and principles you have been studying relate to the issue of quality in health care.

■ A HISTORICAL VIEW

A bit of history might be helpful to frame your picture of an organization's interpretation of standardization and compliance. No doubt, you learned in previous courses that the American healthcare system evolved from an apprentice structure to its current level of sophistication. This evolution occurred in a market-based rather than social-based context, making it unique among other industrialized nations. In its early stages, the healthcare system was exclusively controlled through its professionals. External regulation or community accountability was not part of its structure (Shi & Singh, 2008). Factors such as the development of insurance, increase in government involvement, advent of advanced technology, and rising costs of care brought about a greater need to demonstrate accountability. These factors spawned the increase in external regulation in various forms including "voluntary" accreditation. Even though accountability was not founded in legal obligation, it soon became linked to financial and even state licensure requirements. For example, beginning in 1965, accreditation of hospitals became linked to reimbursement from government programs (Joint Commission on Accreditation of Healthcare Organizations, 2008a). However, many in the system deeply resented government encroachment on their autonomy; this resentment persists today.

The type and style of healthcare regulation has also evolved. In 1918, the American College of Surgeons began a program to standardize practices in hospitals. Other organizations joined in this effort and formed the Joint Commission on the Accreditation of Hospitals. In 1987, it changed its name to the Joint Commission on Accreditation of Healthcare Organizations (JCAHO). Through its ability to accredit, it influences the practices of healthcare services such as ambulatory care, assisted living, home health, behavioral health, laboratories, long-term care, and office-based surgeries.

Initially, JCAHO's accreditation process involved the construction of a set of standards to measure a hospital's capacity to perform its functions. The standards were meant to identify acceptable hospital practices and to protect the community's interests. The healthcare organization was required to document its compliance. Regulators trusted that the documentation presented an accurate and correct picture of the facility's capacities. Accreditation visits largely consisted of a review of the documentation and conferences with key leadership. Accreditation centered on trust between the accrediting bodies and the organization.

However, even at this stage of accreditation's evolution, organizations struggled to comply with the many standards that they often saw as unrealistic and intrusive. Many hours of staff time were devoted to determining the correct wording and placement of information. Because the standards were not always clear, problems arose in the areas of omission and commission. Administrators were concerned about the value of this paper trail, but they also worried about their hospital's rating and image if a "bad" site visit occurred.

Some nonethics-based organizations took advantage of the vagueness of the standards and the lack of actual performance verification. For example, they "fudged" the data to make things appear better than they were or they attended to standards only when a site visit was due. Employees would joke that, "We're going to have a site visit; this means the walls will be painted, and the carpets will be cleaned." These organizations perhaps even viewed themselves as ethical because they did not see the value of excessive paper documentation. It seemed to them that paperwork took time away from patient care.

As the process of regulating healthcare organizations became more sophisticated and expanded to include entities beyond the hospital, JCAHO began to change its method of assessment. In 1986, it began to explore a process of evaluating quality indicators rather than capacity standards. The switch to performance indicators and the measurement of actual performance evolved over several years and actually changed the survey process itself. In 1995, JCAHO began its new survey format, and the **ORYX®** **system** of documenting performance outcomes was initiated in 1997. During its 50th anniversary (in 2001), JCAHO began an emphasis on patient safety and decreasing medical errors, which continues to be an area of assessment (JCAHO, 2008a). In addition, the organization has an initiative to improve all of the standards used to evaluate healthcare organizations beginning with hospitals and home care. This includes its development of E-edition manuals so that accreditation customers can have easier access to updated information and yearly standard changes.

JCAHO decided on another major shift in the way healthcare organizations are evaluated (JCAHO, 2008a). It conducts its regular surveys on an unannounced basis as a continuation of its Shared Vision-New Pathways initiative. The change was pilot-tested in 2004–2005 using all types of organizations that volunteered to participate. The idea behind this radical change was to move organizations beyond just-in-time compliance (i.e., getting ready for announced visits) to one of continuous compliance. It also increases the credibility of accreditation by observations taking place during normal operations, and it decreases the costs incurred from preparation for announced visits. You can imagine the impact of this change on the organization and operations.

JCAHO continues its efforts to improve the quality of health care through its yearly updates on standards for healthcare organizations. In addition, its online Quality Check program provides the public with access to information about community facilities. JCAHO also provides information to healthcare facilities and the community through its public policy reports. In addition, it created the Gold Seal of Approval program so that consumers can easily identify certified organizations (JCAHO, 2008b).

■ THROUGH THE ORGANIZATION'S EYES

Just how is accreditation viewed by the organizations? Has there been a change of attitude during its evolution? First, remember that JCAHO is not the only game in town when it comes to regulation. Healthcare organizations are scrutinized by a variety of federal and state agencies, other accrediting agencies such as the NCQA, coalitions, and the public sector. Each of these groups sees itself as either protecting the public's well-being or protecting its own interests against the awesome power of the healthcare system. However, their many demands for accountability often conflict with each other. Administrators frequently see themselves as drowning in a sea of regulations, paperwork, and site visits. Just as in the early stages of JCAHO, administrators view this process as unjust punishment and a huge waste of time. Hours and hours are spent checking the appropriate boxes on forms and sending electronic submissions. Staff are concerned that the facility is focused on minutia and not on making patient care better. They even question the ethics of being pulled away from patient care to verify documents or reiterate the mission of the organization (Fitzpatrick, 2003).

For some healthcare organizations, the accreditation process is not flexible enough to deal with the market forces that they face. In addition, the cost of gathering the required structural and process information continues to increase while profit margins decrease. Resistance to accreditation is increased when the redundancy and cost of multiple accreditations and surveys is added (Ransom, Joshi, Nash, & Ransom, 2008). According the authors, healthcare administrators (HCAs) should also consider the standards used by accreditation bodies. In order for most providers to achieve accreditation, standards are set at a minimal level of acceptability. While many organizations exceed these minimums, those that do not may have serious patient-care quality issues but still be in business as accredited institutions.

Information technology has also affected administrators' attitudes toward accreditation. The good news is that accreditations agencies such as JCAHO are beginning to make data collection easier through web-based systems. However, healthcare consumers are demanding easy access to data that affirms quality and safety. Data collected to conform to accreditation standards may not provide what consumers want to know, but an effort is being made to provide information through online report cards and Web sites. However, the quality and specificity of information are areas of concern.

It would appear that, like health care itself, the accreditation process is undergoing change. The move from capacity measurement to performance documentation and real-time evaluation through unannounced surveys should move the system to focus more on quality. However, documentation quality and documentation cost issues are always part of the picture. Some organizations have responded to the change by building layers for protection. While they have encouraged staff ideas for quality improvement, these ideas must now be filtered through a plethora of boards, committees, task forces, and officers (Roth & Taleff, 2002). Ideas are reviewed, evaluated, prioritized, and delineated before any action is taken. The message can be, "We like your ideas, but we are still in charge," or "JCAHO is nice but this is business as usual" instead of staff empowerment and collaboration. It is hoped that timely surveys and new ways of regulating health care will cause organizations to grow beyond "business as usual" to creative problem solving. However, a change this radical will not happen overnight. It must be reinforced by successes in financial and other arenas.

■ GOING BEYOND COMPLIANCE: EFFORTS IN QUALITY

The public already assumes that you are providing high quality service. In addition, it is becoming more aware of what used to be a secret business. Television and the Internet have opened formerly arcane healthcare treatments and practices. Consumers are more knowledgeable about the system and question more. They want to be a partner in their treatment rather than a sycophant. This change, coupled with the responsibility for health and healing inherent in the healthcare systems, makes the need for quality assurance paramount. To begin to understand this need, you must first be able to define quality as it applies to health care.

Quality Definitions

As you can see by the title of this section, there is more than one definition of quality in health care. In fact, the definition tends to be different depending on who is trying to define it. For example, clinical professionals think about quality care as being able to provide desirable health outcomes to patients. Their performance is related to quality and the appropriate use of technology can assist with this performance. In contrast, payers, such as insurance companies and the government, view quality in terms of cost. If care is not efficient, then it is poor quality care. If care is not cost effective, then it is poor care. You can already see a conflict here between professionals and payers. Professionals see quality as the best outcome for the patient, while payers are more concerned with the overall cost of that outcome (Ransom, Joshi, Nash, & Ransom, 2008).

HCAs have a different view of quality. They are responsible for the setting of services, quality of the patient-provider encounter, efficient use of resources, and appropriate access to care. In order to assure that there is equity in each of these areas, administrators need to view quality as efficiency, cost containment, waste reduction, and appropriate distribution. Finally, and most importantly, there is a patient and societal definition of healthcare quality. Because health care is a trust-based business, patients assume that clinical professionals have the expertise to treat them. They also assume that the mission of health care is to facilitate their healing. Therefore, quality for health care is defined in terms of their experience with the system or provider. This includes the interpersonal relationships, respectful and courteous treatment, convenience, and attractiveness of the facility.

How can you address quality in health care when the definitions are so varied? Is there any common ground? **Donabedian** (in Ransom, Joshi, Nash, & Ransom, 2008) identified three major components of quality that can serve to provide a common ground. He said that you can measure quality by looking at the structure of an organization including the education of its professionals, staffing, equipment, and organization. In addition, you can evaluate the process of providing care. This element would include the provision of care and patient outcomes. It can also include interpersonal relationships and the patient experience. Finally, Donabedian suggests that you measure the outcome of patient care. This would include patient satisfaction, cost-benefit, and health status improvement. This model can serve as a beginning for the formulation of a definition of quality that could be adapted to a specific aspect of healthcare delivery.

Efforts for Quality Improvement

Quality improvement for the healthcare system is still being developed and perfected. However, many stakeholders are increasingly concerned with determining how to improve the quality of health care for patients in society. These forces serve to push the quality agenda and include payers, regulators, professional organizations, advocates, and patients. It would be helpful to examine examples of their efforts in order understand the complexity of healthcare quality assurance. This understanding will also assist you in applying ethics theories and principles to the concept of quality assurance.

Payers   It seems logical that those who pay for health care would have the biggest stake in assuring the quality of the services that they purchase. For example, the **Centers for Medicare and Medicaid Services (CMS)** pay for more healthcare services than any other entity in the United States. Therefore, it is not surprising that it has become a leader in quality care assurance. Since the CMS pays for services in several aspects of health care, it has been able to launch programs that have the potential to make major improvements in that care. In ambulatory care, for example, CMS began a program to engage physicians in voluntary reporting of quality data through their Physician Quality Reporting Initiative (PQRI). Physicians can earn bonus money by successfully achieving identified quality standards. In the area of home health, CMS collects quality data from its certified agencies. Called the Outcome and Assessment Information Set (OASIS), this tool evaluates how home health improves patient outcomes including activities of daily living (Ransom, Joshi, Nash, & Ransom, 2008).

The **Agency for Healthcare Research and Quality (AHRQ)** is another federal agency that has a major emphasis on quality in health care. As part of the Department of Health & Human Services, this agency gives support for research about evidenced-based health care, quality efforts, access to health care, and costs. Quality improvement programs such as research on patient safety are among its many funded projects. In addition, it is responsible for assessing the consumer experience in health care through the Consumer Assessment of Healthcare Providers and Systems (CAHPS®) program. These efforts even include television public service commercials to increase patient awareness (AHRQ, 2008).

In addition to the federal government, other payers are concerned with the quality of health care. Through their influence and financial incentives, they are trying to improve the quality of the health care that they purchase. Since profit is affected by healthcare costs, many corporations added employees who evaluate health benefits with respect to cost and satisfaction. Businesses are also forming national and regional coalitions to influence the quality of care and its cost.

Advocates   In addition to payers, the general community is interested in assuring that quality health care is provided to its citizens. Some of the interest began with the Institute of Medicine's 2001 report entitled *Crossing the Quality Chasm: A New Healthcare System for the 21ˢᵗ Century.* The findings of this study demonstrated that criteria for evaluating health care should include safety, effectiveness, and emphasis on the patient. Organizations such as the American Medical Association, the AARP, The Robert Wood Johnson Foundation, Institute for Healthcare Improvement, and the National Patient Safety Foundation have supported efforts to both improve quality in health care and inform the public about quality efforts.

Using the **Institute for Healthcare Improvement** (**IHI**) as an example, you can see influence of these organizations to create change for quality improvement. The IHI was founded over 20 years ago as a not-for-profit organization whose focus was to affect the lives of patients by implementing the Institute of Medicine's goals for healthcare improvement. This organization is also dedicated to improving the life of those who serve patients through its goal to increase the number of professionals entering the field. They also want to increase the "joy in work" for those who choose to be part of the healthcare system.

IHI works through collaboration with major hospitals and foundations, and cites the 100,000 Lives and the 5 Million Lives campaigns as part of its successes. It also works to improve healthcare practices and implementation of evidence-based medicine through collaboration with the Veteran's Health Administration and the Robert Wood Johnson Foundation. This collaboration contributed to many improvements in the delivery of health care. Finally, IHI worked with the American Organization of Nurse Executives and other organizations to empower patients and staff to partner in patient care. This collaboration contributed to increased patient satisfaction, quality indicators, and decreased patient safety issues in participating facilities. By using the model of collaboration, the IHI is making a difference in the quality of healthcare services (IHI, 2009).

Adapting from Other Industries   In addition to using the input from government agencies and advocates, many healthcare facilities have adapted programs that are used in other industries. For example, hospital systems and large clinics have participated in the **Malcolm Baldrige National Quality Award.** Even if they do not apply for the award, these institutions use its criteria and scoring system as a way to assess and improve quality.

Another quality improvement system that has been adapted to health care is the **Lean system**. This system was developed by the Massachusetts Institute of Technology to improve mass production methods by decreasing errors and time in production. The Lean system involves the PLAN-DO-CHECK-ACT cycle popularized by Deming (Tapping, 2008). This cycle allows participants to analyze performance and make improvements that increase quality. Various quality assessment tools are part of the Lean model including cause and effect or fishbone diagrams, control charts, storyboards, and checklists. In addition, the Lean model allows organizations to use the principles of Kaizen to enable employees to design processes for reducing waste and improving quality.

It is important to remember that any effort toward quality improvement used by another industry requires care adaptation. The nature of health care is very different from that of manufacturing or technology. When selecting a model or tool, HCAs must always keep the patient at the center of the decision. The goal should be to find the best way to continuous improve the quality of healthcare patient service.

Patients   As you remember, patients see health care differently. They assume that the facility hires competent people who are functioning on high levels of ethics. They assume that their safety is guaranteed and that appropriate efforts are made to assure their healing. When they determine that these assumptions are violated, they begin to lose trust in the system. They are advised to have an advocate when dealing with the healthcare system.

For the patients, health care is not about achieving the appropriate benchmarks or making a score on the Baldrige scale. It is personal. When you are frightened or in discomfort, you want to be assured and to have the discomfort alleviated. At the time you are being treated, you want to be the most important person to your care provider. You also want to have a safe, clean environment with amenities that assist you in your healing.

One way that patients are beginning to address quality is self-education. As you read in Chapter 8, the Internet has made education about the healthcare system much easier. While this vehicle is not bias-free, it does increase the patients' information level and allows them to ask appropriate questions. In addition, there are articles and books available to assist patients in their knowledge about quality. *Don't Go There Alone!* (Kalina, Pew, & Bourgeois, 2004) is an example of such a publication. It offers specific information for patients and their advocates about the inside workings of a hospital and how to assure quality care. As HCAs, you should know that patients might not remain compliant and silent. You should be prepared to address their quality concerns and work to understand their view of quality.

■ ETHICS OF QUALITY PROGRAMS

At first glance, the issue of the relationship between healthcare quality assurance and ethics should be an obvious one. If you read many of the mission statements in this industry, you will find that quality service is featured in almost all of them. Certainly, quality care is supported by ethics theory. For example, those who support Kant's view of ethics see quality as a moral duty. They might even think that it passed the categorical imperative test, given the amount of power and trust placed in health care. Providing quality care to all patients regardless of their ability to pay also recognizes Kant's theory that all humans have value and deserve quality. Buber and Frankl also would support this position.

The utilitarians would actually agree with the Kantians here but for a different reason. They would say that providing quality healthcare services is a way to achieve the greatest good for the greatest number of persons affected and to avoid the greatest harm to the greatest number. For utilitarians, ethical decisions should be weighed against their potential consequences. In this case, the consequences of not providing quality care could adversely affect individuals and the organization. For example, failure to provide such care could cause harm to the organization through poor patient satisfaction rates, loss of revenue, or even lawsuits. Would any healthcare facility like to be known for its poor quality? Quality assurance practices are just plain good business.

Rawls would also support the provision of quality service because it is in the self-interest of both the community and the organization. Using Rawls's theory, you always want to protect those in a lesser position (the patient) because you could also be in that position. How would you like to be treated if you were a patient in your facility? Perhaps, this question should be a part of the management decision-making process. In addition, organizations tend to be judged by how they treat their patients, and the community's expectations are high. An organization's image can be severely tarnished when quality is compromised and this action becomes public knowledge.

The principles of ethics studied in previous chapters also apply to the ethics of quality assurance. For example, the principle of nonmaleficence certainly applies. Giving poor quality service and making medication and patient identification errors can do harm to your patients. The sister principle of beneficence is also involved because you want to act with care and compassion in your treatment of patients.

How do the other principles relate to your actions? First, you give your word through your mission statement that your organization practices quality care. Failure to live up to this mission statement is a failure of truth-telling and promise-keeping. Your veracity and your fidelity come into question. Quality assurance also involves justice. Do you have a duty to provide quality service to everyone or just to those who have insurance or deep pockets? The community can say that you are not being ethical if you provide dramatically different services to people who have the same or similar conditions but different financial resources.

These arguments make sense in the big picture, but how do they relate to the view from the organization? First, you have to look at the ethics of competing resources here. The extensive resource commitment in money and time that is needed for JCAHO, CMS, and other mandated quality assurance efforts is often viewed as a resource drain. This is often seen in smaller and/or rural hospitals where budgets are especially tight. Some question the ethics of spending money on data collection and analysis, computers, electronic systems, and reporting when it could be spent on actually improving or providing patient care.

Still other organizations think that they are already engaged in providing quality service and find it difficult to justify all of the expense and paperwork involved in proving it to an outside evaluator. In addition, they question whether the measures are really a reflection of quality as the community sees it. Even so-called evidence-based measures can be questioned if you understand the nature of the studies on which they are based. Were the original studies valid and reliable? Do they measure quality or would more qualitative measures do a better job? Would patient interviews or administrative rounds (similar to medical rounds) be better ways of gathering accurate information?

Even though organizations take funds from government agencies and from insurance companies, some administrators do not think that they should have to account for their practices in such detail. They view the mandated quality improvement programs as an infringement on their autonomy to practice medicine. This can be true even if they are currently using the techniques outlined in the measurement benchmarks. The source of this irritation may well stem from the history of the system, as government and business regulation is a relatively new practice. Some of the milder comments that you will hear are that this is the equivalent of "Big Brother is watching you" and that they are asked to practice "cookbook medicine." Some practitioners believe they cannot be an advocate for their patients when practices are mandated. They should be free to choose what is best for the patient based on their years of education and experience and not on the mandates of an outside bureaucracy. As an administrator, you will have to be able to explain why this oversight is necessary and why you need the staff's support. This might not be an easy task.

What about the quality assurance programs from industries such as Malcolm Baldrige or Lean? In this case, the organization is not mandated to use these self-assessment methods but makes a choice to do so. These programs are not replacements for other external efforts but add to them. Again, there is an issue of the ethics of competing resources.

Money, time, and staff must be devoted to training, data collection and analysis, and effecting culture change over and above that which is designed for government- or industry-mandated reviews. Funds needed for these programs might explain why they are used mostly in larger facilities, rather than system wide. However, even in a small facility, the programs can be viewed in a positive light because they can be designed to assess issues that are specific to an individual organization and are under the control of that organization. For example, the simple act of filling out the Malcolm Baldrige Award application can yield valuable insight into improving service quality, even for the smallest facility. That said, before any organization decides to implement these programs, it must carefully consider the benefits versus the costs and make sound ethical and business decisions.

Summary

Providing quality care is not just good ethics; it is good business. However, quality cannot be assumed. It requires that an organization comply with both the mandates and the intent of the regulations posed by external evaluators. It also requires that organizations exercise their ability to self-police so that quality practices become the norm. In this chapter, you were able to see how quality assurance programs from other industries might be used to assist health care in this effort.

This chapter also addressed the ethics behind quality programs including application to Kant's, Rawls's, and Mill's theories. You should also be able to see how the many principles of ethics also apply to quality assurance. Understanding how ethics forms a basis for quality assurance should assist you to counteract arguments against it. In addition, this knowledge can be a tool for successfully administering quality assurance programs.

Cases for Your Consideration

The Case of the Obstinate Orthopedist

As you read this case, consider the following questions. Responses and commentary will follow the case.

1. What was the ethics foundation for adding quality measures to the CMS Hospital Quality Project?

2. What ethical arguments did Vice President Gormal make in asking for staff cooperation?

3. What ethical argument did Dr. Cathal make in response to her request?

4. How would you handle this situation?

Case Information

Although the medical staff at Dagma Memorial Hospital (DMH) grudgingly conformed to the annual CMS Hospital Quality Initiative, the new additions to this year's indicators posed some serious concerns for Erin Gormal, Vice President of Operations. DMH was a 100-bed facility that had a strong commitment to meeting the needs of its community, even with its limited staff of specialists. The additional indicators involved surgical infection prevention (SIP), which made good sense from a quality standpoint. In fact, the facility was already complying with most of the new indicators. However, Ms. Gormal knew that collecting the additional data would stretch the resources of her clinical and administrative staff even thinner. She believed in providing the best possible care and in "living the mission" of DMH. Still, she dreaded the upcoming informational meeting with her medical staff.

Vice President Gormal carefully prepared for the session. In the meeting, she presented the indicators and explained the rationale for them. However, when she got to the section on knee surgery and the quality indicator suggestions for presurgical medications, the orthopedic surgeon, Dr. Sean Cathal, became highly emotional. He slammed his fist on the mahogany table and said, "How dare CMS tell me how to practice medicine. What right do they have to dictate which medications I give to my patients?"

At that point, Pandora's Box was opened. Many of the physicians agreed with Dr. Cathal's view and expressed frustration with yet another government mandate. They demanded to know why the administration did not fight against this outrage. The climate in the room went from discontented acquiescence to outright hostility.

Although Ms. Gormal was prepared for some displeasure, she was somewhat surprised by the hostile reactions. The Chief of Medicine intervened and brought the meeting back to order. Ms. Gormal then calmly explained that the list of medications was not mandated but was included as a suggestion to assist in documenting the quality measures. Of course, the patient's medical history must be considered concerning which drugs would be used. She also pointed out that the guidelines for SIP were similar to those already collected by JCAHO. They should not be a significant addition to the data collection process. She also stressed that CMS was basing its measures on clinical evidence from many studies. This information was provided in the package she prepared for each physician. Finally, she pointed out that if DMH wanted to continue its certification for Medicare reimbursement and avoid fines for noncompliance, it had to document these measures.

After another lengthy discussion, the physicians agreed that, while still hating the "Big Brother" approach from CMS, they did not want to lose certification. However, they hoped that this infringement on their expertise as professionals would not continuously increase from year to year. Vice President Gormal breathed a sigh of relief as she returned to her office.

Responses and Commentary on Questions

1. What was the ethics foundation for adding these quality measures to the DMH CMS Hospital Quality Project?

   Vice President Gormal viewed the new requirements from a broad ethics framework that included DMH and the larger community. First, she knew that DMH was already part of the CMS system for data collection as part of its commitment to maintaining certification. JCAHO had already asked for similar data, so the burden of additional staff time would not be too great. She had no desire to tax staff that were already overburdened but committed to caring for patients. In taking this approach, she exhibited what Buber would call an "I-You" ethical relationship because she valued the staff as people, not as just the means to the end of data collection.

   Ms. Gormal was also able to view the situation from CMS's viewpoint. They were not out to punish DMH but rather to work toward the utilitarian principle of the greatest good for the greatest number. By trying to ensure that all of their certified facilities used evidenced-based practices, they were hoping for consistent quality. From the hospital's view, this could mean better patient outcomes, shorter lengths of stay, less use of resources, and higher patient satisfaction. Providing the greatest good for the greatest number would be a winning combination for both the community and the business.

   She could also see some Kantian ethics in the CMS decision. Each patient, not just those who were Medicare-eligible, was to be counted in the data collection. This meant that patients were important even if Medicare did not pay for their services. Buber and Frankl would also agree with this position. Although a new set of measurements might bring up issues of conflicting resources, Ms. Gormal could see that it would serve to protect those in a lesser position by making sure they received the same quality services as those who were better off economically and socially. Her critical issue would be to convince others of the merit of this addition.

2. What ethical arguments did Vice President Gormal make in asking for staff cooperation?

   At first, Vice President Gormal tried to appeal to the rational nature of her physician group. Rational people would see that it is in everyone's best interest to provide care based on the latest evidence of good practice. After all, if any one of them were a patient at DMH, he or she would want the gold standard of care. In addition, she tried to appeal to their science-based nature by providing copies of the studies used to justify each measure. She hoped the Rawlsian ethics might prevail but did not anticipate the emotional aspects of this addition to the CMS requirements.

What she did not understand was how this change could be viewed through different "ethics eyes." Even though JCAHO had already required the collection of similar data, Dr. Cathal saw the new measures as an attack on his expertise and right to autonomous practice. As a scientist, he was taught to question reliability and validity of studies and to express a healthy skepticism. Perhaps he just felt overwhelmed by the increase in external regulations, which seemed to be growing almost daily. His colleagues echoed his dissatisfaction. They found the idea of control of their practice autonomy by nonphysicians and external regulators to be an infringement on their authority.

Maybe Ms. Gormal should have discussed her ethics rationale with the Chief of Medicine to get his input and assistance before the meeting. She might have been able to have greater anticipatory insight and to prepare an ethics and financial argument that would have avoided some of the emotional response. In the end, she was able to use ethics and fiscal data to obtain some level of support.

3. What ethical argument did Dr. Cathal make in response to the physicians?

Another side of the autonomy issue comes into view when you consider Dr. Cathal's response. Often in health care, you have a conflict of autonomy. Whose authority is more important? Is it more important for the practitioner to be able to use his or her professional judgment or should the autonomy of the patient be primary? When you decide to become a member of the health profession, you understand that in all things, the patient comes first. While it is true that these measures limit some of Dr. Cathal's autonomy in practice, his obligation is first to his patients. First, he must determine medically if the evidence-based practices are appropriate for the patient. If they are not, he must be prepared to provide medical justification for his decisions. In this case, his autonomy is not violated. However, if he fails to support the requirements of CMS in total, the organization could be faced with losing its ability to admit Medicare patients. Whose autonomy would suffer in that case?

4. How would you handle this situation?

To answer this question, remember that you have the benefit of hindsight. Although the meeting was tense, Ms. Gormal was able to achieve her goal in the end. How would you have handled this? You can see the benefit of "homework" in this case. The more you can anticipate concerns about an issue and prepare a response, the more likely you are to obtain consensus. It is also a good idea to get support from a champion who is respected by the group you are trying to influence. In Ms. Gormal's case, the Chief of Medicine could have been approached ahead of time for his buy-in. They might have even shared in the presentation of the information to indicate a united approach.

Think of a positive approach when preparing to deliver challenging news. Of course physicians want to be seen as practicing quality medicine. You can even reinforce how they are already using some of the practices that have been identified. You are more likely to get support if you ask for it by using a velvet glove rather than an iron hand. Finally, you must always be in charge of your emotions. If you lose your cool in such situations, you add to the problem instead of solving it. Since you are only human, emotional control takes practice, but it is worth the effort.

The Case of the Self-Assured Employee Assistance Program

As you read this case, consider the following questions. Responses and commentary will follow the case.

1. What assumptions were made about quality at Rampaire Manufacturing?
2. What actions did Mr. Rampaire take to ensure quality?
3. What was his ethics reasoning for taking these actions?
4. What was the result of his action?

Case Information

Background. This case is about an area of health care that is not currently regulated by JCAHO or CMS on a mandatory basis. Nevertheless, the owner and human resources director of the company featured in the case were concerned about the ethics of quality. The owner chose to go the extra mile on behalf of employees and their families. His action led to important decisions for quality assurance.

The case. Rampaire Manufacturing was a 2000-employee company, internationally known for its manufacture of self-cleaning lavoratories. The owner, Frank Rampaire, prided himself on his Buber-centered ethics and demonstrated caring concern for the employees in a number of ways. Recently, with the assistance of his human resources (HR) director, Ruth Washington, he negotiated a contract with a firm for an Employee Assistance Program (EAP).

The contract with Work/Life Associates (WLA) guaranteed certain quality assurance features. For example, all telephone triage would be done by licensed counselors or master's level social workers (MSWs). WLA would maintain records on current licensure for all staff and keep up-to-date directories for appropriate referral to practitioners in the local area. It provided data on usage and referrals on which identifiers would be used to protect the privacy of the employees and their families. The EAP also agreed to annual onsite visits from Rampaire or its designee for quality assurance purposes. Mr. Rampaire believed he had negotiated the best quality EAP for his employees.

After the program had been in place for seven months, Mr. Rampaire was satisfied with the utilization reports he received but wanted some assurance about the quality of WLA's daily operations. He consulted with the HR director about a site visit to the WLA facility. She suggested that the best way to obtain information would be to contract with a licensed professional counselor who could judge both the quality of the quality measurements and the actual performance of the EAP functions. Mr. Rampaire, seeing the merit of an expert outside evaluator, consented to pay a consultant's fees and travel expenses for a two-day assessment.

When the consultant returned from her visit, Mr. Rampaire was surprised by the findings. WLA had one MSW on duty during the observed telephone triage sessions, but the rest of the intake personnel were students from a local university. The records for licensure and credentialing of counselors and MSWs were not current. In addition, lists of practitioners who were available for referral were not up-to-date and contained incorrect telephone numbers. Mr. Rampaire contacted WLA's president about this situation. He saw the situation as reported to him as a violation of his contract and unethical practice. He was assured that this was not their usual way of doing business and that the situation would be remedied. However, when the WLA contract came up for renewal, Mr. Rampaire did not feel comfortable with the ethics of this EAP firm and declined to renew.

Responses and Commentary on Questions

1. What assumptions were made about quality by Rampaire Manufacturing?

   Mr. Rampaire assumed that a business based on helping those who are experiencing problems in work or in life would have a high-level commitment to both professional and business ethics. He believed that they would exercise fidelity and be self-policing in their quality assurance efforts. By stressing features such as group data reporting, using well-prepared practitioners for triage, maintaining credentialing records, and being open to onsite visits, WLA gave the impression of being an ethics-based organization. Mr. Rampaire assumed that truth-telling would be critical to their business and that this organization would share in his respect and concern for employees. He entered into the contract based on these assumptions.

2. What actions did Mr. Rampaire take to ensure quality?

Because there was no external evaluator for this organization, Mr. Rampaire decided to go the extra mile to be sure that his employees were getting the service that they needed and that he had funded. He knew that neither his HR director nor he had sufficient expertise to assess the actual performance of the intake staff and the quality of the recordkeeping. He was willing to spend extra funds to have a qualified person make the site visit and assess the situation. In addition, the counselor was licensed and would not divulge any information she heard while observing the intake process. Therefore, his employees' autonomy and privacy would be protected.

3. What was his ethics reasoning for taking these actions?

Mr. Rampaire was working on many ethical levels here. He wanted to make sure that his employees were treated appropriately, using the best quality care. His quality assurance efforts can be seen as applied Kantian ethics in that he wanted each person to be treated as valuable. He also wanted there to be a categorical imperative that services provided would be quality for all. You can also see some utilitarian ethics here in that he was trying to avoid the greatest harm to the greatest number. If an EAP does not provide quality services, it has the potential to cause even more distress for his employees and their families. Imagine if an inexperienced student gave a distraught employee inappropriate information or made an incorrect referral. The potential for harm was great.

From a business standpoint, he had a fiduciary obligation to his organization to be sure that he was spending funds appropriately. Paying for services that were not rendered or a contract that was not honored could violate his own business ethic of fidelity to his company. Because there was no outside evaluator for this organization, he felt ethically bound to spend some funds to get a more accurate, hands-on report of the performance quality.

4. What was the result of his action?

The first result of his action was that he learned that his contract with WLA was not being honored. This information allowed him to contact its president and voice his concerns from a position of information. His immediate response triggered action to remedy the situation. However, the breach of trust left him with an unsettled feeling about WLA, and he was careful to question all of their reports. In the end, he decided to discontinue business with them because he did not trust them to be involved with the mental health needs of his valuable employees.

Web Resources

··

Agency for Healthcare Research and Quality
http://www.ahrq.gov/

Centers for Medicare and Medicaid Services
http://www.cms.hhs.gov/default.asp?

Institute for Healthcare Improvement
http://www.ihi.org/ihi

Joint Commission on Accreditation of Healthcare Organizations
http://www.jcaho.org/

Malcolm Baldrige National Quality Award
http://www.quality.nist.gov/

References

··

Agency for Healthcare Research and Quality. (2008). *AHRQ profile: Quality research for quality healthcare*. Rockville, MD: Author.

Fitzpatrick, M. A. (2003, April). The JOINT is jumpin! [Electronic version]. *Nursing Management*, 34(4), 4.

Institute of Medicine. (2001). *Crossing the quality chasm: A new healthcare system for the 21st century*. Washington, DC: National Academy Press.

Institutes for Healthcare Improvement. (2009). *20/20 vision: 2009 progress report*. Cambridge, MA: Author.

Joint Commission on Accreditation of Healthcare Organizations. (2008a). *A journey through the history of the Joint Commission*. Available at: http://www.jointcommission.org/AboutUs/joint_commission_history.htm. Accessed January 19, 2009.

Joint Commission on Accreditation of Healthcare Organizations. (2008b). *The Joint Commission*. Available at: http://www.jointcommission.org/. Accessed January 19, 2009.

Kalina, K., Pew, S., & Bourgeois, D. (2004). *Don't go there alone! A guide to hospitals for patients and their advocates*. Kansas City, MO: 33-44-55 Publishing.

Ransom, E. R., Joshi, M. S., Nash, D. B., & Ransom, S. B. (Eds.). (2008). *The healthcare quality book* (2nd ed.). Chicago: Health Administration Press.

Roth, W., & Taleff, P. (2002). Health care standards: The good, bad, and ugly in our future [Electronic version]. *Journal of Quality and Participation*, 25(2), 40–45.

Shi, L., & Singh, D. A. (2008). *Delivering health care in America: A systems approach* (4th ed.). Sudbury, MA: Jones and Bartlett.

Tapping, D. (2008). *The simply Lean pocket guide*. Chelsea, MI: MCS Media, Inc.

CHAPTER 12

Patient Issues and Ethics

Private patients, if they do not like me, can go elsewhere; but the poor devils in the hospital I am bound to take care of.

—John Abernethy

Points to Ponder

1. What is the impact of paternalism on how the organization views the patient?
2. How does society's view of illness and health affect the organization's attitude toward patients?
3. What are the ethical issues involved in measuring patient satisfaction?
4. What is meant by patient-centered care?
5. What is the ethics connection in patient-centered care?

Words to Remember

The following is a list of key words for this chapter. You will find them in bold in the text. Stop and check your understanding of them.

human interaction   paternalism   patient-centered care
Planetree Model   self-treatment
sick role   societal stigma

■ PATERNALISM, OR "WE KNOW WHAT'S BEST"

The American healthcare system's historical roots lie in two traditions: medical practice and medical ethics. In medical practice, the system has been dominated by professionals, most specifically by physicians. Even though this profession stemmed from apprenticeship and proprietary education, it transformed itself into the controller of the medical system. After World War I, the power and prestige of the medical profession became so great that it controlled both the supply of medical care and the demand for its services. Little external control was placed on these "medical gods." In addition, they were able to restrict those who entered their ranks through medical school admission standards and licensure laws. This power base enhanced the physician group ethos of, "We know what is best for you," and the idea of patient compliance as a part of medical practice. These attitudes and practices established **paternalism** as norm in health care.

Two principles of ethics were also involved in the healthcare paternalism. First, health practitioners were taught that they had a moral duty to avoid doing harm to their patients (nonmaleficence). However, many of the procedures used, including those practiced today, had the potential to produce harm. For example, surgery has the power to cure and the power to kill. Professional judgment was required to make decisions about the risks versus the benefits of this or any treatment. As a response to their expert judgment, patients began to trust the wisdom of the practitioner with almost blind acceptance. The physician knew best because he (pronoun used deliberately) had the knowledge to protect you from harm. Further, it was his ethical responsibility to do so.

Practicing nonmaleficence also involved professional decision-making concerning the amount of knowledge the patient could have and the timing of knowing. For example, physicians withheld information from the dying so that suffering would be minimized. The idea was that knowing that patients were close to death would cause them greater harm than remaining ignorant about their condition. Of course, family members also appealed to practitioners not to inform their loved ones about the seriousness of their conditions so that they would not lose hope or suffer too much. Loving concern was the impetus for "don't tell Grandma," but no one asked Grandma what she wanted.

The sister principle of beneficence is also a part of paternalism in health care. In the beneficence-based view, practitioners have a moral obligation to use their knowledge for the reduction of pain and suffering for individuals and the community. While their superior knowledge of disease and treatment regimes should not be minimized, they were often ignorant about the patient's view of his or her own illness. This resulted in the paternalistic definition of "doing good" without consideration of whether that action was seen as "good" by the patient. Again, there was a conflict of paternalism versus autonomy, and paternalism seemed to be the winner.

What happened to change the system's paternalistic view, and how does it connect to ethics? There are several factors at work here. First, the increase in the number of people covered by insurance from various funding sources shifted the control for demand of care. Because of their expertise, physicians still diagnose and treat disease but the others, including the federal government and insurance companies, control payment for services. Those who control the money are beginning to demand accountability and fair value for their payment. Increasingly, they are defining what quality medicine is, right down to what drugs to prescribe and when. This strange business relationship leads to what some physicians see as a loss of control of the practice of medicine. They lament that, in order to be paid, they have to practice medicine "by the book." They feel their authority is lessened by bureaucrats who never went to medical school and who are keeping them from practicing the art and science of medicine.

The rise in the use of technology has also been a force to reduce paternalism. The increasing use of the Internet has led to a dramatic increase in the medical sophistication of the public. Patients use Web sites to shop for physicians and learn about their practices. They prepare for their visit to their physicians by checking the Web and printing out information that may or may not be accurate or even relevant. There is an expectation that the physician will know all about these data. While not all patients have access to computer-based information, those that do are becoming more vocal about their role in their care.

Technology, insurance, and an increasingly more sophisticated patient base have begun to make the shift from paternalism to consumerism. It has changed the patient–physician relationship to of a consumer partnership rather than a dictatorship. On the downside, it has eroded trust in the system. For example, some physicians resent the intrusion of technology on their practice and view it as a threat to their authority. Others relish the collaboration of the patient in his or her treatment and are open to discussing Web information.

You should also note that the consumer-driven phenomenon of integrated medicine (IM) has also influenced the change from paternalism to consumerism and patient-centered care. Because IM emphasizes prevention, holistic healing, and partnerships between practitioners and clients, those who use it are more active in their treatment. They assume responsibility for their own health and listen to the wisdom of their bodies. In turn, clients expect to have a similar experience in the healthcare system and try to share their involvement with their physicians. Although many physicians are coming to accept and even use IM approaches, many do not welcome this change. IM is viewed as a threat to their medical sovereignty and to their paternalism. The results are that some physicians either do not listen to their patients, or even ridicule their practices (the word "quack" may even be used). When such messages are sent, a "do but don't tell" practice becomes the norm, often with disastrous results.

Regardless of the source of the challenge, paternalism, while certainly not dead, has been challenged by the new healthcare consumerism. The new healthcare system might require a shift from an emphasis on professional control and paternalism to one of collaboration between physicians, administrators, payers, and patients. This strange set of bedfellows will make health care interesting and ethically challenging in the future as it attempts to meet the health needs of the patient.

■ THE PATIENT HEALTHCARE EXPERIENCE

To understand the differences between how the patient sees the healthcare experience and how it is viewed by the professionals, you first conduct a systems and culture check (Press, 2002; Shi & Singh, 2008). As you read this section, think about the last time you had a health system encounter and see if your experience parallels what has been codified by the experts. Begin with patients. First, they are not patients until they are defined as such, and they do not have diseases until they are given a diagnosis. People can have a symptom or set of symptoms which, given a logical explanation for their cause, they might ignore. For example, if you just completed a marathon, you might experience muscle pain. In this case, you would not run to the physician's office. You would attribute the pain to its source.

What would you do if your symptoms persisted or repeated? Would you call for a medical appointment? Unless the symptoms are severe, you might not. Press (2002) believes that you try to figure out what is happening or form a self-diagnosis. Many variables can be a part of this analysis and diagnosis including your culture, life experiences, and medical knowledge. For example, suppose you studied all night and forgot to eat. Now you are taking your exam and your head feels like it will implode. You do not assume that you have a brain tumor; you use your life choices to explain your headache.

The next stage in a person's illness experience is to try to take care of the problem, what Press (2002) and others have called **self-treatment**. This can involve taking over-the-counter medications, changing lifestyle behaviors, or consulting your trusted family healer (Mom works well here). Because almost 80% of illnesses are handled by the healing ability of a person's own body, self-treatment is successful, and people go on with their lives. They do not become patients in the healthcare system.

What happens if self-treatment does not work? If symptoms persist even after you have self-medicated and consumed doses of Mom's chicken soup, and they are beginning to affect your daily life, you decide that you are sick. This puts you into what medical anthropologists identify as the **sick role** (Press, 2002; Shi & Singh, 2008). What does this mean? In families and society, when you are in the sick role, you have special benefits and responsibilities. For example, you will not be expected to attend classes but are expected to stay home in bed. Those around you might give you special treatment so that you have time for recovery. However, your responsibilities in the sick role include remaining true to your sickness. For example, if you have a migraine headache, you do not recover in 20 minutes and then go to the mall. Such behavior would be viewed as faking illness and being dishonest. You are also supposed to be compliant, participate in activities to promote your speedy recovery, and seek appropriate professional help for your condition. The specifics of how you interact in your sick role are influenced by your culture and family relationships and, to some extent, by your gender. Sick role behaviors are reinforced or diminished by their level of reward provided by these groups.

Your overall responsibility in this sick role is to get well as soon as possible and return to being a productive member in your family and workplace or school setting. Notice that this responsibility includes seeking out assistance from an appropriate professional and then complying with the treatment provided. Seeking professional assistance means that you must be willing to enter the alien world of medical care with its strange language and rituals. You are expected to share your most personal information right down to your body functions with an absolute stranger. In addition, you are expected to do this in an efficient manner so his or her time is not wasted. In fact, Press (2002) says that if you can present your symptoms in an organized way using appropriate vocabulary, you can receive a higher level of respect, more time in assessment and, by implication, a more accurate diagnosis. Being placed in an environment that, at best, is sterile and uninviting further exacerbates this potentially humiliating experience. Because of this encounter, you are given a diagnosis, declared to have a disease or condition, and become a patient.

You are now a part of the healthcare system. Some would say that you have indeed become a stranger in a strange land. Press (2002) prompts that you are in a closed system whose function is to treat your body and get an appropriate outcome. It treats only what it labels as disease. Illness, which is the patient's experience, is not recognized because the system is centered on reductionism and the mechanics of cure. A set of protocols is defined for treating each disease, which is supposed to be appropriate for all groups of patients with a few minor considerations for age and perhaps ethnicity. Professionals run this system and have many levels of power. They have certain expectations for patients who enter their system.

Patients come from an entirely different system, what you might call the illness system. In their open system (Press, 2002), sickness is deeply personal and affects not only their bodies but also their sense of self. They now have to add the identity of a sick person and a patient to their list of roles. Disease challenges their emotions, their faith, and even their relationships to others. It can change their lifestyles and threaten their ability to earn a livelihood. They also bring a set of beliefs, assumptions, and hopes about the medical system and its healers that influences their perception of the encounter. It is not surprising that such an encounter can create anxiety and a host of emotional responses including embarrassment, discomfort, and fear.

When you go beyond the realm of physical health into that of mental health, the dynamics change even more dramatically. Not only do you have to go through the stages of ignoring symptoms until they affect your life, trying self-treatment, and assuming the sick role, but you now have a **societal stigma** about your illness. To complicate matters further, you have the responsibility of deciding whether you need to seek the help of a psychologist, psychiatrist, counselor, or priest. This decision is supposed to be made when your mind is already confused and frightened. Then, assuming you choose to do so, you are expected to tell a complete stranger information that you would not tell your own mother. Then you must take whatever medication a psychiatrist prescribes or do any follow-up counseling. To fail to comply is to risk being labeled "uncooperative." It is not surprising that clients are often uncomfortable or even wary of the mental health field.

You can already see that the patient is becoming part of a situation where a clash of cultures is inevitable. Professionals in health care also bring their own roles and concepts of appropriate behavior to the encounter. Through professional socialization, they are taught their professional role and expectation about patient encounters. Often, they also make moral judgments based on how the patient acquired his or her disease. Some healthcare professionals place patients into categories of "good" or "bad" people based on whether or not their life choices are viewed as moral or immoral. For example, a nonsmoker who is diagnosed with lung cancer might be given greater value than one who is a lifelong chain smoker.

In addition, patients are expected to exhibit certain behaviors. They are supposed to be grateful, suffer without too much complaint, and be properly humble. They are not to cause problems for the staff or upset others by their reactions to pain or bad news. In other words, they are to be stoic and have a high threshold for physical pain. Patients who do not follow the "rules" are often given labels such as "frequent flyer" (too many visits to the emergency department [ED]), or "drama queen" (e.g., too much noise during labor).

How does this clash of professional and patient culture affect the patient's view? Patients judge care from their personal system and not from the professional's system. They assume that the technical aspects of care, which are the center of your view, are provided by competent people. Those interactions that demonstrate your ability to care and communicate are seen as indicators of the quality of care. As you will read later, the ability to understand the patient's experience will enhance trust and patient compliance. In contrast, if the patient is treated as an inconvenience or worse, he or she will judge your care as poor, even if it demonstrated great technical excellence. This view should remind you of Chapter 1 where Buber's ideas of I-YOU and I-THOU were presented. Minimally, the patient wants an I-YOU relationship with you but hopes for an I-THOU. The true skill is to provide this ethical relationship day after day to patient after patient.

■ MEASURING THE PATIENT EXPERIENCE

Are your patients satisfied and why should you care? As an organization, it makes good business sense to have a solid record of patient satisfaction. This credential can lead to better status in the community and increased patient referrals to help your practice grow. Press (2002) also says that patient satisfaction is linked to your employee satisfaction. High levels of patient satisfaction can actually mean decreased turnover and absenteeism and be a boon to your bottom line. Of course, patient satisfaction numbers are a significant area of review for your external evaluators (e.g., National Committee for Quality Assurance, Joint Commission on Accreditation of Healthcare Organizations [JCAHO]). In fact, the data are often translated to "report cards" that provide surface information about what is going on in your organization. These report cards find their way to various Web sites and publications. Individuals and businesses use them to make judgments about how you treat patients.

How do you measure whether your patients are satisfied? There are actually many ways to do this, as you will read later in this section. However, some form of a survey or questionnaire is the most commonly used method. The instrument can be prescribed by an agency, purchased through a company that specializes in measuring patient satisfaction, or created in-house. Any format presents some limitations that can also create ethics concerns. First, you need to remember that measurement tools do not measure actual real-time patient satisfaction (Press, 2002). Because surveys are often conducted weeks or even months after the actual encounter, what you are getting are data about perception and memories. In addition, your responders might be reluctant or even fearful to tell the truth. This means that the numbers can be based on a biased sample size and are often inflated. Yet, these same numbers are used to reward or punish staff through various incentive programs that could be viewed as an issue of justice.

There are several other ethical issues to consider in using survey data alone for measuring patient satisfaction. First, you have all of the statistical concerns such as sample size, random sampling techniques, population representation, and data manipulation. Knowledgeable and less-than-ethical staff can conduct surveys that are designed to make the data say only positive things about your institution. This "good news" can then be used to market your facility to an unsuspecting community. Even simple things like how you word your questions (or select the wording) can produce "halo type" results. In addition, ordinal or rank data can be treated as if they were arithmetic numbers and subjected to "numbers mania." This can lead to all types of data manipulation to make your scores look better than they truly are. A strong ethical foundation for the whole survey process is needed, especially when bonus money relies on the results.

Along with the ethics of collecting the data, you need to consider what happens to them when they are collected. What is the ethics of patient satisfaction measurement if it is only for the "books"? What is the financial and ethical cost of just shelving data and never using them for any real purpose? If so, is it possible you are spending funds to conduct this useless evaluation that could be used on something more productive?

Of course, questionnaires are not the only way or even the best way to identify the root cause of patient satisfaction issues. Press (2002) and others encourage you to use the data collected through surveys as a spark for discussion and beginning the process of root cause analysis. However, you might also need data from other sources to make a real difference. For example, you can gain valuable insight into the real problem by practicing management by walking around. Observation is a powerful tool, even if it is not quantitative. Consider talking with patients, staff, and practitioners to get a better sense of how things happen in real time. Good administrators have been known to sit in the ED waiting room and talk with patients. They get a much better sense of the "ED experience" by being a part of it. Still others actually become mock patients and go through the admissions and work-up process. You can imagine the insight this brings. Some administrators make it a point to talk to the housekeeping staff because they are often a source for real information about operations.

Press (2002, p. 36) emphasizes that, "measurement is not management." Regardless of its source, data alone will not change anything or bring about improved patient satisfaction. You will have to be engaged in some form of problem analysis and problem-solving strategy to make a difference in this area. To paraphrase the Serenity Prayer, you need the courage to change the patient interactions that you can control, to accept the elements that you cannot change, and the wisdom to understand the difference. Remember to always use the internal experts (the people who really do the job) as part of your problem-solving team so that the plan becomes a reality and not just another piece of paper.

■ HOW DOES MEASUREMENT RELATE TO ETHICS?

You can conclude that measuring patient satisfaction is good for business, but is it good ethics? From a Kantian view, you have a moral duty to treat patients with respect because they are fellow human beings. In fact, this duty passes the categorical imperative test because it should be a universal feature of your practice. It fits the Golden Rule in that you would want to be treated with respect if you were a patient. In order to ensure that you are being true to this Kantian imperative, you must evaluate your practices even if this is not mandated by an external reviewer. How else will you know if you are acting in accordance with your Kantian mandate?

From a utilitarian view, you must provide the greatest good to the greatest number or cause the least amount of harm. Your actions have consequences that must be measured in order to determine if you are providing for the greatest good. Policies are created (rule utilitarianism) to ensure that your treatment of patients provides this greatest good. Collection of data from multiple sources assists you in obtaining a more accurate picture of what is really happening in the patient's care experience and how you an improve it.

Rawls would also agree that gathering data on the patient's experience and satisfaction enhances your ability to provide ethics-based care. Despite different diagnoses, patients are all in the same position. They want the best possible outcome from their medical experience. This is always true—even when the outcome is death. Patients wish death with dignity and without overwhelming pain and trust that you will be able to provide this outcome. The Rawlsian principle of protecting the least well off relates to your need for assessment and improvement of the patient experience. Because you want to be known for your compassionate care and not just for your profit margin, you must be able to make informed decisions about how best to provide this care.

When you consider the founding healthcare ethical principles, you can also see a connection to measuring the patients' experience and satisfaction. For example, the principle of autonomy stresses the patient's ability to own his or her body and make decisions about what happens to it. Infringement of this principle should occur only when it is in the best interests of the patient and he or she provides consent. Measuring the patient's view of autonomy and your impact on it should help you to provide appropriate care and respect the patient's boundaries. If you understand the patient's view, you should also be able to move from paternalistic, professionally driven care to patient-centric care with greater ease.

Consider the sister principles of nonmaleficence and beneficence and their relationship to patient satisfaction. Perhaps you are causing harm unintentionally because the patient does not understand your procedures or intent. Understanding of the patient's experience may help you prevent harm by creating greater understanding. You also have a moral obligation to provide benefit, which should be easier to accomplish if you understand what the patient sees as beneficial. As you read earlier, there are different definitions of benefit depending on who is defining it. Finally, consider the principle of justice. How do you know that you are being fair and just to patients if you have no information? Patient satisfaction data from multiple sources help to determine your fairness and assist you in making any necessary policy and procedure changes.

■ PROVIDING CARE THROUGH A DIFFERENT VISION: PATIENT-CENTERED CARE AND ETHICS

Influences including access to information, an educated and involvement-oriented patient base, and mandates from external agencies have created a new focus on **patient-centered care**. Healthcare organizations including hospitals, clinics, and long-term care centers are re-examining their missions in light of this interest. Should this be surprising? When you give this idea some thought, you should surmise that all healthcare organizations should want to be patient-centered. Can you imagine a healthcare mission statement that excludes the patient? However, just writing that you are patient-centered does not make it so. There is work to be done to make this goal a reality.

In today's healthcare world, the challenge is to provide patient-centered care and still maintain a profit margin. How do you change a paternalistic environment to one that is patient-centric? How does this action relate to ethics? These are among the many questions that cause concern for healthcare organizations. Fortunately, they do have assistance in finding answers through the **Planetree Model** (Frampton & Charmel, 2009) and the Leebov's advice (2008).

The Plantree Model has been attempting to create a patient-centered environment in healthcare organizations ever since its inception in the late 1970s. Its beginnings were based on the patient care experience of one woman, Angela Thieriot. Her hospital experience was one of "Alienation, fear, hopelessness, loneliness, and dehumanization" that lead her to feel that, "I would never get out alive" (Frampton & Charmel, 2009, p. xxviii). After this experience, she began an extensive qualitative research through literature search and interviews to determine what was needed to make the patient's experience more humane and healing.

Through her research and experience, she identified nine major areas that were needed to bring health care back to its roots of holistic patient-centered care. Using this information, she founded a nonprofit organization named Planetree in honor of Hippocrates. Over 2000 years ago, he sat under a sycamore tree ("planetree") and taught his students that a patient's environment is an important part of healing. In 1985, she opened the first Planetree Model hospital unit with the assistance of Kaiser Foundation and other grants (Frampton & Charmel, 2009). Physicians, nurses, and other staff participated in this unit and agreed to function within the Planetree philosophy. An architect assisted in the physical design and created a space where the holistic care could be provided.

Since that original effort, many other facilities have chosen to embrace the Planetree Model for patient-centered care. Some have completely revamped their facilities and practices while others have chosen to implement the changes in increments. Many others have adapted ideas from this model and created their own patient-centered hospitals, clinics, and long-term care centers. As you would expect, the model was challenged from both the medical and administrative components of the healthcare system. For many, it was just too radical a change to be accepted without resistance. Keep in mind that healthy skepticism is a good practice when the patient's well-being is at stake, but taken to extreme, it can impede positive change.

The business sector, while understanding that patient-focused care appeared to be the right thing to do, questioned its effectiveness and return on investment. They wanted to see randomized studies that demonstrated cost savings and direct benefit to their profitability. Fortunately, studies that address the business case for the model are being conducted. Because of the broad scope of the model and its influence on operations, research data indicates that it contributes to shorter lengths of stay, lower costs per patient, and a lower cost for higher-cost registered nurse (RN) services. In addition, patient satisfaction rates were higher than average (Frampton & Charmel, 2009). In addition, facilities that use the Planetree Model exceeded the performance requirements for Medicare and Medicaid services in all ten areas of patient experience.

How does the medical community feel about Planetree? The champions of the Planetree Model have traditionally been nurses and other practitioners and not physicians (Frampton & Charmel, 2009). This might be because these professionals have more of the daily contact with patients, while physicians see them only briefly throughout their hospital stay. In addition, because of their scientific background, many physicians view this model as having insufficient empirical foundation and being unrealistic in terms of today's economic situation. They also see too much emphasis placed on the softer side of patient care and worry that it might diminish the scientific rigor in which they practice. However, this attitude is changing. Recent studies on physician satisfaction found that physicians preferred Planetree units for their treatment of patients.

At this point, you might be asking, "Just what is this Planetree Model?" This model has evolved into a patient-focus care delivery plan that includes Thieriot's nine key areas (Frampton & Charmel, 2009). Areas include a focus on human interactions, emphasis on information, inclusion of social support networks, and an emphasis on nutrition as part of healing. In addition, the Planetree Model addresses the spiritual needs of patients, includes integrative medicine as part of the healing process, and recognizes the role of the arts in healing. Finally, the model considers the environment and the community as part of the patient care experience. The following is a brief summary of these key areas.

Human interaction is a key area in the Planetree Model because it reflects the essence of the patient care experience. As you read earlier, patients who are admitted to the hospital enter an alien culture where their life functions and dignity can be taken away. They are to assume the compliant and noncomplaining sick role and behave in a way that is convenient for the caregiver. Human interaction involves the relationship between the practitioner and the patient and the practitioner and other practitioners. It should center on kindness, concern for patient needs and comfort, and inclusion of the patients in their own care. Trust is built and satisfaction increased when quality interaction occurs. In addition, staff satisfaction increases because they make a difference for the patients and their families (Frampton & Charmel, 2009).

Providing health information has always been a focus of the Planetree Model. In fact, one of the first accomplishments of this model was the provision of information to patients who were often limited in their access to accurate and unbiased data about their own health. Today, with the increase in Internet usage, patients seem to be in information overload, yet there is still a need to have trustworthy sources. The Planetree Model includes a policy for open access to the patient chart. This is suggested as a way for patients to be informed about their treatment and status. While this feature of the model has been somewhat uncomfortable for staff, it has been found to increase trust. Some patients even add their own comments to the record. In addition, hourly nursing rounds are suggested. This action provides for compassionate care and addressing patient concerns in a timely manner. The Planetree Model also addresses the need for community education and provides for easy-to-use libraries.

The concept of a healing partnership is important in the Planetree Model. The family is part of the healing process in this model of patient-centered care. However, a family member does not have to be a direct relative but can be someone who is important in the patient's life.

Many strategies involve healing partners including care partner programs and unrestricted visitation. Some facilities choose to share clinical guidelines for treatment with these care partners. This action enables care partners to be an extra pair of eyes and alert the staff about potential problems. Facilities have also made room for family members by providing for overnight stays in the patient's room or at a nearby facility (Frampton & Charmel, 2009).

Food and nutrition are also part of the healing process in the Planetree Model. Diet is tied to health outcomes and food service personnel are regarded as caregivers. They are empowered to assist in improving the patient experience with food and nutrition. This includes having the correct menu arrive at the correct temperature and at the correct time. Because food is more than just fuel, innovations such as pantries on nursing units, improved cafeteria design and service, nutrition education, and personalized menus have become part of this model. In addition, some facilities use aromatherapy by baking cookies or bread on the floor to decrease hospital smell and increase the comfort level of the patients and their families (Frampton & Charmel, 2009).

The power of the spirit is also included in the Planetree Model. Despite the increase in double-blind studies about the power of prayer and spirituality, many healthcare facilities still cling to the separation of body and spirit model, which was first proposed by Descartes. However, the Planetree Model agrees with Frankl and others that humans are more than their bodies. The model addresses the differences between religion and spirituality and includes both in patient-centered care. To implement this feature, Planetree-based facilities actively involve hospital chaplains in inpatient treatment, conduct spiritual assessments, provide counseling, and honor rituals. Some have included interfaith chapels where patients and their families can go for solitude and prayer. Where Native American healing traditions are part of the culture, efforts are made to respect and include these practices in healing (Frampton & Charmel, 2009).

The benefits of integrative medicine are acknowledged in the model. Modalities such as massage, aromatherapy, and acupuncture are offered as ways to personalize the hospital environment. For example, massage is provided on the same day as surgery on acute care floors and in cancer centers. Some hospitals include infant massage programs and others even offer massage to employees. This service provides an improved patient care experience, which may relate to improved healing and reduced length of stay (Frampton & Charmel, 2009).

The healing arts are also included in the Planetree Model as a holistic way to increase the patient experience. This practice is older than the Hippocratic system when beauty, from many sources, was deemed necessary for healing. In modern times, Florence Nightingale also endorsed the power of beauty as part of healing resources. In the Planetree

Model, the importance of the arts is reflected in facilities that conduct research to select healing-support paintings and sculptures for public areas such as lobbies and activity rooms. In addition, patients are allowed to select art for their rooms from "art carts" or to participate in an art therapy program. These programs are often very inexpensive because they use volunteers and donated equipment. Most important, they provide a "time out" from the stress of illness for patients and their families. Examples include artists-in-residence for the visual and music arts, concerts by local groups, pianos in the lobby, and portable CD and DVD players (Frampton & Charmel, 2009).

Planetree Model facilities are also known for their attention to the total healing environment. Details in facility design and construction are not merely cosmetic. They are rooted in the concepts of holistic healing. Through careful choices in design, the hospital becomes a place where practitioners and patients work together for healing. The facility design makes this process easier and adds a more positive element to the patient care experience. The hospital becomes less sterile and foreboding. It is viewed as a healing place. Attention to patient safety, noise controls, lightening, and use of space contribute to a design for patient-centered care. In addition, the idea of wayfinding is addressed so that patients, families, and visitors have a greater sense of control and less stress (Frampton & Charmel, 2009).

Finally, beginning in 2002, the Planetree Model included an emphasis on healthy communities (Frampton & Charmel, 2009). It encourages organizations to address the biologic, social, intellectual, environmental, and spiritual health needs of communities that they serve. Working to improve community health is not just an ethical thing to do; it has business benefits. First, if the organization is nonprofit, it must demonstrate benefit to justify its tax-exempt status. Actively engaging in community health improvement can assist in this justification. Second, in this age of competition, healthcare organizations need to maintain a strong positive image in their communities. This image is enhanced if organizations genuinely care about the health of the communities that they serve. Finally, it makes financial sense to improve the overall health of a community. Since healthcare resources are limited, it makes sense to prevent as much illness as possible. Using community input and creativity, healthcare organizations can take the lead in improving the community's health.

Leebov (2008) offers practical advice for administrators who want to increase patient-centered care in their facilities. First, she suggests that you increase your level of empathy. It is easy to forget the patient in the busy world of finance and forms. However, patients are the reason for your existence. Therefore, she suggests that you make time to walk through your facility and see it through the patient's eyes. You might even take a ride on a gurney or interview visitors for their insight.

Communication is viewed as an essential part of patient-centered care. Therefore, you should educate personnel to provide information with attention to patient feelings and anxieties. This might include taking time to carefully explain each process and provide follow-up information through handouts. In some cases, scripts may be required to assure that employees are consistent in providing information. In addition, communicating appreciation and expressing thanks also increases patient-centered care (Leebov, 2008).

Leebov (2008) also suggests that, like the physicians, administrators need to make rounds. In this case, random patient room numbers could be assigned to a member of the management team. This individual could then visit the assigned room on a weekly basis. The purpose of the visit would be to understand the true patient experience and gather information about areas like patient comfort, privacy, communication, and staff treatment. Of course, follow-up on this information would be necessary. However, follow-up could lead to positive actions such as writing a thank you note to an employee for his or her service and solving problems in timely way. In addition to sending a message to patients that you care about their experience, you are also show the staff that your mission is more than words; you put it into action.

Is ethics a part of patient-centered care? The answer is, emphatically, yes. All of the ethics theorists whom you have studied would support this effort. You can see evidence of Kantian ethics throughout the nine key areas you have just encountered in the Planetree Model. The emphasis on true patient-centered care acknowledges that each patient is individual and to be valued. Planetree advocates see patient-centered care as a moral duty so that optimum care can be given for optimum healing.

Does utilitarianism support patient-centered care? It would support the Planetree Model because it attempts to provide the greatest good for the greatest number and avoid the greatest harm for those affected. Even minimal adaptation of this model seems to increase patient satisfaction and feelings of empowerment. When patients feel that they are in control of their own bodies, they tend to be calmer, more cooperative, and more appreciative of their care. Employees and the community also express greater satisfaction with the facility; this has a positive impact on its image and support. While patient satisfaction may not dramatically increase your revenue stream, studies are now showing that it does affect your bottom line through decreased length of stay and increased patient and staff satisfaction.

Summary

This chapter described how the patient is viewed by the healthcare facility and its employees. At the negative end of the continuum, patients are seen as whining interruptions to the flow of the day. If they do not remain in a state of quiet suffering and cooperation, then they are labeled noncompliant and avoided whenever possible. On the other end of the continuum, you find the Planetree Model and other efforts for patient-centered care. In this view, patients are partners in their own care and their needs are central to the existence of the facility.

The ethics of measuring patient satisfaction are integral. If you consider this logically, you can see that, like any business, you need information about what is working and what is not. You cannot improve what you do not know. Therefore, it makes good business and ethical sense to acquire as much accurate data about the patient care experience as you can. However, the point is not just data collection. You have to determine the best way to use these data for ongoing improvement of your practices. Failure to use the data collected creates an ethics issue of wasting funds for useless surveys that could otherwise be used for patient, employee, or business benefit.

Today, there is an effort among healthcare facilities to move toward more patient-centered care. The Planetree Model was created because of one person's experience with the alien culture of health care. Each of the key features in the model is founded in good ethical and business practice. These keys will assist your facility making the patient the center of care in a time when resources are already strained and change is an almost daily event. However, the pressures of the increase in baby boomer consumers and greater scrutiny from the media should assist you in making the argument that these changes are good for business. They certainly make good ethics.

Cases for Your Consideration

The Case of Kelly Beth's Mother

As you read this case, consider the following questions. Responses and commentary will follow the case.

1. What factors contributed to Kelly Beth and Caitlin (her mother) O'Brian's experience?

2. What ethics principles are illustrated by this case?

3. If you were the administrator at Dagma Memorial Hospital, how would you handle this situation?

Case Information

Three-year-old Kelly Beth O'Brian was brought into the ED at Dagma Memorial Hospital (DMH) by her mother Caitlin. Radiographs revealed a lateral fracture of the left femur that would require several weeks of traction before a cast could be applied. Naturally, Caitlin was beside herself with worry. The information about Kelly Beth's prognosis and treatment was frightening in itself, but she had other concerns that were troubling. Caitlin was a single mother who needed to keep her job to support her family. She knew that her department did not allow any time off for family illness, and she had no one to help her with this situation. What was she going to do?

Somehow, Caitlin worked out a schedule that allowed her to spend maximum time with her daughter. She went to the hospital early enough in the morning so that Kelly saw her when she woke up. She took her lunch hour to check on her daughter and returned immediately after work. At night, she left only when Kelly was asleep. This schedule became a way of life and, although exhausting, helped Caitlin feel like she was able to keep her job and be there for her daughter.

Several days into this routine, Caitlin arrived at the hospital a little late, after lunch was served. When she kissed Kelly Beth and adjusted her bed, she found that Kelly was lying in food. It was in her hair, which was matted and filthy. When she asked Kelly Beth about this, the child said, "Mommy I tried to eat my lunch but it was too high and everything kept falling," and then she began to cry.

Of course, Caitlin was extremely concerned about this event. Therefore, after comforting her daughter, she went to speak to the nurses. Although she was upset about her daughter's treatment, she made a conscious effort to control her feelings about the situation. The nurse who responded to her said, "We don't have time to feed your child; that is your job. If you are not here, we just leave the tray. You are also responsible for washing your own child's hair. You should bring the supplies and figure out how to do it. That's what good mothers do."

Caitlin was stunned. Not only was this response rude but also no one had told her about all of these rules. She knew she was being a good mother by juggling her schedule to be present at every possible moment, but now she was accused of neglect. She just assumed that because nutrition was important to Kelly Beth's healing, someone would make sure that the child could eat. She also assumed that the nursing staff would help to maintain hygiene as well as changing the sheets. How was she supposed to know that her assumptions were wrong?

Caitlin called one of her nurse friends to find out what supplies she needed to wash Kelly Beth's hair while she was confined to the bed. She also made sure that she never missed a meal again to ensure that her daughter did not go hungry.

When Kelly Beth was discharged in her body cast, Caitlin had mixed feelings about DMH. While she was pleased with the technical care her daughter received there, she was not at all happy with the quality of the support care. In fact, she considered sending DMH a bill for patient care services.

Responses and Commentary on Questions

1. What factors contributed to Kelly Beth and Caitlin (her mother) O'Brian's experience?

   In this case, you need to consider the situation from two viewpoints. First, consider what was happening for Kelly Beth and Caitlin. Kelly Beth was only three years old and had no experience with what she was supposed to do in a hospital. Her mother had not arrived yet and she was hungry. Being a resourceful child, she tried to feed herself but because she was so little, and in traction, her efforts created a mess. Had she been an adult or even an older child, she might have known to ring the call button and get help. However, the nurses had not taught her how to do this.

   Imagine Caitlin's experience. She was trying her best to be there for her daughter and to keep her job so she could pay her bills. She happened to be a bit late for the lunch service and found her daughter lying in her lunch. When she inquired about the situation, she was treated with a rude response that increased her "mother guilt." Now she felt like everyone knew the rules but her. While she was annoyed at the nursing staff, on some level she felt guilty because she was not holding up her part of the care burden. She did not know this was her role in the process. She even made the effort to learn how to wash her daughter's hair. Once her daughter was recovering at home, she became angry at the lack of support from those she trusted with the care of the most precious thing in her life. She wanted to do something about this but felt that nothing she could do would make a difference.

   How did the staff view this situation? The nursing staff felt overwhelmed by the serious tasks of caring for ill children. They had to complete all of the physician's orders, document their nursing notes on the computer, and take care of their own sanity. Here was a "Nervous Nelly" mother who was complaining about food in her child's hair and one missed lunch. The nurses thought somebody should tell Caitlin how she was supposed to take care of her own daughter, and one of the nurses did just that.

   There might been some other messages going on in the nurse's response. Because she had "seen it all," she might have assumed that Caitlin was just another one of those uncaring mothers who are not at their children's bedside at all times. After all, how important can Kelly Beth be to this woman if she pops in and out all day? If she really cared so much, she would take off from work and be there 24/7 for her daughter. The nurse had no idea about the difficulty of Caitlin's situation. Perhaps the nurse just assumed that mothers were with their children in the hospital at all times, because she had seen that in the past.

Regardless of which view you take, there was a serious lack of communication and kindness in this situation. Rules regarding the responsibilities for Caitlin and the nursing staff may have existed but were not communicated. In addition, the simple act of kindness was forgotten. All the nurse had to do was to explain the rules to Caitlin in a nonjudgmental way. She could have taken a brief moment to instruct Caitlin on how to care for her daughter's needs and what supplies she needed to purchase. On the other hand, with even greater compassion, she could have assisted with the first shampooing of the child's hair with the understanding that Caitlin was responsible for this care in the future. Such an action would have led to a much different patient care experience for both Kelly Beth and Caitlin.

2. What ethics principles are illustrated by this case?

It is easy to see issues with all of the major principles of ethics in this case. First, the idea of nonmaleficence should be considered. The hospital staff's obligation in treating Kelly Beth was to do no harm. Certainly, a missed meal and dirty hair are not as harmful as a medical error such as amputating the wrong limb, but the lack of attention to the needs of the child and mother did cause some damage. Kelly Beth was probably humiliated by not being able to feed herself and making a mess. She was worried because her mother was late. She was hungry. None of this enhanced her ability to heal.

When a child is the patient, the family is also part of the picture. Did the staff cause harm to Caitlin? Again, this is a matter of degree. While no physical harm occurred, the response to her questions caused psychological damage to the conscientious mom. The tone of the nurse's message implied that Caitlin was not following the rules and therefore was not being a good mother. Perhaps the harm was not intended, but it certainly was felt.

How does the sister principle of beneficence fit here? Did the staff act with kindness and compassion in this situation? Obviously, they did not. It is true that they were extraordinarily busy, but letting a three-year-old struggle with a lunch tray that is placed out of her reach borders on cruelty.

The actions of the staff nurse toward Caitlin did not even resemble beneficence or respect for her autonomy. The nurse might have been acting from "compassion fatigue" and not from a lack of kindness.

Nonmaleficence was also violated in this situation because the hospital experience caused harm to the mother and the daughter. It was unjust to expect a parent to care for her child's hygiene when she was not informed of that fact. In short, all of the principles that form the basis of ethical healthcare behavior were violated on some level in this patient care experience.

3. If you were the administrator at Dagma Memorial Hospital, how would you handle this situation?

This seems like a facility that could benefit from the Planetree Model and from some lessons in communication. As an administrator, you have the obligation to consider the situation from both sides before taking action to prevent further incidents of this kind. Process improvement for the patient's needs is your primary mission. What could you have done to increase Caitlin and Kelly Beth's comfort level within the alien culture of DMH?

First, it might be helpful to include both written and oral communication about the expectations and responsibilities of staff and parents when a child is admitted to the facility. This could be accomplished through a brief conference coupled with an appropriate handout or pamphlet. Some facilities even include this information on their Web site.

You could also employ the principles of Planetree to find out more about Caitlin's experience and her struggle to meet her daughter's needs before passing judgment on the staff. When the situation is correctly assessed, you could try to provide appropriate support services. To do this, you could involve social services, pastoral care, or even a family support group. Perhaps there is a way to provide respite services for Caitlin when she has to be late and nursing services are too busy. The Planetree Model includes volunteer care partners for patients who are alone. Perhaps this option could be adapted to Caitlin's situation. The driver for your efforts would be to try to secure the best healing environment for Kelly Beth.

The nontangibles offered through the Planetree Model would also enhance this patient-care experience for mother and daughter. Kelly Beth and Caitlin needed a mechanism for asking questions and voicing needs without fear of staff retaliation. For example, showing Kelly Beth how and when to use the call button would have made a major difference in her care experience. It could also alter her mother's negative perception of the facility.

Other nontangibles like spirituality, touch, and the healing arts could be useful in improving this care experience. For example, Caitlin could have been taught how to provide massage for her child to help in pain management and sleep. Perhaps some complementary and alternative medicine (CAM) such as pet therapy or aromatherapy could be used to improve Kelly Beth's healing process. Some of the healing arts like storytellers, clowns, or play therapy could also decrease Kelly Beth's discomfort and assist in her healing.

Consider Planetree's emphasis on the physical environment. Could the addition of a more home-like design have helped this situation?

What about accommodations so that Caitlin could spend the night if she wished to do so? Think about the stress reduction potential of simply providing a bed or sleeping chair in the room.

In considering the patient's viewpoint, you must also include Plane tree's emphasis on empowering the patient. There might have been a different outcome had Caitlin been educated about the rights and responsibilities of a parent whose child is hospitalized at DMH. Instead, without complaining she took on a burden of care that could have been shared or supported by staff. However, she left the facility with a deep resentment over the treatment that was received. She felt that Kelly Beth was treated with indifference and disrespect when she deserved so much better. The potential was great that Caitlin would voice her negative impressions to the outside community.

Consider the staff in your decision-making. Surely, their intent was not to cause harm to a helpless three-year-old. However, they might have been placed in a situation where they were stretched beyond their limits so compassion fatigue became normal. Planetree principles, which also apply to staff, might have been useful in preventing this situation. The model stresses the way staff are treated and the way that they treat each other. For example, in this model employees receive care and support as well as the patients. This might be as simple as increasing the number of volunteers so that "extra hands" are available during busy patient care times. Caring for staff might include creating a physical environment that supports their health along with that of the patient. The model also includes areas where staff can go to regenerate their spirit and enjoy a respite.

Professionals also need to understand that they are valued and respected. Planetree stresses that they have a need for touch and a spiritual connection. As a way to demonstrate this, you could choose to provide chair massage to staff members during certain times in the week. Including staff in educational programs about CAM practices might also be helpful. Staff can enjoy the same music and art that you provide for patient healing.

Finally, good staff-patient communication cannot be overemphasized. You could begin this process by conducting a policy audit regarding proper communication methods. Perhaps it is time for a change or reinterpretation. If the policy is appropriate, you need to stress the ethical principle of "first do no harm" as part of patient communications. Acting with kindness and compassion in communicating messages could go a long way to prevent future situations like that of Caitlin. In other words, the same message conveyed with empathy might have had a very different result.

The Case of the Ardent Administrator

As you read this case, consider the following questions. Responses and commentary will follow the case.

1. Why did Dorothy Dee find the Planetree Model attractive for implementation at DMH?
2. What was the CEO's reaction to Dorothy's proposal?
3. What ethical principles were involved in the implementation decision?
4. What benefits were derived from this decision?

Case Information

Dorothy Dee, RN and VP of Nursing Services at Dagma Memorial Hospital (DMH), read something extraordinary in her latest nursing journal. A hospital adopted something called the Planetree Model, where patients were the center of their business. She read, at first with disbelief, about the changes this facility made based on the principles of the model. After reading about a hospital where patients are respected and the environment was dedicated to healing, she wondered how they were able to make such a complete change.

Becoming more curious, she found the facility's Web site and located the name and number of her counterpart. She called and had a long conversation about the accomplishment of the Planetree effort. She also learned that workshops were available at the Planetree Annual Conference. There were even manuals to assist organizations that wanted to try this patient-centered model. Dorothy really wanted to know more and if this model might work for DMH.

Fortunately, she had a chief executive officer (CEO), Christopher Higgins, who was open-minded. In fact, he prided himself on being community-centered and progressive. When she told him about Planetree and the documented increase in patient satisfaction scores and employee retention rates, he agreed to support her attendance at the conference and workshops.

Dorothy was amazed at what she learned at the workshop sessions. She even purchased the manuals and stayed up many nights reading them. She began to consider how the model could be used to make DMH a more patient-friendly environment and one that could enhance healing. Because this model made sense to her on many levels, she used her nights and weekends to develop a proposal for submission to Mr. Higgins. It included everything from changing the color of the wall paint to different modes of lighting. There were ideas for integrating music and art throughout the facility. She even had a plan to update the nursery using local art talent and staff assistance. She researched the budget to make these changes and attached it to her proposal. True, her plan included some costs, but they seemed minimal when compared to the potential benefits.

Dorothy submitted her ideas to Mr. Higgins and made an appointment to discuss the document. Because she knew his history of innovation and community service, she had hopes that her ideas would be accepted. Mr. Higgins told her that he had read the proposal carefully and that it did contain some promising ideas. However, it was just too radical and he worried about the reaction of the physicians. This much change might just be too much for DMH.

Dorothy was disappointed but, having learned to have a Plan B, she asked if she could take alternative action. What if she put together a team and created a feasibility study using the short-stay unit only? She would keep the budget to bare bones and provide documentation that the changes produced a positive result. Would he green light such an effort?

Knowing that Dorothy had the knowledge and skills to deliver on her plan, he consented. She assembled a team, making sure to include a physician champion. Other members included representatives from housekeeping, materials management, dietary, nursing, patient services, and other involved staff. After providing an information session, she said, "What if we changed short stay into a patient-centered environment? What would it be like?"

The group became enthusiastic about the chance to change things for the better. They came up with a way to get the rooms painted, add bedspreads and drapes to each room, and even provided aromatherapy by having cookies baked on the floor on Friday afternoons. Local artists were asked if they would like to donate healing art for the halls. The biggest change was in the family waiting room. It now housed a small resource center with a computer, a fish tank, and plants. They also included a "Kids Nook" with bright-colored walls and children-sized furniture. The transformation, which was supported by all of the team, was nothing short of amazing and finished on a very limited budget.

Almost immediately, Dorothy noticed a change in the routine of the short-stay unit. Patients were surprised by the nonhospital environment and quickly appreciated it. Instead of being negative about the change, staff seemed to embrace it and want it to work. Their attitude seemed to be more positive with patients and each other. In fact, they seemed to want to be scheduled for short-stay rather than traditional floors. Family members were also pleased to be able to learn more about how to care for their loved ones through the computer programs offered in the waiting room. The children used their own area and were less of a distraction.

Somehow, the local paper found out about this patient-focused care effort, and Mr. Higgins was featured in an article as a community-caring administrator. The print article sparked the interest of the local TV station, which ran a human-interest piece. DMH was given the title of a "Hospital That Cares." Mr. Higgins was so pleased with the results that he gave the green light to Dorothy's next innovation idea. Onward to the nursery and bunnies on the walls!

Responses and Commentary on Questions

1. Why did Dorothy Dee find the Planetree Model attractive for implementation at DMH?

   The first question to ask is why Dorothy chose nursing as her profession. Even in her student days, she wanted to make a difference in the health of her patients. She understood that healing was a process between the patient and the professional. Her current position at DMH seemed so far removed from her original vision of nursing. She struggled with scheduling, JCAHO reports, staff complaints, physician complaints, and community issues. Where was the healing environment she had hoped to create? She was experiencing quiet discontent when she found the journal article on Planetree and its philosophy.

   Being a realist, she knew that this would be a major change for the physicians, her nursing staff, and the other professionals. Yet she believed that if she were able to communicate the model well enough, most of the professionals would want to try it at least. She knew that patients and their families would appreciate being treated with respect and allowed to be part of their own care decisions.

   While her initial proposal was not well received because it was too far reaching, tackling the change in small steps and demonstrating positive results seemed to work. Her data showed that staff morale increased, as did patient satisfaction. An added bonus came when the press and TV media found the change newsworthy. DMH received priceless marketing through its improved community image.

2. What was the CEO's reaction to Dorothy's proposal?

   Mr. Higgins's response was not surprising. In fact, it was almost predictable. Although Dorothy had done a good job showing cost-effectiveness for the change, Mr. Higgins had to consider the political element. The last thing he wanted was a staff revolt because they were asked to move too far out of their comfort zones. He worried that the physicians would not be behind this and a disaster might result.

Still, the idea had merit. Therefore, when Dorothy asked to pilot a more limited version of the model with a fixed budget, he gave it the green light. As it turned out, she was right. The staff seemed to rally around the project, and the patients and their families were full of praise for it. The press coverage was excellent and several board members called to congratulate Mr. Higgins on his foresight.

3. What ethical principles were involved in the implementation decision?

There are many ethical principles at work here. From the patient side, autonomy is central to the whole model. Patients were treated as valued people and not as noncompliant nuisances. As a result, there were actually fewer patient complaints on the unit. Certainly you can see beneficence and the sister principle, nonmaleficence at work in this model. Everything from the physical environment to the staff interactions was designed to provide compassionate care that produced an optimal healing environment.

Justice was provided by this model for staff and for patients. Plane tree stresses the value of both. While improving the physical environment for the patients was a clear goal, the process and the results also improved the environment for the staff. They were enthusiastic about work again because they were engaged in a process that respected their knowledge and allowed them to make a difference that could be seen. In fact, short-stay became the place to be among the hospital staff. Dorothy felt certain she would have their support for other Planetree-type changes.

Web Resource

Planetree Information
http://www.planetree.org/

References

Frampton, S. B., & Charmel, P. A. (2009). *Putting patients first: Best practices in patient-centered care* (2nd ed.). San Francisco: Jossey-Bass.

Leebov, W. (2008). *Wendy Leebov's great patient experiences: No nonsense solutions with gratifying results*. Chicago: Health Forum Inc.

Press, I. (2002). *Patient satisfaction: Defining, measuring, and improving the experience of care*. Chicago: Health Administration Press.

Shi, L., & Singh, D. A. (2008). *Delivering health care in America: A systems approach* (4th ed.). Sudbury, MA: Jones and Bartlett.

The Inner Circle of Ethics

■ INTRODUCTION

This section completes the circle model that you saw in Figure 1. As you strive to live ethics and function as an ethics-based health care administrator, all of the outer circles exert their influence. Given this fact, your ability to practice eudemonia and practical wisdom in your professional and personal life will not be easy. However, making the decision to be a person of character and virtue can provide you with a level of integrity that will last for your entire career in the field of health administration.

The format of the chapters in the last section is slightly different. Because this inner circle is more personal, the text is written in the first person. In this way, I can talk to you as a future colleague in our profession. In addition, case studies are not used in this section. Instead, I will pose some challenges that I hope you can use toward the formulation of your own position on how you will apply ethics in your career.

This last section comprises three chapters that focus on your quest to find a way to practice ethics as the foundation of your practice as a health care administrator. Chapter 13, *Moral Integrity*, presents ideas about what it means to be moral administration in the challenging healthcare environment. The chapter begins with definitions of morality and its relationship to ethics. From there, you will explore expert views on practicing morally centered administration in a health care environment. You will also learn what happens when professionals lose their moral center. Finally, there some specific challenges are included to help you formulate your own position on morality.

In Chapter 14, *Codes of Ethics and Administrative Practice*, there is a discussion about professional codes of ethics and their relationship to healthcare administration. Your professional code as an administrator (the ACHE Code) is detailed and its application is featured. Because many administrators have other codes that govern their actions, this chapter also looks at codes from several professional groups to analyze their themes. By the end of this section, you should be able to understand how a "code clash" can occur and how to deal with it. To provide a balanced view, criticisms of codes are also discussed.

Chapter 15, *Practicing as an Ethical Administrator*, presents the core management functions and the relationship of ethics to each of those functions. It should assist you in applying ethics to your daily functions as an administrator. The chapter also includes information on ethics challenges you might face based on anecdotal data from practicing administrators.

Chapter 16, *Where Do We Go from Here?* provides a summary of the subject matter that you have encountered by studying this text. It also looks to the future and discusses examples of challenges you will be facing. Finally, it encourages you to write your administrative ethics statement in a way that is suitable for framing. If you do not wish to hang it on the wall of your office, you can keep it on your desk for reference.

CHAPTER 13

Moral Integrity

I have often thought morality may perhaps consist solely in the courage of making a choice.

—Leon Blum

Points to Ponder

1. What is moral integrity?
2. How do the experts' views of moral integrity differ?
3. What temptations will you face in choosing moral integrity as a basis for your professional actions?
4. What is the best way for you to maintain your moral integrity?

Words to Remember

The following is a list of key words for this chapter. You will find them in bold in the text. Stop and check your understanding of them.

administrative evil
evil
labeling
personal morality

deceit
extermination camps
moral integrity

■ DEFINITIONS OF MORALITY

What does take to be moral in a world that challenges morality? What does the idea of **moral integrity** mean for your role as a practicing healthcare administrator (HCA)? What is the relationship between morality and ethics? The answers to these important questions begins with an exploration of the meaning and concepts of morality. As we have seen with other ethics concepts, there is no absolute definition of the term morality, but experts seem to agree on certain themes. Purtilo and Criss (2005) define morality as everyday behaviors that allow us to live successfully with one another. They include concepts like values (what we cherish) and duties (actions that we are required to do).

How does morality relate to ethics? Purtilo and Criss (2005) explain that ethics is a way to examine moral problems by using a systematic and theory-based process. It allows you to analyze a situation using what she calls ethical reflection. This reflection can lead to resolution of the situation through appropriate action. Ethics differs from morality in that morality entails a course of action based on reasoning rather than one based on habit.

Purtilo and Criss (2005) further divide morality into personal, societal, and group categories. **Personal morality** includes those values and duties that you hold independent of work or social groups. For example, if you say, "I honor myself and give others the same honor," you are expressing part of your personal morality. Societal morality is influenced by culture, geography, religious foundations, and even legislation. It is the values and duties that reasonable people expect of each other and allows for a secure and peaceful society. An example of this morality is the statement, "All people are created equal." Because health care exists within a society, it is affected by its society's definition of morality. This means that its business practices must conform to society's view of a moral organization. For example, you are expected to make a profit and treat those who are least well off in a society with dignity.

Finally, Purtilo and Criss (2005) introduce group morality. They point out that subgroups such as those found in healthcare facilities often codify their own set of values and duties. These desirable actions are expressed through policies and procedures so that all group members have an understanding of the subgroup's definition of acceptable behaviors. You will learn more about this process when you study codes of ethics in Chapter 14.

Aristotle (Summers, 2009) also teaches about morality when explains how to apply ethics to daily living. Through the idea of practical wisdom and eudaimonia, he makes us aware of the need to apply ethics and behave in a moral way. We develop our moral character so that we use our knowledge of ethics to address challenging new situations. Ethical principles become the center of our lives and we apply them as virtue-centered administrators.

Frankl (1971) can also add to our definition of morality. Remember that he was concerned with the idea of choice and responsibility. This idea is in keeping with practicing as a moral agent (Darr, 2005) for your community and organization. In this role, you must be able to make personal and professional choices that have a foundation in ethics. Exercising your choice means that you take ethics beyond discussion to action. Frankl also reminds us that with choice comes responsibility. Therefore, you must not only make the best moral choice for the situation, you must be responsible for it. Given the challenges that you face as an administrator, making a choice and being responsible for it will not be easy. However, if you practice this aspect of Frankl's theory consistently, you will build a reputation for being a person of character and integrity.

■ WHAT DO THE EXPERTS SAY ABOUT MORALITY?

Now that you have a baseline definition, your next step is to study expert views about this topic. This will prepare you to address and solve the challenges posed for you later in this chapter. It should also allow you to deal with the real problems that you will encounter in your career. The following information comprises a survey of the extensive literature available on this topic and is condensed into palatable "wisdom bytes." I have also included my own observations, interspersed with those of the experts.

To begin, I will offer general ideas on how to combine leadership and morality from Parker Palmer (2000). More specific concerns raised by Johnson (2009) and Gilbert (2007) will also be discussed. Ideas from Dye (2000), Hofmann (2006), Gilbert (2007), and Johnson (2009) will be used to show the effect of the immoral or amoral actions on health care and other areas of society. The discussion will be followed by advice on keeping your moral center while being successful in the dynamic, temptation-ridden healthcare environment.

Palmer (2000) believes that, because we all live in a community, we are all followers or leaders depending on time and circumstance. To be a respected leader, you must practice what he calls authentic leadership. This form of leadership stems not from the profit/loss statement, but from the heart. As a "co-creator" of the world in which you exist, you must make choices for positive moral action. Nowhere can the impact of these choices be seen more clearly than in your choices as a HCA.

Your leadership actions should be geared toward producing good and avoiding harm, which Palmer calls light versus shadow. In other words, as morally-centered leaders, you are to "cast less shadow and more light" (p. 85). To accomplish this, you must be willing to explore your inner or spiritual life including your moral center. This exploration can be conducted through activities such as keeping a journal, allowing time to reflect or meditate, participating in discussions, and using prayer. Palmer also asks you to assess the role of fear in your decisions. While everyone who assumes a leadership role has fears, he or she should not be used as a basis for making decisions. You will need to draw on your knowledge, skills, and moral core to lead from a position of strength rather than one of fear.

Johnson (2009) devotes an entire chapter in *Meeting the Ethical Challenges of Leadership* to your character as a leader. His content is based on national and international research concerning characteristics of model leaders. These characteristics or virtues include courage, integrity, humility, reverence, optimism, and justice. The author feels that these characteristics are more than "talking points"; they are integral parts of your inner life and behavior. For example, courage means that you are willing to do the right thing even when it makes you unpopular. Integrity happens when you are consistent in your public statement and your private actions. Humility happens when you have an accurate view of your strengths and weaknesses. You are not seduced by praise and are not likely to be co-opted by power. Optimism helps you to expect good things from the future, and justice gives you a duty to treat people with equality and fairness.

Practicing morality as healthcare leaders requires a commitment to lifelong learning and personal growth. Johnson (2009) suggests that you find role models who can be examples of morality in leadership. These leaders can teach you how to act when there morals are challenged. They can also instruct you how to make a difference when moral action is needed. Reading and reflecting about actions of moral leaders whether fictional or actual can also assist you to enhance your character. In addition, Johnson (2009) suggests that you can extend your moral character through experiencing difficult situations and overcoming them. This deep learning could come from suffering a traumatic event such as an illness or divorce, dealing with difficult employees, or making a business mistake.

With respect to moral action, I often ask ethics students, "What is your personal bottom line? Over what issue or action would you be willing to quit your job?" When the questions are at this basic a level, these students struggle with the reality and fear of unemployment versus what they feel to be morally correct. However, when I turn the situation around and ask, "What are you worth? Would you be willing to sell your integrity for a paycheck?" a different vision appears. By going along with something that the students know is morally wrong, they are endorsing the action. While the immediate consequences might be negligible, the long-term effect could be extremely damaging. It is hoped that you will never have to face such a difficult situation in your career, but it is always important to formulate your fallback position should it occur.

Gilbert (2007) discusses your personal integrity as function of your legacy, mindfulness, and choice. You need to be aware that, as an administrator, you are building your future legacy by your words and your actions. Your actions and even your inaction reflect your ethical stand on issues and is noted by employees and superiors. Building a positive legacy requires a commitment to going beyond discussing ethics. It means that you are living eudaimonia.

Mindfulness is also a part of your personal integrity (Gilbert, 2007). It involves your inner thought processes and the ability to practice ethical wisdom. Mindfulness allows you to be aware of ethical issues and decide what to do about them. You make these decisions by evaluating your biases, gathering information, and using a system to evaluate possible options. It also includes the feelings that you have when you have made an appropriate decision and when you have made the wrong choice.

Choice is the next major factor in your integrity. Every day you will be given the choice to make ethical decisions. These choices do not have to be about major events; they can be in your attitude, treatment of fellow employees, or creation of the work environment. When you choose to be consistent with your values, you create a sense of personal peace. In addition, your employees know that you are true to what you say. In other words, your actions match your statements. Remember that you always have a choice in what you think, say, and do. However, with choice comes responsibility. Ethical administrators own their choices and do not try to palm them off on others (Gilbert, 2007).

Gilbert (2007) also offers advice on how to build your personal integrity. For example, if you want to have a positive legacy, he suggests that you make your career matter. Work is a way to make a difference and not just something to be endured. You also need to be the example of an ethics-based administrator and not lose faith in the future. Concerning choice, he cautions us against making snap decisions that seem right in the short-term, but may be disastrous in the future. However, even if you do fail to make the best decision, it is possible to learn from this mistake and avoid it in the future. Keeping mindful of your choices and their effect on you and those around you is essential in building your personal integrity and expressing in both in work and in your personal life.

Morality Ignored: What Happens When the Compass is Broken?

What happens when moral integrity is ignored in the administrative practice? Are there any consequences for being an immoral administrator? Dye (2000) speaks about behavior where normally effective leaders choose behaviors that are destructive and result in poor performance. He calls this phenomenon "managerial derailment" (p. 170). This management failure is attributed to negative or immoral behaviors such as pessimism, dependency, low self-esteem, laziness, lying, and excessive egoism. Unfortunately, these traits cannot be detected during the hiring process, but they can seriously affect employee morale and the organization's bottom line.

Dye (2000) stresses that future and current employees should be assessed for their moral integrity beyond surface questions at an interview. You also need to be aware that a seemingly "good" administrator can be tempted by any of these negatives. Be sure to take the morality pulse of your staff from time to time. Most important, do not forget to monitor your own behaviors in these areas.

Hofmann (2006) agrees with Dye (2000) and suggests that we evaluate potential employees for their ethical integrity and ability to fit within the moral environment of the organization. He suggests that we not rely on reference letters or resumes alone to discern a future employee's integrity. Rather, he suggests that we ask questions about how candidates have handled ethical situations in the past. You could also ask candidates to read one or two ethics cases and respond to them. He also stresses that the number of group and individual interviews should be considered to assess compatibility. Your goal is to hire a person who exhibits personal integrity and can decrease the likelihood of derailment within your department or division.

Gilbert (2007) introduces the idea of "ethical erosion" which he defines as "a pervasive and subtle, negative dynamic to which we are all vulnerable, organizationally and personally" (p. 13). Ethical erosion happens when we slowly move away from the positive values that we hold. We make small decisions that are expedient, but may undermine our mission and values. Over time, these practices can become part of who we are as an organization or as a person. They become acceptable and we do not even see them as unethical.

Ethical erosion can have disastrous consequences. We can begin to think that what is commonly done is also ethical. This allows us to practice unethically while thinking that we are being ethical. Gilbert (2007) suggests that the counterbalance for ethical erosion is the application of ethical wisdom to alert when our values are compromised. Ethical wisdom can be applied in organizations through their culture, structure, leadership, governance, and integrity. For example, when examining the culture of an organization, erosion can be prevented if that culture allows employees to voice ethical wisdom, hear us the concerns of all individuals, works to resolve situations, and provides a legacy of quality.

Johnson (2009) presents a view of the dark or shadow side of leadership and its effect on your moral center. All leaders have both a light and dark side. They must struggle to master the darkness and not let it be a dominant force in their administration. Leaders in health care are particularly at risk because of their tremendous power and prestige in the community. Johnson addresses qualities that can make you a bad administrator (ineffective and/or unethical). He also discusses the concept of **evil**, and the ability to overcome it.

When you exhibit certain qualities, you have the ability to create an adverse affect on your employees and your organization. A few of these qualities include overriding ambition, inflated ego, and arrogance. If you are greedy, cannot discern right from wrong, and are reckless, you can also cause great harm. Not understanding problems and issues, and unwillingness to make difficult decisions, along with general incompetence can lead to personal and organizational downfall. These destructive behaviors contribute to violations of employee rights, unethical or illegal actions, creation of scapegoats, promotion of incompetence, and a toxic work environment. It is easy to see how such noxious administrative qualities can lead to personal and organizational disasters.

How can you keep from becoming a bad administrator? Johnson (2009) suggests that you address the administrative shadows of power and privilege. First, you cannot do your job without power. As you know from your management courses, it takes many forms, each with its own use. Of course, these power sources carry with them the potential for abuse if they are used inappropriately or excessively. How do you avoid the shadow of abuse of power? Johnson (2009) asks you to consider how you use each type of power and whether its use is appropriate. Be sure to balance delegated power with power that you own. Becoming impressed with your own sense of power can cause a loss of perspective leading to behaviors that can harm yourself and others. After all, you really do not have power unless people choose to give it to you and thereby comply with your plans and direction.

Because you assume a leadership position, your power is also linked to certain privileges. You receive more money, benefits, and status than others in the organization do. This is supposed to be compensation for the extra responsibility and accountability that you bear as an administrator. How much privilege is fair? Can you misuse privilege? Are you guilty of hoarding wealth and status, or feeling that you are better than others are? Introspection to answer these questions should help you to avoid being overcome by the privilege shadow.

You learned in Chapter 2 that fidelity is an important part of your autonomy as a HCA. However, the dark side of deceit is also part of your choice in this position. You have access to greater sources and levels of information than others in your organization. This makes sense because you must be "in the know" to do your job, but your knowledge power can also add to your ethical burden. For example, as you saw in Chapter 2, you sometimes have information that could adversely affect your staff, but you might not choose, for whatever reason, to disclose it.

Deceit does not have to be as direct as lying. You can practice deception by denying that you have particular knowledge, withholding information to sabotage others (as in bullying behaviors), or using information for your own benefit. Deception, once uncovered, undermines trust from your staff and your community. Once you have lost their trust, it can take years, if ever, to be restored.

The idea of having favorites—known as "ingroup/outgroup" management—is also one of the possible administrative shadows. Johnson (2009) considers this choice to be a lack of consistency. Because you are human, you will find some people more appealing than others. However, in the workplace, you have to strive for consistency of treatment. A way to avoid the temptation or even the perception of favoritism is to be careful about your lunch partners. If you lunch with only those you like, you have identified an "in group," even if this is not your intent. Your rule should be to have lunch with everyone or no one. Similarly, be very careful about socializing outside of work, particularly dating behaviors. Dating subordinates not only sets up the temptations of favoritism, but it can backfire if "love goes bad." In the worst-case analysis, a spurned subordinate might retaliate with claims of sexual harassment that can ruin your career. Indeed, it is lonely at the top.

Loyalty and responsibility are also key areas where shadows can overtake light in leadership. You have multiple loyalties as a HCA that can often conflict. Your first loyalty should be to the patient and the community that you serve. Obviously, you also want to be loyal to your boss and your staff. However, this loyalty cannot be absolute. For example, you must be willing to take appropriate action if your boss is engaging in behaviors that jeopardize the organization or the community. This is your moral Catch 22. You want to be loyal to your boss, but if you say nothing, you are supporting his or her behaviors. When you feel compelled to report your boss, you must always have appropriate documentation and go through the organization's channels. Keep in mind, however, that if you decide to go over your supervisor's head, you might shatter your career if you are labeled as a whistle blower. It is hoped this awesome decision will never be one that you have to make.

Responsibility is linked with loyalty. You are held accountable for your own actions and for those of the members in your department. You act irresponsibly when you do not do all that you can to prevent inappropriate staff behavior, blame others for your decisions, or expect more from staff than you are willing to do yourself (Johnson, 2009). Again, assessment of your level of responsibility and the expected accountability will help you maintain your moral integrity. It is also critical that you hold your staff accountable for their decisions and behaviors.

Before we move to the next section that will provide some ideas for maintaining moral integrity, we need to examine your most difficult challenge—facing evil. Johnson (2009) presents aspects of this threat to your moral integrity. He also presents ideas on how to combat it. First, you must acknowledge that evil exists and define it from an administrator's view. Evil is a force for the destruction of health, happiness, and community. It causes human suffering on many levels and destroys dignity. In order for you to understand the impact of evil, Johnson (2009) organizes it into categories including perverse enjoyment, deceit, and bureaucratic-approved injury and destruction. He also provides information on the role of choice and situational factors in the practice of evil. How do these categories relate to evil?

Evil can express itself as perverse enjoyment. For example, boredom can create situations where people seek alternatives that are more exciting or fill voids in their lives. They may seek enjoyment from the power of inflicting pain on others or having lives full of secret practices. Great harm can result if this behavior is exhibited by a member of the health-care profession.

Self-deception can also lead to evil behavior. For administrators, this could happen if they think of themselves as the higher force, as perfect and all-powerful. Controlling others' behavior and bending them to the administrators' will reinforces their **deceit**. However, their self-deception of omnipotence leads to actions that can destroy individuals and even the entire organization.

Bureaucratic or **administrative evil** happens when faith in technology, science, and the power of reason—devoid of compassion or conscience—becomes the driving force of a group, organization, or society. Ultimate faith in technology and science serves to remove you from the human part of your decisions and makes it easier for evil to exist. This belief also allows you to engage in daily operations that produce great pain and suffering for others without any sense of guilt or remorse.

Administrative evil has existed throughout time and explains many destructive actions in history. The classic example of this practice in modern times is the **extermination camps** that existed in World War II. Through daily operational functions (e.g., providing on-time transportation, building campsites, collecting taxes, and compiling records), civil servants supported and enabled the death camps to execute their deadly work. These citizens did not view their role as evil at all. They were merely doing their jobs with business as usual and paying attention to their profit margin.

Caplan (1992), in *When Medicine Went Mad*, brings the role of administrative evil in the holocaust even closer to home. He presents the case that certain elements of German society went beyond compliance with government policy. The medical community, through its scientists, physicians, and administrators, actually designed and implemented many of the government's destructive programs. These endeavors were focused on racial hygiene and extinction of whole populations. The medical community viewed these programs as highly ethical since they were designed to prevent the degeneration of the human race via genetic contamination. Sterilization laws, euthanasia, ghettos, and eventually the death camps were all part of this effort. Technology made this evil much more horrific because it increased efficiency; more people could be killed with less gas, thereby improving the bottom line. It also removed people from the process so that they could deny its existence even when it occurred in their villages and towns.

Johnson also presents the category of "evil as sanctioned destruction" (2009, p. 107). In this view, evil occurs when you give direct or implied permission to victimize others. Victimization is deemed acceptable when the group or individual is not viewed as a valued member of society. Such action violates all of the ethical principles you have studied. However, if you are not careful, it can be business as usual for health care. It is not always easy to treat each person with dignity when you see pain and suffering every day. You might experience compassion fatigue and grow angry about the choices people make that imperil their health. It is especially frustrating when these choices also adversely affect your bottom line. Without reminders that your true mission should recognize the worth of all human beings, it would be so easy to deny care or treat only those whom you decide are the "deserving poor." Johnson (2009) reminds you that even small dose of this evil, such as **labeling** those you find undesirable (e.g., GOMER, Frequent Flier). can lead to a loss of dignity. Even if you never use any of these labels, if you laugh at them among yourselves or remain silent when you hear them, you are supporting sanctioned destruction.

Johnson (2009) also notes that evil occurs through a series of choices rather than just one event. Even small choices can have large moral consequences. Therefore, it is imperative that you determine why you are choosing one option over another and think about the consequences of your choices. A rush to decision can lead to a wrong action that is both morally and fiscally unsound. However, as you build your moral integrity, it will become easier to discriminate between a good choice and one that can have negative consequences. As in any skill, practice makes positive choices easier to make.

■ MAINTAINING YOUR MORAL INTEGRITY

The previous section demonstrated that moral integrity is not genetic. It is developed through education, experience, self-assessment, and decision-making. As in other areas of administration, you must create a lifelong commitment to cultivating and supporting your moral base. The following are suggestions from a variety of experts to assist you with this process.

Griffith (1993), a well-respected leader and educator in health administration, believes that you can be moral and still be successful in healthcare leadership. This is particularly important as you advance in your career and assume higher administrative positions. When you achieve these higher positions, you will serve as a moral beacon for those who follow you and for your community. You will not have the option to hide your commitment to doing what is right, and you will be known by your moral convictions.

Griffith also challenges you to administer your department or organization in a way that fosters integrity. This includes designing policies and procedures that encourage doing the right thing. Make it easy and nonpunitive for staff to identify and report problems, and be willing to act on these reports. Build working groups who do not jump to the first solution, but take the time to ask, "What is the right thing to do?" Be sure that you are not a moral hypocrite and that you truly put patients first instead of just writing it in your mission statement.

He encourages you to use true participative management. This means truly delegating both the task and the responsibility to your team. It also means that you provide rewards to those who deserve them and not just give them to those who curry favor. Certainly, Griffith (1993) asks much of you, but the benefits for your organization and your career are worth the effort.

Purtilo and Criss (2005) devote an entire chapter to advice on how to survive in health care and keep your moral integrity at the same time. The principle of beneficence means that you must act with kindness and charity for others. This also means that you should treat yourself with kindness. Therefore, you have a duty toward self-care that, if honored, will enable you to function at your optimum level of moral integrity. This duty also entails giving yourself permission to care for your own needs as well as those of others. While the necessity of taking care of you might seem obvious, many find it difficult. Perhaps, the professional socialization process has been too effective. Healthcare professionals can feel guilty when they address their own needs. Some have even been known to come to work when they are ill. While this might seem to be noble, it actually is not. They are in fact increasing the risk of illness for their colleagues and patients.

You are also challenged to strengthen your personal moral integrity (Purtilo and Criss, 2005) through what I will call personal quality improvement (PQI) efforts. For example, take responsibility to engage in activities that improve who you are as a person. This will not only make you more interesting but also increase your resources when your integrity is challenged. You should also think about all the time you spend at work or thinking about work. Is it in balance with the time you spend on other aspects of your life? What are you doing to recharge your moral batteries? Do you spend enough time doing what you really love or being with those you truly love?

I am reminded of a remarkable person who came to speak to my students. He was a chaplain in a hospice program and spoke to the class about his work. At the time, his clients ranged in age from 4 to 98, and he spoke about how he supported each of them through the end of their lives. One of my students asked him, "How do you deal with all of this as a person? How do you keep a sense of balance?" His answer is still with me. He said, "When I play, I play. I take time to be away from work physically and emotionally. I use the time to recharge." When was the last time you played? Even a small "time-out" can help you gain better balance and a chance to maintain your moral integrity. From my research and observation, balance is critical to maintaining your personal and professional integrity. Without balance, the stress of your job can lead you to make those snap decisions that can lead to ethical erosion and shadow-side leadership.

Be vigilant about your moral integrity—never take it for granted. Be careful to take time for self-assessment and think about your strengths, weaknesses, and moral bottom line. This process should help you avoid being deluded by self-deception. Self-deception is not just about lying to yourself. It includes decisions like choosing to be ignorant, ignoring the unpleasant, becoming emotionally distant, and rationalizing your behavior. Being true to yourself is not easy, but it has great long-term payoffs for a life well lived.

Summary

This discussion provides some insight into moral integrity and its maintenance difficulties. Our culture does not always reward those who maintain moral integrity, but I am hopeful. As I write this, the news is filled with stories about the "miracle on the Hudson." Stories abound about how the captain of the doomed plane not only glided it to a safe landing, but also made sure that all passengers were off before he left. He is being honored for his skill and his integrity.

As a HCA, you have the power to affect something important. If you believe what you have read, you will agree that trust is the basic commodity of your business. Because you are the organization to the community, you can help to restore trust in the healthcare system and its organizations through your actions as an administrator. Admittedly, it will not be easy. You will have to make a conscious choice on a daily basis to cultivate and maintain your moral integrity. You will have to be courageous enough to do what is right even if you do not personally benefit from that decision. You will also have to be willing to base your reputation on the moral position that you take. You can help to create a working environment where moral integrity becomes the norm rather than the exception. The last section of this chapter gives you challenges and ideas to assist in maintaining your lifelong efforts to serve health care as a moral leader.

Ten Challenges for Maintaining Moral Integrity

The following 10 challenges are designed to assist your process of refining and maintaining your professional moral integrity. Each of the challenges requires introspection and a time commitment to reap positive benefits. I have included some comments under each of the challenges to give you additional insights and encouragement. This list is one that you can revisit at different stages of your career and use to confirm or re-establish your moral center. It will also help you with the final challenges that are part of Chapter 15.

1. Prepare an answer to this question, "Why do I want a career in health administration?

   Comments

   On the surface, this seems like an easy question. Some of my students would jump to an answer and say, "So I can earn the big bucks and buy fast cars." Obviously, no one chooses a career in health administration to be poor—not even those who serve in public health where salaries are historically low. However, the "material goodies" do not compensate for having a job that does not satisfy you or, at the worst, one that you hate.

   Your reasons for wanting to be a part of this enormously challenging career are as individual as you are. However, when you get to the essence of most people's decisions to choose and remain in a career, you see two powerful forces. The first is to make a difference through service and the second is to engage in meaningful work.

   We can start with making a difference. What would happen if you chose a different career? Are there things that you can contribute through that job that will make a difference to your staff, your organization, and your community? When I consider these questions, I recall the root of the word "vocation." It actually means having a calling rather than finding a job. If you are called to health administration, it means that you are willing to stay there even when things are not so pleasant. It means that you are willing to make a commitment to prepare yourself intellectually and ethically so that you can make a difference. It also means that you are willing to go beyond the minimum or "duties as assigned" to accomplish what is needed. Your goal is to create a better organization for your staff, patients, and community and really make a difference.

   Of course, Frankl (1971) would encourage you to consider how your work contributes to your life's meaning. Meaning, he tells us, comes from what you take from the world, what you give to the world, and what you choose to love. When service becomes a focus of your work, you are more likely to view it as a source of meaning rather than as drudgery. In contrast, if you view your work as meaningless and see yourself as just another cog in a great bureaucratic wheel, you can exhibit poor performance, unnecessary stress, disloyalty, and even depression. It is easier to be a shadow leader or even to succumb to evil when your work has no meaning.

The key becomes how you find this meaning and a way to make a difference on a daily basis. First, as Frankl (1971) reminds us, you must always remember that you have a choice. You can choose to take even small actions that create a positive work environment. You can choose to be a role model for moral integrity through your actions. You can choose to make a lifelong commitment to moral integrity. It is also helpful to remember how important you really are to your staff and your organization. Although your profession does not get its own TV show like the clinical staff does, your actions make saving lives possible.

2. Conduct a personal moral integrity cost/benefits analysis.

Comments

Does this sound strange to you? First, I am not suggesting cost-benefits analysis in its traditional definition where dollar values are assigned. In my version, you assign a career "cost" to a decision to help you decide if it "benefits" your moral life. For example, you can draw up a table to help you make a decision whether or not to accept a job promotion. Then, by filling in the blank cells, you can do cost-benefits analysis to help you arrive at the best decision for your moral health. Your table might look list this.

Decision: State what you plan to do.

Moral costs for making the decision	Benefit for making the decision	Moral Costs for NOT making the decision	Benefits for NOT making the decision

Notice in my example that I included columns for not accepting the promotion. The cost-benefits analysis of not choosing an action can be just as beneficial to your moral health as choosing the action, but this option is not always considered.

A simple self-brainstorming technique can help you think about possible benefits and costs. Remember to think "big picture" and include your family in the benefits and/or costs. They are often the beneficiaries or bear the emotional and financial burdens of your decisions. You can also use this technique, in addition to your fiscal and risk analysis, to assist in making organizational decisions that involve moral issues.

3. Define your "moral bottom line."

    Comments

    This challenge is worthy of a television reality show. You are asked to establish the criteria that, if met, would cause you to resign from your job. It asks you to identify what you are really worth. Will you compromise when you know that your boss is doing something illegal? What if his or her action is legal but immoral? You might struggle with this for a while, but it is important for you to assess this area for your life career. Having this information can also help you decide whether to take a position in the first place. For example if, after doing your homework and participating in interviews, you detect something that would compromise your bottom line, your decision is easy. Do not take the job.

    Your moral bottom line does not have to be solely about things that would cause you to resign. You need to identify those principles that will cause you to take action or speak out in meetings, even if it makes you unpopular. Because no one wants to be known as a complainer—or worse, a snitch—this is also a difficult assessment to make. The thing to remember is that failure to speak up or to provide a different view can actually lead to disaster. In several textbooks, this failure is called groupthink. It exists when no one wants to say anything that might offend the leader or appear to be disloyal. The result is a decision based on incomplete or erroneous information and can be a disaster for the leader and the organization. So, it becomes very important for you to assess and articulate these principles. The last thing you want to have to say is, "I knew and I should have said something."

4. Engage in directed activities to build and maintain your moral integrity.

    Comments

    There is a variety of options available for taking on this challenge. However, all of them are useless unless you make a choice to do them. In your already busy world, it might seem unreasonable to take on yet another "thing to do," but the payback is worth the effort. Remember to start small and simple so you will make this practice a part of your daily life (just like showering or brushing your teeth).

Palmer (2000) suggests several techniques that can be used for moral integrity. First, you can try keeping a journal. This technique is a variation of "freedom of speech." You are free to write anything without any censor or restriction. You do not need any special books or tools, just paper and pen or computer. You do not have to write in your journal every day. However, it is a good idea to set aside time to write an entry at least once a week.

You can use a rhetorical question to gear your journal toward your moral integrity issues. Any question or issue that is of concern to you will do. You can ask yourself, "What is morality to me?," "What is the moral way of dealing with this situation?" or, "Who could be hurt if I make this decision?" Then just write. Keep writing until you have captured all of your thoughts about your question. I usually set my journal aside for a day or so, then go back, and read it. There is often some practical wisdom in my musings that can really help my decision-making. I also save my journals and read about former areas of concern. This review helps me see how much I have grown as a person.

Reflection is also a way to foster growth in moral integrity. Reflection usually requires a trigger event or source to guide it and gear it toward moral issues. You can use actions of others and think about what you would have done if faced with that situation. You can use events in the news and reflect about the moral issues that relate to them. Certainly, with all of the corporate and personal scandals that have eroded trust in American business, sports, and even churches, you should not lack sources for moral integrity reflection.

Sources for reflection do not have to come from the work setting. The arts can provide some great reflection opportunities. For example, photography captures a point in time and can lead you to muse about morality and growth. You can look at the photo and ask, "What would I have done or felt at that point in time?" Similarly, movies can illustrate many areas of moral and immoral behavior for consideration. In fact, Johnson (2009) features many movies in his book and provides ethical thematic analyses of them. His suggestions include *Dead Man Walking*, *Twelve Angry Men*, and *Schindler's List*. I am sure you can find many more examples, including movies that relate specifically to health care such as *Patch Adams*. Regardless of your choice, take time to reflect on what critical moral decisions the characters experienced and what they did. How did the decisions affect the person and the organization? What would you have done in that situation?

Do not neglect the power of literature to create areas for reflection. I particularly like poetry because it can affect me emotionally as well as intellectually. One of my favorites is *A Brave and Startling*

Truth by Maya Angelou. I have also had great conversations about moral integrity that centered on novels and short stories. You can find book clubs that reflect on the moral issues presented in a specific novel. If you do not have time to read for "fun," then use your journal entries to spark this process. The main idea is to think about your moral integrity and its practice. You cannot assume integrity will be there without taking direct action to help it grow.

5. Identify a moral mentor.

Comments

Do you know a person whom you consider a highly moral leader? Is there someone who could serve as your moral mentor or as a role model for you? You have already heard about the benefits of mentoring in some of your courses. Perhaps some of you have completed internships or residencies where you were assigned a mentor. This person taught you the inner workings of the organization and made your transition easier. A moral mentor, however, is someone who is willing to go beyond sharing information about how things work. He or she is willing to hear and understand your deepest professional concerns in confidence and provide guidance without judgment.

Because the healthcare system increases in complexity almost daily, it will be normal for you to have concerns and questions about the right thing to do. It is possible that you do not want to "lose face" by expressing them too publicly. This is where a moral mentor can be invaluable to your career. He or she will let you think through your options and conduct a verbal moral cost/benefits analysis. Your mentor will not solve your problem for you but will guide you in selecting your best plan of action.

How will you find a moral mentor? First, be observant. Observe how people interact with their staff. Are their behaviors consistent with their words? Can they be trusted? Second, when you identify such a person, take time to get to know him or her. See what he or she is like in a variety of settings. Is this someone you can trust?

If the answer is "yes," make an appointment to talk with this person. Ask if he or she will be your moral mentor, and observe the reaction. If there is any reluctance, do not pursue it further. It has been my experience that if you choose carefully, the person will be honored to be your mentor. However, keep in mind that your mentor has many other duties. Do not abuse the privilege of having a personal adviser by engaging in "whine sessions" or "pity parties." Instead, come to your mentor with the tough decisions and listen to his or her wisdom. The advice you receive will be a valuable asset to cultivate and maintain your moral integrity.

6. Examine your life experiences (successes and failures) and find their moral lessons.

Comments

This is a difficult challenge. It is easiest to start with your successes. You all have had shining moments when you achieved your goals and made yourself and your family proud. List those accomplishments and next to them write the moral lessons you learned from them. For example, one of my shining moments was the first time my major professor called me, "Dr. Morrison." Because I was working full-time and raising a family, completing my doctorate was not easy. So this moment meant a great deal to me. My moral lessons were that everything has a price, but the price was worth it. I also learned to follow my heart, even when I was tempted to give up.

Now look at the areas of which you are not so proud. All of you have actions you wish you had not taken, decisions you wish you had not made, or words you wish you had not said. For this part of the challenge, you need to list at least some of these areas. Because they are in your past, you cannot change any of them. However, some good can still occur from these experiences. Beside each item on your list, think about a lesson that you learned from this experience and write it down.

Finally, go beyond just writing. Use these lessons, regardless of where you learned them. They can help you in the future by teaching you what to do and avoid doing. In taking this last step, you can increase your moral integrity through the analysis of your own experiences.

7. Design a prevention plan to avoid moral derailment.

Comments

As you increase your success in your career, unfortunately there will be increased potential for moral derailment or moving closer to the shadow side of leadership. All of us have aspects of our personalities or behaviors that can cause us to derail as administrators. You need to have a plan to avoid derailment and understand its causes.

First, you need to think about who you really are as a person. For example, how do you feel about power? You already have it or will have it. Without power, you could not be in an administrative position. However, what will happen when your power increases? Will power become the center of your life, or will you maintain your judgment and humility? Will you use your power to help others or to benefit yourself alone? The answers to these questions need to be formulated before power becomes an issue, and they should come from introspection, as you look deep into your heart.

What about the privileges that stem from your position? They can be a great temptation if you put too much value on them. They can also lead to shadow leadership if you see your possessions as a reflection of who you are. How much is enough for you? Are you what you wear and what you drive? While you will no doubt live comfortably as a HCA, you are part of a culture that puts great emphasis on externals rather than people. You might be tempted to buy the latest car or the best piece of real estate.

One of the many lessons that the events of September 11, 2001, taught us is that impressive creations and material possessions can be taken away in an instant. However, as the death toll rose on that tragic day, what turned out to be of utmost importance were compassion, service, and heroism. These remained even when buildings were rubble. Perhaps there are moral integrity lessons to be learned from the loss of privilege as well as from gaining it.

Another way to move toward the shadows of leadership is through deceit. However, it is not just about lying to others or covering up the misdeeds of those in higher positions. Sometimes we practice self-deception as leaders. McGinn (2005) expresses the caution that the ability for self-deception is almost limitless. You will be required to make difficult decisions when the solution is not easy to implement. In order to be successful in these cases, you must be able to stand up to pressure, motivate yourself, and have courage. Practicing self-honesty instead of self-deception requires that you take time to think. Ideally, you should have a minimum of 30 minutes per day to be alone and practice self-reflection. While this can seem like just another demand on your time, it pays off in terms of more effective and morally sound decisions for yourself and your organization.

McGinn (2005) discusses another shadow area that can easily trap you—complacency. When you become too comfortable with your job, you can cause yourself trouble. Complacency, he asserts, happens when you are too confident and become saturated with your success. It can also happen when you stop paying attention to the signs that warn you of trouble. When you are complacent, you think everything is just fine when, in reality, you might be in a downward spiral.

McGinn suggests that you stay away from the shadow of complacency by pushing yourself to make a difference and not just to do a job. You need to find a way to measure your success and use obstacles as challenges and opportunities. I agree with McGinn that caring about your work to the point of being passionate about it helps you avoid complacency. If you are passionate about the work, you will always want to learn more and strive for higher goals. Frankl (1971) would ask, "What makes your work meaningful?" Finding the answer to that question will help you avoid complacency because, if your work is part of your life's meaning, you cannot take it for granted.

8. Engage in PQI.

Comments

You remember that PQI is my morality version of the total quality improvement/continuous quality improvement process. Think of your life beyond the work environment. Do you have a life fully lived? Do you work to live or live to work? McGinn (2005) suggests that you need a "work/life synergy" (p. 59) where your life and work augment each other. Your life experiences contribute to your overall moral integrity by providing physical, mental, emotional, and spiritual resources. You can bring these resources to your job.

Just how does this happen? Start with the most obvious: your physical health. Because you have only one body, you will want to keep it as healthy as possible for as long as possible. However, your body cannot accomplish this task without your cooperation. It means that you must do what you counsel others to do: eat in moderation, exercise, take time to rest, and sleep. Yet, too often we think of physical selves as the exception. We ask our bodies to function without even the minimum of care. The truth is that you cannot take time for moral reasoning (or any kind of reasoning, for that matter) when you are tired, hungry, and out of shape.

Consider your mental and emotional health. Are you learning and experiencing new things, or fighting to keep everything the same? In health care, we have no choice but to be lifelong learners. The changes happen too fast not to be on an active learning curve. Consider your emotional side. Health care makes demands on you in that area as well. Yet, you cannot afford to get too blue, lonely, and stressed. Your effectiveness as a leader would surely be compromised.

To rejuvenate your emotional resources means to take time out for recreation. Do you remember my story about the chaplain? He took time to renew his mind and his emotional health through play. When was the last time you played? Hemsath and Yerkes (1997) created an entire book called *301 Ways to Have Fun at Work*. Their examples come from highly successful corporations and illustrate the impact of fun on morale and productivity. You have a life beyond work. What activities can you do to renew your resources? My students are able to create long lists of these activities. Actually doing them becomes their challenge.

Social health is also a component for building moral integrity. We all learn from our friends, especially those who know us well enough to be caring and honest. You might not always like what you hear, but when it comes from your friend's heart, it is worth hearing. Friends listen even when they have heard you talk about something many times. Having this empathetic sounding board is critical to your moral development because it lets you process your thoughts in a nonjudgmental and supportive environment.

There is a caution here. You cannot have this level of friendship without investing time and energy with your friends. It cannot be one-sided. Sometimes this means that you have to be the one to listen even when you do not feel like it. It can also mean that you have to show up and support someone when you would rather do something else. For true friendships to exist, they must be cultivated.

There are so many writings about emotional health and its care that we would need another book just for this topic. There are two concepts that have been especially helpful for me in my roles in health administration. One is a phrase from a Beatles song: "Let it be." Sometimes you just have to let go of whomever or whatever is causing you emotional stress. This is especially true if it happened in the past, because you cannot change the outcome. I try to ask myself, "Did I do everything I could about the situation that was so stressful?" If my answer is "yes," then I know that I should let it go. I also use the phrase, "It is not about me," to remember that there are always at least two sides of a situation. This realization helps when you get a reaction that is not expected or when people say things that are rude or hurtful. Maybe they are having a bad day and the reaction has nothing to do with you. Try not to take it personally; this axiom is often used in business. Often, this is easier said than done, but reminding yourself that you might not be the source of the problem does help with maintaining positive emotional health.

9. Have a rich and varied spiritual life.

Comments

I mentioned spiritual health as a component of PQI. Your spiritual well-being is so tightly connected to maintaining your moral integrity that it presents its own challenge. Johnson (2009) gives a model for your spiritual maturation that is similar in some ways to the Kohlberg model of moral development. This model gives insights about the process you can use to become spiritually centered. Reflecting on your beliefs, understanding your part in the world, and learning to deal with life's struggles and disappointments are all part of this process. Johnson also gives some specifics for exploring your internal and external spiritual health.

Spirituality that you practice in private can be enhanced through contemplation using either the Western tradition (connecting to God) or the Eastern (opening your mind). Prayer or connecting to a higher spiritual center, or what Frankl (1971) calls the ultimate meaning, is also a part of this process. Prayer helps you to concentrate on your spiritual issues and learn patience. Johnson (2009) includes study as part of private spirituality. This technique helps you to concentrate and explore various concepts related to spiritual health. Study includes reading and being present in nature as inspirational sources.

Spirituality that you practice in public can get you back to basics. If you can learn to bypass the glitz and dig deep into what is important, you can have a deeper spiritual experience. For some, this can mean divesting themselves of things that once seemed so important, but that now feel like burdens. Living more simply allows more time and energy to live more spiritually.

Johnson (2009) suggests that you spend time alone, in silence, and in service as techniques for spiritual growth. The discipline of solitude is very difficult for most Americans because we live in such a sensory-saturated environment. Still, the effort to find time for solitude can reward you with insight and ways to maintain your spiritual balance. Service is a major component of your public spirituality. Johnson defines it as putting others first when you are not rewarded for doing so. Your motivation is not recognition. Instead, you practice altruism in the fullest sense of that word. When you are engaged in service just because it is needed, you will find gratitude for the experience and be humbled by what you learn.

10. Work to create a climate of moral integrity.

Comments

This last challenge asks you to go beyond yourself and provide an opportunity for others to experience their own moral growth. You can provide a workplace where moral action is considered the way things are done. Such a workplace might be counter to our current culture. Those who strive to become better people or to treat everyone with respect might be viewed as trying to be "holier-than-thou." Conversely, they might be considered naïve for not taking advantage of their power. Cheating, dishonesty, and other moral flaws are sometimes mistaken as good actions when they get you ahead of the next person. However, can you imagine trying to manage a department where everyone is out to get everyone else? Where would that lead?

Part of the creation of a morally centered workplace starts with you because, as the leader, you model the actions that you expect from others. Your behavior sets the climate for what is acceptable and what is not. For example, if you say you believe in diversity, then you must put together teams with this in mind. While you might not get much ego stroking from this, you could get answers to problems that really work. If you say that patient care is your real mission, you must do all you can to make this a reality.

Johnson (2009) advocates using practice-based "servant leadership" as a way to increase moral integrity in your department. This means that although you are a leader, you are also a servant to your staff in that you care, listen, accept, grow, and build community. Viewing staff as an asset instead of a liability can go a long way toward creating the trust needed for a morally centered workplace. Some bosses will criticize you for being a servant leader because they think you will lose control over "your people." These leaders (and bullies) prefer to use intimidation and fear to keep staff in line. The use of force and fear are only productive for a limited time and as a tactic do not work for all employees. The best way to lead is to understand the people with whom you work. Then you can choose the best way to work together so that goals can be met for the benefit of patients and the organization as a whole.

These 10 challenges are not easy ones; they will take time and thought. I hope that you will continuously work on them after you complete your course and enter the workplace. The ideas that these challenges generate will assist you with the major challenges that are presented in Chapter 15. Remember that this is a process, so be patient with yourself and others. The rewards for making this journey can be life affirming and life giving.

Web Resources

The Holocaust and Administrative Evil
http://www.ushmm.org/

A Brave and Startling Truth, by Maya Angelou
http://www.inspirationpeak.com/poetry/bravetruth.html

References

Caplan, A. L. (Ed.). (1992). *When medicine went mad: Bioethics and the holocaust.* Totowa, NJ: Humana.

Darr, K. (2005). *Ethics in health services management* (4th ed.). Baltimore: Health Professions Press.

Dye, C. F. (2000). *Leadership in healthcare: Values at the top.* Chicago: Health Administration Press.

Frankl, V. (1971). *Man's search for meaning: An introduction to logotherapy*. New York: Pocket Books.

Gilbert, J. A. (2007). *Strengthening ethical wisdom: Tools for transforming your health care organization*. Chicago: Health Administration Press.

Griffith, J. R. (1993). *The moral challenges of health care management*. Ann Arbor, MI: Health Professions Press.

Hemsath, D., & Yerkes, L. (1997). *301 ways to have fun at work*. San Francisco: Berrett-Koehler.

Hofmann, P. B. (2006). Evaluating ethical fitness. *Healthcare Executive*, 21(3), 34–35.

Johnson, C. E. (2009). *Meeting the ethical challenges of leadership: Casting light or shadow* (3rd ed.). Thousand Oaks, CA: Sage.

McGinn, P. (2005). *Leading others, managing yourself*. Chicago: Health Administration Press.

Palmer, P. J. (2000). *Let your life speak*. San Francisco: Jossey-Bass.

Purtilo, R. B., & Criss, M. L. (2005). *Ethical dimensions in the health professions* (4th ed.). Philadelphia: Elsevier Saunders.

Summers, J. (2009). Theory of healthcare ethics. In E. E. Morrison (Ed.). *Health care ethics: Critical issues for the 21st century*. Sudbury, MA: Jones and Bartlett, pp. 3–40.

CHAPTER 14

Codes of Ethics and Administrative Practice

In the arena of human life the honors and rewards fall to those who show their good qualities in action.

—Aristotle

Points to Ponder

1. Why do professional groups and associations create codes of ethics?
2. What are the key features of your professional code of ethics?
3. What can you learn from the codes of other health professionals?
4. What are the limitations of codes of ethics?
5. How can you apply your professional code to your practice as a healthcare administrator (HCA)?

Words to Remember

The following is a list of key words for this chapter. You will find them in bold in the text. Stop and check your understanding of them.

ACHE Code of Ethics
professional socialization

ethical policy statements
self-regulating

■ INTRODUCTION TO CODES OF ETHICS FOR PROFESSIONALS

Why you need to have a code of ethics if you are a professional? Are you not a moral person who knows what is right and wrong? While you may have excellent ethical wisdom in most cases, practicing as an administrator in health care will present new ethical quagmires. You will need resources to assist you in making the best decision when these situations occur. One of these tools is a professional code of ethics.

In addition, you should remember that healthcare professionals have great power over people. Because of this power, codes have been developed, based on ethics theory and principles, to delineate their responsibilities. This delimitation is an attempt to prevent the abuse of professional power. Codes have also been used to describe the necessary characteristics for membership in a professional group. For example, in addition to describing acceptable moral conduct, a code may tell you the appropriate title for you to use. It may also spell out how or when you can advertise. In health care, professional codes of ethics do not replace those developed by the organization in which you are employed or those mandated by external organizations such as the Joint Commission on Accreditation of Healthcare Organizations and the American Hospital Association. Rather, they provide guidelines for your deportment as a professional within an organizational setting.

The major code of ethics for your practice as a HCA was developed through the American College of Healthcare Executives (ACHE), and it defines expectations for your ethical conduct as a professional. You will study the features of this code including its practice guidelines so that you are more aware of the expectations for assuming the title of HCA. You will also survey features of examples of codes from other groups of professionals and consider their wisdom for your own field of practice. To balance the discussion, you will review the limitations and criticisms that have been made about the professionals' codes. Finally, you will be presented with five challenges that will help you define what a code of ethics means to your future practice of administration.

■ WHY BOTHER WITH CODES OF ETHICS?

In healthcare administration, you will continually face situations where an ethical course of action is not clear. In fact, these gray areas can be so disturbing that they cause you to lose sleep at night. Codes of ethics are tools that can give you greater guidance and wisdom for making decisions. They are based on the theories and principles of ethics and on experiences of leaders in your profession. Codes of ethics also serve as prevention or "ethics vitamin" that sets boundaries for acceptable behaviors. This should assist you in avoiding some of the quagmires and shadow areas that could jeopardize your career. Of course, this assumes that you know your code and try to live your professional life according to its tenets.

How do you learn to be a professional? First, you must understand what it means to be a professional. The community assumes that, if you are a professional, you are highly competent, well educated, and highly ethical. The process creating you as a professional is called **professional socialization** and requires study, role modeling, and practice experiences. Becoming a professional often requires years of study to master a body of knowledge that is germane to your particular field. It may also require that you pass a comprehensive examination that demonstrates your basic understanding of your profession's knowledge. In addition, being a professional may require meeting the requirements for licensure and functioning under a practice act that limits your actions. Another major component of being a professional is to have a code of ethics. As an aspiring professional, you must be thoroughly familiar with your particular code of ethics.

Worthley (1999) presents information about organizational codes of ethics that can also be applied to your professional behavior. Codes are not just words; they are designed to regulate your actions. This is particularly evident when they are a part of practice legislation for licensure. In this situation, violations of the codes can lead to punitive action including being stripped of the license to practice. As an HCA, you are not licensed and do not currently face this aspect of regulation through codes.

However, Worthley's (1999) second function of codes does apply to you. Codes serve as a standard of practice that assists you in knowing your profession's expectations. This knowledge can be used as a tool for problem solving. Worthley (1999) suggests that there are certain criteria that must be met if these standards are to prove useful in practice. First, as you read earlier, you must know that they exist. This sounds almost silly, but you would be surprised how many professionals are clueless about the standards under which they practice. Second, you must understand what the standard is asking of you and be able to implement it. For this reason, the standard must be based on actions, not just theory, and remain reasonably stable over time. You cannot adhere to standards if they change too rapidly or capriciously. Finally, to be useful, the code must assist you with real practice issues. Without these features, a code becomes just a theoretical document with no relevance for your daily life as an HCA.

Codes are the most commonly used ethical device for professionals (Johnson, 2009). They help to define your position on ethical issues and provide an expectation for those who interact with you. If you use them, codes provide some protection from lawsuits and increasing external regulation. As an HCA, your goal is to be **self-regulating**. This means that you make the choice to maintain high standards of practice because it is the right thing to do. You are not behaving ethically just to avoid an encounter with the law. If you truly self-regulate, the public will put an extraordinary amount of trust in you. However, self-regulation is not absolute. If enough HCAs violate the trust placed in them through a lack of self-regulation, the public will demand that you be licensed like many other health professionals.

Codes of ethics help you resist behaviors that can lead you toward the shadow side of administration (Chapter 13). However, to be effective, they must contain certain features (Johnson, 2009). First, they must explain the minimal standard of acceptable behavior rather than make global statements. For example, the **ACHE Code of Ethics** (2007a) includes specific areas of concern for professional behavior. Supplementary materials called policy statements are also found on the ACHE Web site. These statements delineate the organization's recommended actions for specific situations. The ACHE Code of Ethics is revised frequently, with the most recent major review and changes in 2003 (Squazzo, 2008)

Codes can help you act responsibly when they are designed for everyday practice if they use unambiguous language. They should also be based on moral principles and theories that you can identify. By following the code, you should be able to decide on appropriate action and explain the rationale behind your action. Codes should be living documents you use in your practice and not just something that you memorized for a test. They should be an important tool for operations and discussed frequently with fellow professionals. Finally, codes should be relevant and assist you in formulating your ethics position on issues that affect your profession, organization, and community.

Ethics has not always been the center of healthcare business practices, but self-regulation has always been expected (Darr, 2005). Codes for professionals serve to assist administrators who "want to do the right thing but need help determining what it is" (p. 62). For professional codes to be of benefit, they must be included in the educational process. However, if you are educated about them, but do not use them; they cannot serve as a resource. This is why Darr stresses your need for continuing education and discussion about ethics issues and codes.

In summary, no document is perfect, but the knowledge and use of an ethics code can assist you in determining the standards and expectations for conduct. It allows you to use your title with the full understanding of what it means to those in your profession and in the community. A code also protects you against others who choose not to abide by professional standards and helps you "know them by their deeds." The choice to avoid association with these kinds of HCAs can protect your reputation and that of your organization. It also challenges you to practice self-regulation by not hiring unethical individuals and by taking action against their behaviors when necessary.

When appropriately written, codes provide guidance for decisions in the gray areas of health care. They can be used to foster a more ethics-based workplace by allowing you to be consistent in your actions and to educate others about your standards of performance. Remember that your words and actions have great power and that, as the leader, you set the moral tone for your workplace. If you are consistent with your own professional code, staff will have a better understanding of how you will make decisions and the rationale for those decisions. This understanding should be accompanied by greater support for you as a leader and for the decisions that you make. Finally, codes make it easier for you to avoid the shadow areas of leadership by giving you a fall-back position and a way to avoid future difficulties. They allow you to decide not to take a position on issues that might be a violation of your ethics code.

■ CODE OF ETHICS FOR THE AMERICAN COLLEGE OF HEALTHCARE EXECUTIVES

As HCAs, you can use the ACHE Code of Ethics as a mechanism for knowing the standards and practices of your profession. The ACHE Code of Ethics and Ethical Policy Statements can be found on the Web site listed in this chapter. These documents are reviewed by the ACHE ethics committee and updated frequently. Notice that in the ACHE Code, your primary ethical duty is to serve those who seek health care. You fulfill this duty by working to create a better healthcare system in any way you can. You are also obligated to consider more than the financials when you make decisions. The community's rights and needs must also be a part of your decision-making because you serve as a "moral advocate" (ACHE, 2007a, para. 6).

The Code (ACHE, 2007a) divides your responsibilities into eight areas involving the needs of your profession, patients, organization, employees, and community. Further clarification of your responsibilities and behaviors is included under each area. For example, you have a duty to your profession to act in a manner that honors it. You must also be careful not to use your power and knowledge to further your own finances or betray professional confidences. Avoidance of conflicts of interest is also expected.

As part of your duty to the patient, you are supposed to protect individual rights and resolve the conflicts when patients' and staff values differ. Protecting patients' rights also means that you preserve autonomy, protect confidentiality, and do not tolerate abuse. Quality assurance is also viewed as part of your duty to the patient because it serves to provide an environment where the best patient care is possible.

You also owe a duty to the organization in which you are employed. This involves being truthful in your communications, implementing a code of ethics for the organization, and providing the resources for the staff when ethics issues arise. You are to be vigilant about your accounting practices to avoid fraud and abuse. When considering employees, you have an obligation to create a place where ethics is the norm. You must also protect employees from harassment and create a safe environment where they can use their talents to benefit patient care.

Finally, the Code (ACHE, 2007a) provides examples of your duty to the community. You are to provide information that allows the community to make informed decisions about your services. There is an obligation to assess the community's healthcare needs and work to provide access to needed services. While maintaining a strong fiscal position, your organization is supposed to be an advocate for actions that improve community health.

You can certainly see that the ACHE Code demands much from you as a professional. These demands are made because you have a great deal of influence and power and you represent both your profession and your organization to the public. When you are a member of ACHE, you are held to standards defined by this organization. Complaints about ethics violations can be made against you, and the College has a detailed process for dealing with complaints. The ACHE Ethics Committee has several actions it can take, including censure and expulsion from the organization. While these actions do not carry the same weight as a loss of the licensure, they can have a negative effect on your career. For example, you might not receive positive consideration for new positions, particularly those in higher levels, if you are not in good standing with the College.

The ACHE goes beyond the code to provide you with **ethical policy statements**. These statements serve as "mini white papers" on issues that affect your personal and organizational ethics. They define the College's position on each issue and give recommendations for action. One example that I find particularly interesting is their statement about ethical decision-making (ACHE, 2007b). This document reinforces the expectation that you will be a leader who practices eudaimonia and ethical wisdom. It encourages you to foster ethical decision-making in your healthcare settings and offers suggestions for practice. These include offering educational programs on ethical practice and decision-making, maintaining an ethics committee with members who have diverse views, and evaluating processes for addressing ethics issues.

In addition to the Code and Policy Statements, ACHE offers several other ethics resources through its Web site. These resources, called the Ethics Toolkit, include a self-assessment instrument. This scale measures the frequency with which you engage in behaviors that reflect compliance with the Code. Any answer that falls below the "usually frequent" should be given your attention. Of course, as with any other self-assessment, this instrument is only as valid as the honesty with which you answer its items.

In addition, the ACHE Web site provides a list of resources and Web sites to assist you with your ethics concerns. A copy of Nelson's (2005) article on ethics decision-making is included on the Web site. This article is particularly useful because it includes an eight-step process for making sound ethics decisions. Steps require you to clarify the situation, determine affected stakeholders, and research the circumstances. In addition, you should determine the ethics principles involved, consider possible options, and select the best possible decision. Finally, Nelson suggests that you communicate the decision and use it in your organization. Of course, you will want to evaluate the action to determine if it solved the problem. Nelson cites the ACHE Ethics Toolkit and the Web site as resources to assist you in decision-making.

While the ACHE Code (ACHE, 2007a) and the Toolkit provide you with guidance concerning the expected behavior for an HCA, it is not perfect. Some of the eight areas can be too vague to provide you with actual performance standards (Darr, 2005). However, if a code is too detailed, it becomes legalistic and loses its voluntary direction for ethical behavior. The issue in developing a code is to balance specificity with flexibility.

What should you do with this Code? Darr (2005) suggests that your role is to safeguard the public against potential abuse from the healthcare system. To accomplish this mission, you need well-identified, professional standards and the ability to act on those standards. Therefore, you must use the Code as a tool for self-regulation, even if you are not a member of ACHE. Failure to protect the public and to regulate your own practice can lead to loss of licensure and additional regulation by external agencies. Darr also encourages you to use the ACHE Code because professional integrity is essential for your career progress. Adherence to its basic principles will help you maintain employee and community trust. Finally, using a set of standards should help you be a person of integrity even when there is no financial reward for doing so. Darr considers this to be "the right thing to do—it is a principle for life and the profession" (p. 90).

■ LEARNING FROM OTHER CODES

Many HCAs are "bicodal." By this, I mean that they are members of clinical professions as well as being HCAs. In their education, they have learned the Code of Ethics that is specific to their profession. These HCAs must honor the tenets of both the ACHE Code of Ethics and those of their profession, in addition to the policies of the organization where they work. There is always some congruence between the codes, and therefore application may be simple. Areas like integrity, honesty, appropriate communication, respect for others, and confidentiality are common features among virtually all the ethics codes. However, problems can arise if a provision is in conflict with the organization's mission. As an HCA, you must find a way to make the codes compatible with the policies of the organization, in order to arrive at the best interests of the patient and the community.

Darr (2005) and others go on to say that, even if you are not bicodal, you can enhance your job as an HCA by familiarizing yourself with the ethics codes of the many other professionals who work under the aegis of the same organization. The Center for the Study of Ethics in the Professions (CSEP) (2008) cites ethics from hundreds of occupations with over 50 from the field of health care. Their Web address is included in the Web Resources at the end of this chapter. While it would be educational to examine all 50 codes, the following section offers examples from the ethics codes particular to some of the healthcare professions. These examples will be followed by lessons that an HCA can learn and apply to running an organization that is ethical to patients, clinical staff, and the community.

Code of Ethics for Nurses

The Code of Ethics for Nurses from the American Nurses Association (ANA) (2005) has nine provisions, each with detailed subsections on the subject of moral integrity. For the purposes of this text, I will paraphrase samples of the statutes within Provision 5 on what nurses must do to keep a high standard of moral integrity.

In addition to their duty to their patients, the organization, the profession, and the community, nurses are charged with a duty to themselves. This duty includes the practice of self-respect. One of many ways to achieve self-respect is by striving for the highest professional competence at all times. Continuing education and a commitment to lifelong learning are requisite to keep up-to-date on current practices and procedures. Courses, seminars, and workshops often must be undertaken at the initiative of the individual.

Self-respect also comes by respecting others. Nurses must be open to consult with, and seek advice from, other professionals. Respecting the knowledge and experience of others is a form of self-respect. Lifelong learning, expertise on current procedures, and knowledge gained from other professionals result in the best possible care of each patient and the community as a whole.

Under Provision 5, nurses submit to the notion that their personal and professional lives are inseparable. To practice nursing means being a nurse at all times, in the workplace and in the community. Nurses' words, actions, and authority in public and in private lives reflect on the entire nursing profession. Paradoxically, they must separate the personal and the professional when communicating with patients, families, and the community. For example, offering advice, instruction, or comfort to their patients is good. Confiding personal opinions or conveying negative emotions is not.

It is of utmost importance, under Provision 5, that nurses resist the temptation to compromise their integrity during times of stress, whether it is work-related or personal. Certainly, the ability to compromise with others is a necessity to have a well-run department, but they should never violate patient safety or the standards of the profession, even if they are having a bad day. If a nurse finds that his or her professional integrity is at odds with the policies of the organization, Provision 5 states that the nurse can take the stance of a conscientious objector. However, pursuant to that stance, the nurse has the obligation to try to affect change in a respectful manner and working within the system. This is an extreme example, and it places a great deal of responsibility on nurses. They might even have to put their jobs on the line rather than forfeit their moral integrity. Remember, the objective at all times is to provide the best possible care for patients.

Lessons From the Code For an HCA, the following lessons can be derived from examining the Code of Ethics for Nurses. Applying concepts identified from the nurses' ethics code can assist you in becoming a better administrator. For example:

1. As an HCA, you also have the responsibility to respect yourself and to balance your personal and professional life.
2. What you say and do in the community carries additional authority because of your knowledge and position in the healthcare system. Because the community relies on you, you must also be careful about what you say.
3. A foundation in theory or business practice is not enough for your actions. There might be times when you have to risk your pride, and maybe even your job, to protect patient safety or the honor of your profession.
4. Like nurses, you must commit to lifelong learning. On your own initiative, take steps to ensure your own competency by being up-to-date on the latest procedures and taking continuing educational classes. Changes in healthcare systems and procedures are rapid and can sometimes seem chaotic. Do not be caught off guard by changes taking place in health care.
5. You must also be willing to compromise, but never compromise integrity. In times of financial trouble, for example, you might be tempted to indulge in creative accounting or to cut corners. Look for alternative solutions. Compromise, while necessary, should never jeopardize patients or injure integrity—yours or that of your organization.

Code for Dental Hygienists

Health care takes place in many settings and encompasses many professional groups. The following is an example from the dental health component of health care and provides some lessons that HCAs can easily emulate. This example code is for dental hygienists, licensed professionals who, along with the dentist, provide preventive and therapeutic services. The Code of Ethics for Dental Hygienists is actually a series of documents that includes Standards of Practice and Principles of Ethics (CSEP, 2008). The Standards of Practice provides a detailed explanation of the hygienist's role in assessment, treatment planning, implementation, and evaluation. Expected performance in each of these areas is made clear and is the foundation for ethics-based practice dental hygiene practice.

In the Preamble of the Code (CSEP, 2008), dental hygienists are charged with living "meaningful, productive, satisfying lives that serve us, our profession, our society and the world" (para. 1). This statement suggests that dental hygienists are more than "cleaners of teeth"; they have lives that must be fully lived beyond their professional roles. The Code also presents the foundational concepts and beliefs that are used to formulate its recommendations. They include the concept that people should be valued and allowed to make their own choices. In addition, dental hygienists are responsible for the quality of the care that they provide as part of their ethical obligation.

The Code itself is quite lengthy but is based on principles you have studied in this text. Mention is made of the value of trust, autonomy, beneficence, nonmaleficence, and justice. Additionally, dental hygienists are cautioned to avoid self-deception and to work toward their optimal personal health. Responsibility for maintaining professional competence through continuing education is also stressed. The Code spells out the dental hygienists' duties to clients, colleagues, employers, the profession, and the community. This description provides clear direction for providing client services in an ethics-based manner. Finally, the Code includes a section on the ethics of research. Mandates are presented for determining the benefits to subjects and the necessity for communicating results honestly.

Lessons From the Code   The Code of Ethics for Dental Hygienists (CSEP, 2008) is a detailed document. However, it does contain wisdom that can be applied to your practice as an HCA.

1. Again, in this code you see the reference to ethics as part of your whole life and not just your professional one. The code goes further and specifies that you have a moral duty to be physically healthy. Frankl would be proud.
2. Ethics statements for dental hygienists go beyond a code and include standards of practice. While this may seem too detailed for some, it

does help to establish professional boundaries. Efforts to codify practice standards for HCAs have been underway for many years, and someday will be available for both educators and practitioners.
3. This Code demonstrates roots in common with other ethics codes. For example, the ethical principles of autonomy, justice, beneficence, and nonmaleficence are part of its elements. You can use these roots to design your personal ethics code for practicing health administration.
4. Research ethics is prominent in this code. A moral approach to research includes being truthful to the participants in a research project, and to do them no harm. How can you apply this principle to your practice of administration?

Code of Ethics for Counselors

The field of mental health includes unique ethics challenges because these practitioners serve clients who are in their most vulnerable state. Essentially, patients are disclosing their most private information to a total stranger. As you can imagine, counselors have immense power and the potential for great benefit or harm because of their relationship to the client. Obviously, trust and confidentiality are critical. In order to foster a healing environment for clients, the Code of Ethics for Counselors created by the American Counseling Association (ACA) (in Cottone & Tarvydas, 2003) is not just detailed; it is prohibitive.

The code contains eight major sections that contain many subsections to specify expectations for professional ethical behavior. In addition, there is separate document describing the standards of practice for members of the ACA. Examples of professional expectations are found in the Client Relationship Section (A). This section includes guidelines about disclosure, choice, and patient dignity. There is also a section on dual relationships and specific language prohibiting sexual intimacy with clients, an area not found in other codes. This section even spells out how long a therapist must refrain from having a personal relationship with the patient, even when therapy has ended (two years), and defines the nature of those relationships. This can seem to be a simple matter—do not date your clients—but it is actually more complex. What if you live in a small town and attend a holiday party where you encounter three of your clients? What should you do? Your action needs to protect their right to privacy, without causing embarrassment. This section is so detailed that it even prohibits bartering for services, dictates the use of computers, and has strict procedures for termination of a professional relationship.

Because it is so critical to counseling practice, there is an entire section on confidentiality. The section describes gray areas in which counselors can have heavy responsibilities, such as confidentiality when working in groups, dealing with minors, and maintaining client records. This section also includes confidentiality requirements when engaging in research, training students, and consulting with fellow professionals. As a cornerstone of client trust, this area must be given serious consideration.

Other equally detailed sections include clarification of a counselor's duty to maintain professional competence and honor their colleagues. Counselors are expected to seek assistance if they experience personal impairment. They are also cautioned against advertising, providing advice on the media, and using their position for unethical personal benefit (such as financial gain or sexual favors). Counselors also have duties to comply with the moral standards imposed by their colleagues and licensing associations. These include submitting to regular professional reviews, being monitored for professional conduct, and refusing to accept referral fees.

Other sections of the code (in Cottone & Tarvydas, 2003) deal with counseling functions such as client assessment and the use of psychological tests. A section on the responsibilities of counselors who serve as teachers is also included. It acknowledges the unequal power relationship between teacher and student and forbids sexual relationships between the two. It also stresses the responsibility to present a variety of theoretical viewpoints, design safe and effective self-growth activities, and maintain high levels of professional conduct.

The last two sections of the Code (in Cottone & Tarvydas, 2003) deal with the practitioner's responsibility for research and for resolving ethical issues. The research section (G) contains detailed information about treatment of subjects, informed consent, and publication of results. Counselors also have the responsibility to report suspected ethics violations and cooperate with all investigations of the Ethics Committee. Finally, the standard of practice document provides minimum standards for each of the eight sections. This document helps to simplify the complex ethics code necessary fir ethics-based counseling practice.

Lessons From the Code   The ACA Code of Ethics may seem like "overkill" in some cases, but remember the potential for benefit or harm that lies in the counseling relationship. The level of detail most definitely provides a guide to acceptable behavior for the individual practitioner. The code, while based on theoretical principles, also reflects rule utilitarianism. Areas have been included because, in the past, they have caused someone difficulty either ethically or legally. What lessons can you glean from this code of ethics?

1. Respecting the patient's right to confidentiality is a prominent theme in this code. This is also of great concern to you as an HCA. You, too, have access to confidential information about employees, and this confidentiality must be kept sacred. You also have knowledge about your organization that, if disclosed, could lead

to financial losses or consequences that are more serious. You are trusted and your ability to maintain that trust is important to your current and future career.

2. The ACA Code has many sections regarding personal relationships with counselors' clients and students. These sections should make you think about power inequity and the appropriateness of certain behaviors of an HCA. While you are human, you should give great thought to the cost of workplace romances, particularly with your staff. These situations can be awkward at best and leave you open to accusations of favoritism. When they go bad, you are vulnerable to charges of sexual harassment that, even if unfounded, can play havoc with your life and career potential.

3. In this code, you can easily see the burden of competence that is placed on a professional. No one will force you to maintain currency in your field; it is something you should choose to do. There is so much to learn as an HCA that you will need to update your knowledge base continuously. You will be challenged throughout your whole career.

4. The ACA Code parallels the ACHE Code in its inclusion of conflicts of interest as an ethics issue. You will always have access to information that you can use to enhance your personal finances as an HCA. Use of such insider information for personal benefit might or might not land you in jail, but it has the potential to ruin your professional life. The best advice from this Code is to be aware of potential conflicts of interest and to avoid them. This is not always easy to do; you must examine the opportunity with your ethics eyes as well as your business acumen.

5. Counselors, like HCAs, are charged with self-regulation within the context of their professional associations. They must deal with ethics violations when they encounter them and not remain silent. You too have the responsibility to speak out when you find a violation of your code. While this might not make you popular, you can handle these situations in a way that is both professional and compassionate. Remember the management rule of always confronting behaviors in private. However, you also need to be willing to go to the next level if the violation warrants doing so.

Code of Ethics for Acupuncture and Oriental Medicine Practitioners   Since there are an increasing number of Americans who choose to use acupuncture as a form of integrative medicine, the code of ethics of the National Certification Commission for Acupuncture and Oriental Medicine (NCCAOM) is included as an example. The NCCAOM Code (2008) uses the format of a pledge to the patient, profession, and public. With respect to the patient, professionals pledge to respect privacy and dignity, provide high quality service within the scope of their practice, and keep accurate records. In addition, the code prohibits sexual contact with patients while they are being treated. This is prohibited because it would violate the patient's trust.

In addition, acupuncturists promise to honor their profession by practicing with high standards and provide accurate information about their licensure. They also pledge to give the community accurate information about their education and training, advertise only accurate information, and comply with all public health agency regulations. In addition, acupuncturists assure the public that they will respect and collaborate with other forms of health care. The patient is the center of practitioner's actions and ethical code.

Lessons From the Code   Although this aspect of health care is not yet part of the traditional system, there are lessons to be gleaned from the code of ethics of NCCAOM. These lessons include:

1. This code requires making promises to patients, the community, and the profession. Using the format of a promise strengthens the power of the statements. When you state that you will do something it implies a strong commitment to accomplishing what you say you are going to do. As administrators, we should consider our code of ethics as a promise and work toward honoring this commitment.
2. The code includes statements about honest business practices and quality of care in its commitment to both the patient and the community. Certainly, ethically sound business practices should also be a part of our professional commitment.
3. This code also promises that NCCAOM members will respect other healthcare professions and work with them toward the best care for patients. Certainly, this promise should also be a part of our ethics considerations as practicing HCAs. Being respectful of all the professions with which we work should go a long way toward reaching quality care for patients and the community.

■ LIMITATIONS AND CRITICISMS OF CODES

This chapter makes an argument for knowing and using your professional code of ethics. However, the chapter would not be fair and balanced without presenting the limitations of such codes. Experience tells us that ethics codes are often forgotten after a person graduates. Many do not even remember that they exist or how to locate these professional codes. For professionals of high moral character, perhaps a code is not even necessary. They would do their best to serve their clients even in absence of a formal code. Conversely, those professionals who are immoral by nature will not abide by a code.

Darr (2005) agrees and reminds us that a code of ethics, even if it can be enforced, is only a guide for behavior. Those who choose to be immoral can use codes as a way to do what they wish and avoid sanction. If the code enters into legalities, it is too difficult to apply. Therefore, all codes have to walk the line between vagueness and constriction. Even without a professional code, the principles of respect, justice, beneficence, and nonmaleficence should guide your behavior as a professional.

Johnson (2009) also takes the position that ethics codes are popular but not without limitations. His criticisms include elements of their design in the application. He finds most codes to be too vague and more about professional image than moral behaviors. He also cites difficulty with enforcement.

Finally, Eriksson, Höglund, & Helgesson (2008) identify three main problems with respect to ethical codes. They say that there is a problem in interpretation because there is a difference between the statements in the code and actual practice. In addition, the person who must interpret the code needs an understanding of ethical theory in order to fathom its intent. There is also a problem of multiplicity. This problem occurs because there so many codes and guidelines under which professionals operate (my term is bicodal). This situation requires professionals to sort out the commonalities of their codes and determine how to handle situations and stay within them. In addition, there is legalization problem. According to Eriksson, Höglund, & Helgesson (2008) there is a danger that ethical problems may be viewed as legal situations. If this happens, those affected may see the situation in terms of how to meet stay within the law and not as a moral duty.

Summary

As Darr (2005) says, a professional code of ethics helps you know the right thing to do. Certainly, they are not a panacea for all the ethics problems faced by HCAs or any other professional group. In fact, they can even assist those who choose the shadow side of administration to remain on the thin ice without falling in. Unless they are tied to licensure, they are very difficult to enforce.

So why bother? First, a code provides you with a way to understand your professional obligations and expected behaviors. In some codes, these behaviors are carefully delineated. When they are, they definitely help serious ethical and even legal problems. In any case, you can use the information provided in your code as a starting point when making professional and personal decisions.

If codes are responsibly read and referenced, they have a positive impact on administrative behavior. Keeping a copy of your professional code readily available, reading it, and using it as part of decision-making lowers the potential for lawsuits and career failures. Darr (2005) feels that using codes also assists in the success of your career. Codes help you maintain integrity and public trust. Darr (2005) would say that living by the code is just the right thing to do.

Five Challenges for Living in Code

The following five challenges are designed to assist you in becoming more familiar with your professional code of ethics and learning how to use it. You will need to do some research about the ACHE Code of Ethics and to examine at least one other code. Discussing the ACHE Code with other administrators should help you have a better concept of how it can be used in decision-making. Finally, you are challenged to try including the Code in your operational decisions and developing a personal code with the ACHE Code as a starting point.

1. Learn your professional code.

   Comments

   In this challenge, locate a copy of the ACHE Code of Ethics and all of its support documents and read them in-depth. Do not just scan the words on the page. Instead, thoughtfully peruse material and answer the question, "What do they mean by that?" You can get helpful insights just by slowing down as you read the document. It is supposed to define who you are as a professional.

   After reading the code, ask yourself, "Do I believe this, and can I support it?" This will allow you to formulate your position on the Code. Finally, ask, "How can I use this in practice?" The answers to this question will help you identify ways to apply the Code to your daily operation as an HCA.

2. Investigate codes from other professions.

   Comments

   This challenge can be met in a number of ways. First, you can use the CSEP Web site to identify a code that is interesting to you. You might select one from a professional group with whom you work. If you are bicodal, you can investigate one from your coprofession. Try to determine just what this code is asking of its professionals. Read the section on limitations again and see if you can identify some of those mentioned in your study code. Finally, ask yourself, "What can I learn from this Code?"

   Second, after you have learned about the code, have an informal conversation with a member of that profession. Find out if they use the code. If they do, how does it assist them in their practice? If they do not, why do they not find it useful?

3. Ask key administrators about the challenges of living by a professional code.

Comments

This will be an easy challenge if you have already identified your moral mentor. If not, take time to find an administrator who will give you some discussion time. Next, get on his or her calendar and discuss what the ACHE Code means. Why does he or she think that you need a professional code? Does he or she find particular features helpful? You can also ask for cases where the ACHE Code has made a difference to this person. This information will give you insight into the practical application of the Code and assist you with Challenge 5.

4. Try living the code in your daily operations.

Comments

Pick a decision that you must make in your daily operations as an HCA. If you have not begun your career, think of a hypothetical case for this challenge. Next, get out the ACHE Code or the appropriate Policy Statement. Along with the financials and any other data you are using, review the Code and add a question to the decision process, for example, "Would this decision fit with the ACHE's recommendations?" What did you discover?

5. Design you own personal code starting with the ACHE Code as a foundation.

Comments

This challenge is by far the largest of the five. Think about what is expected of you by the profession as presented by the ACHE and what you have learned so far. Next, take your time and put your perceptions into your own words. Make sure that these you are willing to stand by what you write. This process should not be done lightly; make each word count.

By the end of Chapter 15 you will be formulating what some authors call a personal mission statement, or what I call a personal ethics code. It will combine your foundation beliefs about moral behavior, professional codes of ethics, and the application of ethics to practice. This statement should be something that you could frame and put on your office wall. In fact, some of my braver students have done just that. They also review this ethics statement at least once a year to see if they are staying true to their personal morality and their professional obligations.

Web Resources

ACHE Code of Ethics and Support Materials
http://www.ache.org/aboutache.cfm

The Center for the Study of Ethics in the Professions
http://ethics.iit.edu/

References

American College of Healthcare Executives. (2007a). *American College of Healthcare Executives code of ethics.* [Electronic version]. Chicago: Author.

American College of Healthcare Executives. (2007b). *Ethical decision making for healthcare executives.* [Electronic version]. Chicago: Author.

American Nurses Association. (2005). *Code of ethics for nurses.* Available at: http://www.nursingworld.org/. Accessed February 15, 2009.

Center for the Study of Ethics in the Professions. (2008). *Codes of ethics online.* Chicago: Illinois Institute of Technology.

Cottone, R. R., & Travydas, V. M. (2003). *Ethical and professional issues in counseling* (2nd ed.). Upper Saddle River, NJ: Pearson Education.

Darr, K. (2005). *Ethics in health services management* (4th ed.). Baltimore: Health Professions Press.

Erikson, S., Höglund, A. T., & Helgesson, G. (2008). Do ethical guidelines give guidance? A critical examination of eight ethics regulations. *Cambridge Quarterly of Healthcare Ethics,* 17(1), 15–30.

Johnson, C. E. (2009). *Meeting the ethical challenges of leadership: Casting light or shadow* (3rd ed.). Thousand Oaks, CA: Sage.

National Certification Commission for Acupuncture and Oriental Medicine. (2008). *Code of ethics.* Available at: http://www.nccaom.org/. Accessed February 15, 2009.

Nelson, W. A. (2005). An organizational ethics decision-making process. *Healthcare Executive,* 20(4), 8–14.

Squazzo, J. D. (2008). Ethics and excellence: The making of a profession's values, standards. *Healthcare Executive,* 23(2), 30–33. Available at: ABI/INFORM Global database. (Document ID: 14459954410). Accessed February 15, 2009.

Worthley, J. A. (1999). *Organizational ethics in the compliance context.* Chicago: Health Administration Press.

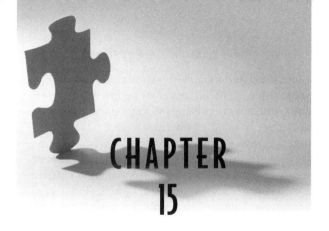

CHAPTER 15

Practicing as an Ethical Administrator

Leadership is a potent combination of strategy and character.
But if you must be without one, be without the strategy.

—Norman Schwarzkopf

Points to Ponder

1. Why is it important to apply ethics to your daily practice as a healthcare administrator (HCA)?
2. How do ethics fit into the classic functions of healthcare administration?
3. How can you better prepare yourself to be an ethics-based administrator?

Words to Remember

The following is a list of key words for this chapter. You will find them in bold in the text. Stop and check your understanding of them.

ethical hypocrisy   ethics of "bossdom"

■ INTRODUCTION

Ethics without action has no value. Just talking about your ethics but never acting on these convictions puts you at risk for **ethical hypocrisy**. Because your staff notice when there is a dissonance between your words and your actions, this hypocrisy can go a long way toward

undermining their trust in you. Without this trust, you will find it difficult, if not impossible, to be successful as an HCA. So, just how do you
integrate ethics into your daily operations? What are some practical
ways to be an ethics-based administrator?

This chapter assists in answering these questions. First, you will
be asked to think about the classic functions of healthcare management. How can you apply ethics to each of them? You will also find
wisdom from the scholars of practical ethics. Finally, the chapter
gives you some anecdotal information from practicing HCAs. How
can their challenges and solutions help you to improve your own
practice? At the end of the chapter, take the three challenges and use
them to refine your opinion on ethics in action for your daily HCA
practice.

■ KEY PROCESSES OF HEALTHCARE ADMINISTRATION AND ETHICS

Many texts define the essential functions of healthcare administration.
In general, the classifications include planning, organizing, staffing,
influencing, and controlling (Dunn, 2006). Three examples of applied
ethics are presented for each of these areas. However, I am sure you
will be able to add many others.

Planning

Planning means setting the future direction of your department or
organization and includes your ability to meet community needs. Planning also includes establishing mission, vision, goals, and objectives
(Dunn, 2006). These steps lead to the development of policies and procedures, rules, budgets, and other operational actions to achieve the
desired plan. While some think of planning as solely an upper management function, all HCAs must engage in this process. Whether you are
a CEO or a supervisor, effective planning allows you to keep your competitive edge, maintain a strong bottom line, and serve those who use
your services. How can ethics apply?

Ethics Applications   When you think about all that is entailed in planning, you can probably identify several areas where the practice of
ethics makes a difference. The ethics of data integrity, information
presentation, and overall communication are just a few areas that
should be considered. With respect to data integrity, remember that
planning decisions ultimately rest on the quality of the data used to
make them. If these data are collected appropriately, honestly

recorded, and fully considered, you have a greater chance of making decisions that succeed.

Ethics has a major influence on the quality and integrity of any data set. You can begin with the ethics of those who are responsible for its collection. If they do not see this task as important, they might be tempted to rush through it. Too much speed can lead to errors and omissions and give you poor quality data. They might also be tempted to fabricate data when their integrity is not stressed. As an HCA, you have a duty to educate your staff concerning the use of the data they collect and the need for integrity. You also need to build time into the work schedules to allow for adequate collection. Finally, you should make it a published policy to conduct periodical data integrity checks so that you can comfortably "stand on your data."

Data integrity is also influenced by how you conduct your analysis. Choosing the correct format is the first step in preserving integrity. While statistical packages assist greatly with creating information, they are only as good as the data you choose to enter. It can be tempting to omit those numbers that appear to be negative, especially when your bonus is derived from your numbers. However, in the end, poor decisions made by faulty data can cost you more than a bonus. Remember that your data can also be qualitative, which can also challenge you ethically. You are trusted to review all of the data, design codes that are accurate, and assign responses appropriately. Be sure that you can explain your coding system and your data. It is often helpful to have a reviewer look at your coding system to help with its construct validity.

The ethics of presentation is an important one for the planning process. You have probably learned in your courses that numbers can be presented to say almost anything. The temptation will be to present your information only in a positive way so that you and your department can shine. Providing an unbalanced account of your achievements by neglecting the whole picture (sin of omission) can serve you well in the short run. However, decisions made on incomplete data can hurt your department and the organization in the bigger picture. In addition, if you try "stacking the deck," you will be questioned. Minimally, you will look foolish and dishonest, and you might even jeopardize your career. Providing a balanced picture does not mean that you only present the bad news and neglect all of the accomplishments. It just means that along with successes, you diplomatically address the goals that have not been reached. This allows you to evaluate what you have done and alter the process as needed.

Presentation also includes the clarity of your information. To avoid addressing the real issues, some HCAs choose to obviate them through data dazzle and presentation confusion. They resort to these tactics because they know that the human brain can absorb only so many numbers. So, they show too many PowerPoint slides at a time (sometimes called "death by PowerPoint"). After a while, people tune out (take a mental vacation). It can be tempting to use a data fog to keep from being criticized, but you are not providing good stewardship for the organization. Leaders need a clear and understandable picture of what is happening to avoid faulty decisions. Therefore, ethics practices mean that you make every effort to be clear, concise, and accurate in what you present. As you prepare a presentation, ask yourself, "Do I understand this, and will my boss get it?"

Applying ethics to communication facilitates successful planning. You can have the most beautifully designed strategic plan but, if no one uses it, it is worthless. First, you must support the plan yourself and communicate your support. You also have an ethical obligation to educate your staff about the plan's purpose and implementation. In order for implementation to succeed, you have to create an environment where individuals feel that they can honestly communicate with you. This climate of cooperation is necessary for you to gain accurate information on the progress of the plan. Without it, "group-think" (thinking only what you are told to think) will rule and you will learn only what your staff members think you want to hear. The result can be disastrous for a strategic plan.

You also need to be careful about "groupspeak" (i.e., saying only what people want to hear) in your communications with superiors. While diplomacy and a spirit of cooperation are important in effective communication, you should not be afraid to express your concerns. No one can see all sides of a decision, so your courage to speak up can actually assist your boss in making the correct decision. Communication needs to be top-down and bottom-up if a strategic plan is to be successful.

Organizing

The organizing function of healthcare administration includes deciding how the work is to be done. It includes the correct placement of activities, materials, and staff to accomplish the objectives of the strategic plan. This process also involves designing specific jobs and educating staff about how to do those jobs. Delegation of authority and assigning accountability are part of the organizing function. You must provide the structure that facilitates the work of your department and leads to the staffing function. As you can imagine, organizing involves many areas of human resources and finance. It also engages much of your time as an HCA.

Ethics Applications   The potential for ethics challenges within the organizing function is great. Examples of these challenges are the ethics of design, matching, and delegation. We can begin with job design and redesign, which are important steps for the success of any organization. Designing jobs to be both effective and efficient also conserves scarce resources by avoiding unnecessary use and waste. In order for this task to be done well, an accurate picture of what is to be done and the best way to do it must be obtained.

One ethics issue in job design is the rush to creation. It is too easy to take a job description or a set of practice guidelines from another facility or Web site, plunk it into a document, and say, "Do it this way." The problem with this action is that there are no clones among organizations; everything must be customized to your workplace. While a draft can be invaluable to jump-start the process, it must be adapted to your particular organization. One way to achieve adaptation is to consult those who actually do the job and ask them to review a draft of the job description for accuracy and omissions. Taking this step provides you with two things. One, you capture a better picture of how the job is done in your organization. Two, you honor your employees and their knowledge by including them in the process. You should also have an easier time with implementation because the design is not just a top-down effort. Staff members are included in its development.

Once you have the job design, you have to engage in the ethics of matching. Part of the art of administration is your ability to match the best person to the job. This is especially critical in health care where many jobs involve higher levels of professional knowledge and skills. While it might be easier to just assign someone the new task, ethics practice asks you to avoid the easy way of dealing with this challenge. To make a decision for the best fit, you should first know the strengths and weaknesses of each of your staff members. Who is interested or educated in this area? Who would have the shortest learning curve if assigned this task?

You also need to take the workload of each staff member into consideration. It has been my experience that when certain staff members demonstrate job excellence, they are often rewarded by being given more work to do. Having a full and varied workload can make your day interesting, but overload can lead to burnout and resignation. Ethics requires that you avoid delegating everything to "old faithfuls" and take the opportunity to challenge someone who might be a "coaster" to strive for career excellence.

You must keep in mind that ethical matching also requires job training. Do not assume that the person you select fully understands the assignment. You have a responsibility to educate that person about any needed specifics. You also should recognize that a person's pride could keep him or her from asking questions or requesting help. Just assume that some level of orientation is necessary for successful implementation. Finally, encourage the employee who takes on additional tasks. Encouragement does not have to be time consuming or expensive. It is often enough to just informally check in with the employee and ask, "How is it going?" If you have established a climate of trust, this management by walking around will head off problems before they happen.

Once a job is assigned, you face the challenge of the ethics of delegation. Delegation is often misunderstood; it is not just giving the "dirty work" to the "worker bees." It is a decision of trust where you are willing to grant the implementation and authority to another person. The key word here is authority. Delegation does not work if there is a person who is responsible for the outcome but who does not have authority to make it happen.

Delegation is based on common trust. You trust the staff to do their jobs to the best of their abilities and to communicate to you when assistance is needed. Staff members trust that you will allow them the autonomy to do their jobs without micromanagement. They also expect that you will recognize and acknowledge their efforts toward accomplishing the department's objectives.

This sounds very easy on paper, but it is often difficult in practice. If you do not trust your staff or believe that they are competent, you will have trouble with delegation. You will wear yourself out checking and redoing everyone's jobs. To avoid the temptation of false delegation, you should first get to know your staff. Can you work with each of them? If not, why not? You might also have to assess your attitude toward delegation and understand that you are not omnipotent. You just cannot do it all. For the jobs to be done and the plan to be achieved, you must be able to rely on staff.

Recognition is also part of delegation. A staff that is working well will make you look like an organizational star. This does not mean that you get to absorb all of the starlight. Ethical and effective administrators know the basis for their success and acknowledge it. They celebrate progress toward goals and thank their staff with humility and appreciation. Making this step part of delegation is not only ethical but it also goes a long way toward making work meaningful for your staff. People who are engaged in meaningful work and receive appreciation are less likely to burn out and resign.

Staffing

Dunn (2006) lists staffing as a separate function of management. This function considers both recruitment and hiring efforts to assure quality employees. It also requires that you balance the need for quality employees with the budget allowed for labor costs. In addition, the staffing function includes assurances of current licensure and training for maintaining competence. Performance evaluations and improvement planning are also included in this management function. Although you might consider this area to be part of your human resources department, you will be responsible for many decisions within this function.

Ethics Applications As you might imagine, the staffing function involves challenges to ethical administrative practice. Three areas to consider are autonomy, justice practices, and responsibility for competence. Autonomy issues begin with the hiring process. As an administrator, you will have access to candidates' transcripts, talk to their references, and conduct personal interviews. Because of these activities, you will have information about them that is confidential. The temptation will be to talk about what you know to those who do not have a "need to know." The "juicy gossip factor" may be tempting, but engaging in this activity may endanger trust. After all, the person hearing this information may wonder, if you are telling confidential information about a candidate, what else would you divulge?

Justice issues and temptations are frequent within the staffing function. To be ethical, you must treat everyone fairly and in compliance with your policies. However, we are all compassionate people and this compassion challenges fairness. For example, if you have an employee who is just returning from maternity leave, you might be more lenient when she is late for work. However, this apparent favoritism will not always be perceived well by those who come on time every day.

Justice must be practiced when it comes to performance evaluations and authorizing raises. However, since there is always room for interpretation in standards, temptation exists. Suppose you have an employee whose personality clashes with yours. This person does excellent work, but does not appeal to you. The temptation would be to reduce his or her performance evaluation score based on an "obnoxious personality." However, succumbing to this temptation could lead to major discord with the employee, your other staff members, and the human resources department.

As an HCA, you are trusted to hire and maintain competent staff. This means that you must know if your staff members have current licenses to practice and are up-to-date on their continuing education. An ethics challenge occurs when there is not a clear policy on who is responsible for maintaining currency. For example, some organizations consider continuing education to be the individual's responsibility and do not pay for any courses. Others offer onsite courses to facilitate currency and control for the costs of staff member absences. As an HCA, you must know the policy for your organization and communicate it to your staff members. Clear communication should reduce issues related to the responsibility for competency assurance.

Influencing

Influencing or directing is the process of getting the work done. It uses the tools of communication, motivation, and education to influence staff to achieve organizational goals and objectives. In other words, you are getting the job done through your employees. This area involves issues like morale, motivation, productivity, and turnover. The influencing function allows you to demonstrate your effectiveness as a leader and create a workplace where employees want to be.

Ethics Applications   Three areas of ethics practice that can affect the directing process are the **ethics of "bossdom,"** staff motivation, and effective teamwork. How do you behave when you are the boss? Do you respect your employees in at least an "I-YOU" relationship? Do you see them as means to an end? How do you feel when you have a staff resignation or termination? To avoid becoming an Idiot Boss (I-Boss) or, even worse, a Bully Boss, you must first consider what being the boss means to you. Along with the benefits of increased salary and status comes the responsibility of using your power astutely. Remember, you have no real power unless your staff members grant it to you. As free human beings, they always have the option to do their jobs well or poorly or even to resign. Power based on respect, honesty, and fairness will take you further toward meeting goals than power based on coercion and fear. This is especially true in the healthcare environment where employees tend to be highly skilled and in demand.

The responsibility of directing also includes employee motivation. To motivate, you must go beyond being an organizational cheerleader. It is more effective to influence people's desire to make the organization's goals their own and work to complete them successfully. Many administrators still believe that the best way to motivate employees to do what they want is to pay them. If you pay staff enough, they reason, staff will do anything. While money is a motivator when people cannot pay their bills, it loses its influence as they become more secure.

What do employees need to motivate them? One somewhat radical way to find this out is to ask them. Instead of planning something that you think will be motivation, why not use management by walking around or e-mails to ask employees for their ideas? Then you can build your motivation strategies on things that might have a better chance of accomplishing their goal. Of course, you can always check current literature for ideas. Research repeatedly shows that recognition, interesting, meaningful work, and loyalty are stronger motivators than cash. From an ethics view, employee motivation begins with an "I-YOU" relationship among you and your staff. Once this climate of trust and respect exists, it becomes easier to keep the mission and goals in the forefront.

Many administrative tasks are conducted by teams. A good example of a clinical team can be found in the emergency department (ED).

Each team member knows his or her job and works together for the good of the patient. Teams also exist in the nonclinical aspects of health care and need to work equally well. Your responsibility is to practice ethics when establishing and leading teams so that each team member will work well with others.

The first step in meeting this responsibility is to consider whether or not a team is needed and who should be on it. Be careful to use teams for important tasks that cannot be done by one or two people. Otherwise, it is just busywork. Make sure you select team members based on their knowledge and ability to contribute to the solution and not just on their title. When you ask a person to serve, acknowledge his or her value and reason for selection. Being asked to serve on a team can be viewed as an honor or a curse, depending on the individual.

Once you have assembled the team, remember all of the key ethics principles. Respect the team's time and autonomy by making sure they understand the task, organizing efficient meetings, and providing follow-up information. Meetings should be conducted to foster open and honest communication so that the best solution can be derived. As moderator, make sure that all voices can be heard and one or two members do not dominate the process. Do not schedule meetings if there is no real reason for them. This is disrespectful.

Teams, like individual employees, need to be recognized for their work. Include team members' names on the final product or document. This acknowledges that the product was not the work of one person, but was the best thinking of the team. The names on the document also provide a source for information when outside staff members have questions. Team members become authoritative champions for the plan that they helped to develop. Finally, from the standpoint of reward, everyone likes to see his or her name in print.

Controlling

The controlling function is designed to monitor activities and ensure that organizational goals and objectives are met. The process includes developing performance measures, evaluating those measures, and taking corrective action if necessary. Financial controls are also part of this function, which include budgets, cost-benefit analyses, and inventory controls. Information systems provide valuable tools to assist with the controlling process if they are used ethically and effectively. Ethics issues related to the controlling function include stewardship, patient and employee satisfaction, and justice.

Making sure that resources are optimally used and not wasted is part of your responsibility as a steward. Controlling waste in healthcare inventory is a serious challenge. A large part of the annual budget in any facility is spent on supplies and equipment. However, managing an inventory this large can be a challenge because of the number and variety of products and supplies that are used. Of course, there are also problems with shrinkage (another word for theft) that must be addressed. You need to determine the best way to conserve resources and still provide quality care. This includes using technology such as computer monitoring systems to assist in the process.

To be a good steward, you must also pay attention to your balance sheets and other financials. Ask questions when you see entries that do not make sense. Of course, you must also be accurate and honest in documenting your expenditures and inventory. Creative accounting might solve your immediate problem, but this quick fix can come with a price you do not want to pay.

Controlling also includes documenting treatment outcomes and progress toward organizational goals. This aspect requires the analysis and evaluation of mandated and proprietary data sets, including those related to patient satisfaction. Patient satisfaction data are increasingly more important and are often surveyed by external evaluators. In addition, individual departments can be granted bonuses using these numbers.

Ethics Applications   Because it can be linked to money and accreditation, patient satisfaction can become an ethics temptation. As you know from studying the research, there are a number of unethical ways to obtain favorable data. First, if you limit the size of your mailings, you will get a smaller return. When this happens, you can make greater claims about patient satisfaction level but they will be based on only a small sample. This is not ethical. For example, if you have only a 5% to 10% return, you are dealing with numbers that have virtually no meaning. However, if they show you in a positive light, you might be tempted to use them.

Timing also affects survey data. If you do infrequent mailing, some of your patients will not remember if they received good treatment or not. Therefore, your data can be inaccurate. The length of the questionnaire also makes a difference. If it is too long, it will be tossed rather than completed, giving you lower return numbers. Questions can also be slanted to provide more positive responses than negative.

To avoid ethical temptations from data collection, healthcare facilities are beginning to use a triangulation method for gathering patient satisfaction data. To improve data integrity, they use multiple methods such as telephone surveys, focus groups, and visits with patients who are still in the facility. While this data collection might be more expensive, it yields information that can be used to improve patient care. In this case, knowledge is power; once you are aware of a problem, you can fix it.

There is also a temptation to "cook the books" to show favorable numbers. After all, who would know? This is particularly enticing when written comments are included. If someone takes the time to write a comment, he or she wants you to have this information. However, it takes time to organize comments into categories for meaningful information and to match comments with the categories. Of course, not all of the comments might be favorable. When there are too many negative comments, you could show yourself in a more positive light if grouped numbers together. For example, you could total every score that mentioned "satisfied" as one number, giving you a higher satisfaction score. In addition to being unethical, this decision robs you of important information for improving patient services.

The ethics of employee satisfaction needs to be considered under the controlling function. What can an ethics-based organization do to provide an environment where employees can engage in meaningful work? Is it important to measure employee satisfaction? Some organizations think that it is not. They take the, "You are lucky to have a job" attitude, while still expecting staff to treat patients and families with care and compassion. This dissonance can lead to poor morale and soaring turnover rates. Employees, like patients, want to have at least an "I-You" relationship in the workplace. As the leader, you have the ability to demonstrate respect and value for your staff. This is good ethical practice and good for business.

The ethics involved with employee discipline and termination is part of the controlling function. These decisions are part of the job of an HCA. While these tasks are unpleasant at best, they can be handled ethically and respect the dignity of the persons involved. For example, corrective steps should always be taken in private and agreements pertaining to necessary improvements should be provided to the employee in writing. Even though it is a frequently used tactic, it is not ethical to drive out an undesirable employee by making the workplace so miserable that he or she resigns. Even if you succeed in getting the desired resignation, you make yourself vulnerable to legal action and you send a powerful message of fear to the remaining staff.

This section has examined a few of the ethics challenges involved in the five processes of administration. You will experience many others in the course of your career. The key to dealing with these challenges is to combine your sense of ethics with sound business practices. Being an ethics-based administrator requires much of you. You might have to risk being unpopular in order to be ethical. However, your conscience will be clear if you try to balance the right thing to do with what is best for business. The challenge of achieving this balance will always make your work interesting—boredom will never be an issue.

■ WISDOM FROM THE MASTERS: ETHICS IN PRACTICE

Where do you go to find advice about how practice as an ethics-based administrator? One source of information will be those who practice this way themselves. You will find some of their wisdom in the next section of this chapter. However, you do not have to be limited to just health care as a source of wisdom. You can so study writers that inspire HCAs. You will be introduced to a few of these experts in this section.

One place to start is with a writer who is part of an ethics dynasty. Steven A. Covey wrote much-discussed works including *The 7 Habits of Highly Effective People* (1989) and *Principle Centered Leadership* (1992). These works have been included on the reading lists for generations of HCAs. In fact, there are whole university courses devoted to their content. Steven A. Covey's son, Steven M. R. Covey followed his father's path and published a book that offers ethics wisdom. This book is entitled *The Speed of Trust: The One Thing that Changes Everything* (Covey, 2006).

In this book, Covey (2006) discusses the concept of trust and its influence on leadership and the global economy. Trust is the core of interaction, but low levels of trust exist in aspects of life and business. Covey tells us that the ability to establish and grow trust is the most critical element to success in a global economy. He presents five waves of trust: self, relational, organizational, market, and societal. His first wave of trust starts with you and your confidence in yourself. The essence of this wave of trust is your credibility as a leader and a person. How do you build this credibility? Covey suggests that you concentrate on four core areas.

The first area of concentration in building credibility is your personal integrity. He feels that integrity is not just talking about ethics; it includes acting on your values and practicing humility. Credibility also means that you do what you say and are willing to stand by your principles. Certainly, Aristotle would agree with this version of eudaimonia.

In addition to credibility, you need to be clear about your motive for your actions and your personal agenda. What do you support and why do you support it? This translates to your behavior. In other words, who benefits when you take action? To increase trust, you should be acting for the benefit of others as well as for yourself. Taking this position means that you are willing to know and communicate your intent, and have the courage to act on it.

Elements of character are not enough to build trust as a leader. You also need to build your capabilities (Covey, 2006). Capabilities can be expressed in the "acronym 'TASKS' or Talents, Attitudes, Skills, Knowledge, and Style" (p. 94). He encourages you to know your strengths in each of these areas and use them appropriately. You must maintain your currency by mastering the knowledge and skills in your field and continuing your education beyond graduation. In health care, the need to build capabilities continually is an absolute must for leadership growth and success.

Finally, to build credibility and trust as a leader, you need to have a record of performance. Covey (2006) states that your ability to make things happen matters in the overall assessment of your credibility. You need to be thinking about the results you have achieved and the results you want in the future. As Frankl would remind you, taking responsibility for your choices and the results is part of your creditability and ethics-based practice. In addition, you must be willing to stick with your plans and not give up when things are difficult. Quitting does not build credibility and trust.

Although Covey (2006) did not write his book specifically for the healthcare business, the information presented in his first wave of trust can provides solid advice to HCAs. If you are known as a person who has personal integrity and acts on your values, you will add to your status as a leader. If your actions are geared toward the benefit of patients, employees, and your organization, you will be trusted to be a leader in a healthcare organization. Finally, if you use your capabilities to produce results, you will gain the trust of your employees and those to whom you report.

Jerry Harvey is another business writer who can offer advice to HCAs. He is well known in the business world for his work *The Abilene Paradox* (1998). In his book, *How Come Every Time I Get Stabbed in the Back My Fingerprints are on the Knife? and Other Meditations on Management* (1999), he provides useful insights on how to put ethics into action. He explains the difference between sitting (doing nothing) and standing (taking principled action) in business settings. He encourages you to avoid sitting and use your energy to find the truth. This means being willing to ask questions and take a stand. Sometimes HCAs avoid taking a stand because they want to avoid being seen as a troublemaker. However, when you make your position known and have information to support it, you can actually enhance your career. You can save others from decisions that could decrease the image or even the bottom line of the organization.

In practicing ethics-based leadership, consider what it means to be authentic and how to use your head and your heart in your practice (Palmer, 2000). While money and measurable results are important to operational success, there are also intangibles that matter. You have to learn to balance the concrete (data, reports, and financials) with these intangibles (integrity and fairness) to be effective. Achieving this balance requires contemplation, conversation, courage, and conviction. You are encouraged to find time for solitude, overcome your fears, and learn to lead from strength. Palmer (2000) believes when you are called to the profession of healthcare administration, you must be able to balance the elements of life, and that will make ethics-based practice possible.

You can learn how to practice ethics by studying those who write about unethical leaders. Two books on this subject I find useful and entertaining are *Dealing with People You Can't Stand: How to Bring out the Best in People at Their Worst* by Brinkman and Kirschner (1994), and *How to Work for an Idiot: Survive and Thrive without Killing Your Boss* by Hoover (2004). Brinkman and Kirschner provide excellent advice on working with staff and others who challenge your patience and your ethics. The authors include general advice on how to get the best from people regardless of their personalities. You should assume the positive when dealing with their actions, make sure you understand them, and take time to listen. You cannot change these people, but you can try to change your reactions to them. They also suggest getting advice from people who seem to be able to work with these people. What are they doing differently from you?

Hoover (2004), a recovering idiot boss, provides a satiric look at administrative ineffectiveness from the employee view. This information is invaluable in assisting you to understand how your staff members view you, and how to avoid idiot behaviors. After identifying boss types (including god, sadist, masochist, buddy, and idiot), he provides information on how to be a good (ethical) boss. First, you need to treat staff the way you would like your boss to treat you (Kantian ethics). You also need to be clear in your communication and ask questions to be sure you really understand. Sharing information and treating staff with respect is also part of being a good boss. You need to be fair in the way you apply policies. Consistent use of these lessons will keep you from becoming an idiot boss and increase your effectiveness.

What healthcare leadership lessons can be gleaned from the examples in this section? First, the idea of choice seems to be a theme. You must make the choice to practice ethics even if there is no immediate financial reward for doing so. You can choose to act on principles or not, become a respected boss or an I-Boss, and base your decisions on ethics or not. Your choices do make a difference.

Communication in its many forms also seems to be a theme. You are urged to use reflection to communicate with yourself and determine your vocation, motivation, and actions. You are also asked to be fair and honest in your communications with others as part of your practice of ethics-based administration. You have to be aware of the power of your communication and use it to reap benefit and to avoid harm.

Another thematic area is accountability. Although you are accountable to many in your role as an HCA, you have to define your ultimate source of accountability. When you identify your life-center and it is bigger than you are, it becomes easier to act with ethics in mind. Of course, you must be willing to spend some time thinking about the ethics of your decisions, talking with trusted colleagues about your actions, and learning.

■ VOICES FROM THE HEALTHCARE FIELD

A number of writers from the healthcare field provide advice on how to practice as an ethics-based administrator. For example, Patch Adams (1993), now famous because a movie was made about his life, offers ethics advice from a patient view. He believes that service, joy, and humor should be part of practice of health care. He also suggests that you should always be thinking about the patient as you conduct your daily operations. Patients should never become just an inconvenience or a Diagnosis Related Group Code; they should be the reason for your job.

He asks you to make a decision to be happy when the world seems to reward you for being unhappy. Choosing happiness means that you grow friendships, remember when to let go, build community in your workplace, and choose wellness. You also need to increase the level of humor, laughter, and silliness in your life. Humor and silliness have not been stressed as part of effective health administration. Yet, they are the forces that assist in healing, maintaining morale, and decreasing burnout. He offers you advice on how to increase your humor levels, such as finding silliness from reading, watching television and films, laughing, and playing (with children, pets, or just by yourself). If you are happy, in Adams's definition, it should be easier to practice ethically.

Purtilo and Criss (2005) also give excellent advice on using ethics in your practice of administration. You should begin by reading and understanding the mission statement of your organization. This knowledge provides you with an understanding of how the organization views its purpose in the community and allows you to evaluate whether or not you can support such a purpose. Assuming that you want to be part of the organization's mission, you must next read and assess its policies and procedures. You should use the key principles of ethics (i.e., justice, beneficence, nonmaleficence, autonomy) to analyze these policies for their ethical foundation. If this analysis indicates the need for alterations or changes, you must work to achieve policies that are rooted in ethics and not just convenience.

Carson Dye (2000) has over 30 years of experience with health care and extensive background in practical health administration. He asks you to begin your practical application of ethics with the American College of Healthcare Executives Code of Ethics. It should be part of your daily operations. He then advocates that you develop your own code and write it down. By writing it, you make it a tool and not just a theory.

He also suggests that when making a decision, you should analyze the costs of not being ethical. You can ask, "What happens when someone finds out?" If the consequences are not acceptable for your organization, your community, or yourself, you should think again, research some more, and make another choice. Avoid playing with the truth (stretching, padding, or bending it) and be sure to honor your promises. He also suggests that you be careful in using your power, take responsibility for your mistakes, and be vigilant in your personal financial management. By this, he means being a good steward of your expense account, perquisites, and benefits.

McGinn (2005), also an experienced HCA, offers advice on practical ethics. His 10 Laws provide assistance in being an effective leader in the challenging healthcare environment. Of particular interest is the First Law, which reminds you of your moral obligation as an HCA. Avoid taking actions that can bring harm to your organization and yourself. Self-deception is a factor that has led several leaders, including those in health care, to cause harm. He cautions you not to delude yourself and trade ethics for money, power, or fame.

Keeping your sense of purpose in mind as you make decisions is important. Have enough courage to act on that purpose when it is necessary. Never forget that you are in covenant with patients, staff, and the community. You are trusted to be doing what is in their best interests. They, in turn, trust you with their finances and even their lives.

Take a moment to consider what you have just read. What common areas did you find? Are there things that you can use? I notice that a great emphasis is placed on mission, either from a personal or organizational view. This makes sense as a source of thinking about practical ethics. If you do not know what you believe and what you are working toward, I think that it would be difficult to have high standards. I also find in the preceding text that there are no simple answers and that many intangibles are included like courage, humility, principles, responsibility, and trust. Think about all of these and find ways to make them a normal part of who you are as an administrator. In fact, consider ethics in the same way you do finances whenever you make a decision. This might require a new way of looking at what you do, but it is worth the effort. Ethics matters.

Anecdotes to Assist

Sometimes anecdotes can bring real insight into practicing ethics. Although anecdotal information does not constitute science-based research, I found that my conversations with practicing administrators included some real-world ethical issues. One recurring issue was balancing money and mission. With managed care and other agencies trying to trim the budgets to the bare bones, there are real concerns about how to keep providing necessary services. The profit margins are so low for some facilities that there is even a fear of closure. Pressure is being exerted on administrators to do more with less and to stretch the salary dollar as far as it will go. This pressure is also occurring at a time when nursing and other professionals are in short supply. One administrator expressed the frustration that the best interests of the patient are becoming lost when the message of the systems sounds like, "Show me the money." This ethics issue becomes even more problematic in times of economic slow down, depression, and impending healthcare reform. Being an administrator in these times is not for the ethical faint of heart!

Money and mission will always be part of your ethics challenge no matter what your position in healthcare administration. Be sure that you do your part by acting as a good steward of resources to avoid mismanagement and waste and by staying current on financial and treatment trends. Always read your financial statements carefully and maintain accuracy of your records. Good financial health involves the bottom of the organization as well as the top. At all times, resist the temptation to forget the reason you are in this business. Practicing administrators remind you that, if service is not your motivation for being an HCA, then you need to find another career. While being an HCA is prestigious, powerful, and even lucrative in some cases, a foundation in service is the only thing that will maintain your career longevity and happiness.

Coupled with this monetary pressure is the growing awareness of consumers and their demand for what they consider quality care. Every time consumers see a new procedure or technology on television or in a popular magazine, the phone seems to ring with requests for the newest miracle. The demand is not just for glamour services. Administrators were gravely concerned about the overuse of their emergency department (ED) services. Patients seem to be using the ED as a clinic with greater frequency, and the problems they present are becoming ever more complicated to treat. This inappropriate use can become an even greater concern as unemployment rates increase and the ranks of the uninsured grow. Administrators are worried about how they will staff and fund these services and what would happen if they had to close the ED entirely.

Administrators also provided me with examples of behaviors that can kill your career. I arranged these examples into what I call the *Suicide Twelve*. They are:

1. Getting drunk at organizational functions.
2. Dating a subordinate.
3. Telling ethnic or other inappropriate jokes.
4. Sending offensive e-mails.
5. Knowingly and repeatedly violating corporate culture.
6. Getting arrested.
7. Getting into a physical fight.
8. Falsifying records.
9. Violating patient or employee confidentiality.
10. Invading privacy.
11. Taking kickbacks from vendors.
12. Giving away proprietary information to competitors.

While some of these 12 would seem to be obvious career killers, they all have occurred in healthcare settings. Remember that, as a leader, your behavior is noted. Often my students tell me that they should be able to do whatever they want in their private lives. They should have the freedom to date whomever they want or drink when and where they wish. In theory, this might be true. However, in an age of camera cell phones and Internet photo sharing, you may have to think about the consequences of your acts before deciding what to do. Remember also that the healthcare administration community is often a small world, so your mistakes may follow you. Practical wisdom makes practical sense in avoiding these career destroyers.

Summary

You might think that health care, with its emphasis on service and compassionate patient care, would be the easiest environment in which to practice ethics. The unfortunate truth is that health care must balance business and compassion. To achieve this balance, you must understand that employees are human, even though they are called to such a noble vocation. Pressure from finance, technology advances, personnel needs, and external evaluators can add to the burdens of finding this balance. Conducting the business of health care that is centered in ethics will never be easy. However, your patients and the community expect nothing less. Trust, the basis for your business, is at stake.

Before you review the challenges for this chapter, I ask you to reflect on the following quote by Ralph Waldo Emerson. For me, it helps define a meaningful, ethics-based life as an administrator.

- To laugh often and much;
- To win the respect of intelligent people and the affection of children;
- To earn the appreciation of honest critics and endure the betrayal of false friends;
- To appreciate beauty, to find the best in others;
- To leave the world a bit better, whether by a healthy child, a garden patch, or a redeemed social condition;
- To know even one life has breathed easier because you have lived.
- This is to have succeeded.

Challenges

The following are your last three challenges. They should assist you in finding your own sources of wisdom to meet ethics challenges now and in the future. Remember that you always have a choice. The key is to make choices that are true to your conscience and benefit your patients, organization, family, and yourself.

1. Ask.

   Comments

   Repeat my informal study. Contact three or more HCAs and ask them my question, "What are your top three ethics challenges?" Listen to their responses and learn. You can also think about what you would do if you faced a similar situation. Having thought about how to behave ethically is the first step in acting ethically when a situation arises.

2. Evaluate.

   Comments

   Conduct an ethics assessment and analysis in your department or organization. Look at the policies that most affect your services and how their implementation. Do you see any ethics gaps? If so, create a team to clarify existing policies and practices so that they are more centered in ethics.

3. Go within.

   Comments

   Bring a notebook and pen and find a quiet place. List all the activities that are part of your daily operation as an HCA. Decide whether you practice ethics when you do each activity. If the answer is "yes," place a letter E by the item. If the answer is "no or maybe," brainstorm some ways that you can use a more ethics-based approach. Here is the challenge. Take your list and use it to make changes in your daily activities.

   All of the challenges in this section should assist you in creating your personal ethics statement, which can be a powerful resource for practice. My students are required to create this statement on one page, suitable for framing. I ask them, "For what do you want to be known?" The brave students actually frame their document and put it in their offices. Minimally, my students keep it handy as a reference for their beliefs and definition of ethical practice. Graduate students also prepare a treatise to explain the foundation for their statements from theory, principles, and practice. Although some students find this a difficult assignment (especially those who are more quantitative in their views), they all report change in their views on and application of ethics in the operation of health care.

Web Resources

··

Patch Adams
http://www.patchadams.org/

Articles by Parker Palmer
http://www.mcli.dist.maricopa.edu/events/afc99/articles.html

References

··

Adams, P. (1993). *Gesundheit!* Rochester, VT: Healing Arts Press.

Brinkman, R., & Kirschner, R. (1994). *Dealing with people you can't stand: How to bring out the best in people at their worst.* New York: McGraw-Hill.

Covey, S. M. R. (2006). *The speed of trust: The one thing that changes everything.* New York: Free Press.

Covey, S. R. (1992). *Principle centered leadership.* New York: Free Press.

Covey, S. R. (1989). *The 7 habits of highly effective people.* New York: Simon & Schuster.

Dunn, R. (2006). *Haimann's healthcare management* (8th ed.). Chicago: Health Administration Press.

Dye, C. F. (2000). *Leadership in healthcare: Values at the top.* Chicago: Health Administration Press.

Harvey, J. B. (1998). *The Abilene paradox.* San Francisco: Jossey-Bass.

Harvey, J. B. (1999). *How come every time I get stabbed in the back my fingerprints are on the knife? And other meditations on management.* San Francisco: Jossey-Bass.

Hoover, J. (2004). *How to work for an idiot: Survive and thrive without killing your boss.* Franklin Lakes, NJ: Career Press.

McGinn, P. (2005). *Leading others, managing yourself.* Chicago: Health Administration Press.

Palmer, P. J. (2000). *Let your life speak.* San Francisco: Jossey-Bass.

Purtilo, R. B., & Criss, M. L. (2005). *Ethical dimensions in the health professions* (4th ed.). Philadelphia: Elsevier Saunders.

CHAPTER 16

Where Do We Go From Here?

In a time of drastic change, it is the learners who inherit the future.

—Eric Hoffer

Points to Ponder

1. What have you learned by reading this text?
2. What key ethical issues might you face in the future?
3. How can a foundation in ethics-based administration help you to deal with ethics issues in the future?

Words to Remember

The following is a list of key words for this chapter. You will find them in bold in the text. Stop and check your understanding of them.

brain drain
toxic work environment

bully behavior
"what if" plans

■ SUMMARY OF PREVIOUS CHAPTERS

How is ethics important for your future success as a healthcare administrator (HCA)? At this point in your study, you have a basic understanding of the key theorists whose work relates to healthcare administration. From this groundwork, you explored the fundamental principles of ethics that are used by healthcare organizations. This exploration included chapters on autonomy, nonmaleficence, beneficence, and justice, with real-world case studies in each of these areas. You should be able to see that these principles are not just words in books, but areas that can influence administrative decisions and behaviors. These theories and principles were included in Chapters 1 through 4.

Because ethics is not practiced in a vacuum, you investigated potential influences that may affect your application of ethics theory and principles to daily administration decisions in your facility. In Section II, you examined sources of influence from outside the organization. In Chapter 5, you looked at the power and influence of the healthcare industry from the community's viewpoint. You might not have realized that health care is so powerful that the community feels the need to be protected from its power. The community attempts to protect its interests through stringent, but often confusing, regulations and limitations on the scope of professional practice. The chapter also introduced you to the thinking behind some of the major regulatory organizations so that you have a better understanding of their purposes. You were also given insight into your responsibility as guardians of the public's health through your duty to advocate, ensure staff competency, and maintain your own level of currency.

Chapter 6 examined market forces that can greatly influence both ethics temptations and ethical practice. While not every influence could be included in this chapter, it did feature two areas that continue to be of concern. Managed care is an influential force on both the finance and practice of health care. You learned about its history, future issues, and the ethics dilemmas it creates. Integrated medicine was also featured in this chapter as a reflection of the change in consumer attitudes and behaviors. These practices were once regarded as pure quackery, but now are being used and studied by well-known hospital systems. They cannot be ignored but there are certainly ethics issues of autonomy, respect, and competence to consider.

Chapter 7 also discussed external influences. In this case, you examined the healthcare system's role in social responsibility. The problem here is to remain compassionate and still have a viable bottom line. The chapter explored the connections between prevention services and your relationship with public health in your community. It also introduced the idea of quality assurance as both an ethics and a social responsibility issue.

Technology is such an influential external force that it merited its own chapter. It has already influenced the provision of health care and increased the number and complexity of ethics issues you must face. Chapter 8 addressed the current impact of technology on the system, including its cost-benefit. Implications of information technology on clinical, consumer, and business practices were discussed. Emergent technologies such as neuroenhancement and ART were introduced. Through this discussion, you were able to identify some of the critical ethics issues that are linked to the use of technology and how theories and principles of ethics could be used to help HCAs deal with these complex issues. This chapter asked the question, "Just because we can do something, does it mean we should do it?"

Organizations also have a great influence on how administrators behave and make decisions. Because of this influence, Section III introduced ethics-related issues from the viewpoint of healthcare organizations. Financial viability is a primary concern of all these organizations. Chapter 9 provided insight into how healthcare organizations can balance the ethics of finance and the organization's mission. This balance challenge is exacerbated as the demands for quality care increases and budgets to fulfill those requirements decrease. Organizations struggle to avoid ethics temptations to cut corners and overwork staff in order to maintain the bottom line. In addition, business practices that are acceptable in other industries tend to be unethical in the business of health care. For example, if we shut down hospitals to save money, we are often seen as being heartless because we ignore community need and increase its jobless rates.

The culture of your healthcare organization can foster ethical practice or discourage it. No administrators would overtly tell staff to behave unethically, but their actions set the tone for unwritten but understood policies. Chapter 10 stressed the importance of culture on your day-to-day decision-making. You will not only be faced with the impact of the overall organizational culture, but will have to deal with potential clashes between subcultures. The problems of cultural ethics are often resolved by inside committees or outside consultants. As an HCA, you will be involved with these ethics committees. You might also be responsible for hiring an ethicist as a consultant and ensuring that the best possible person is chosen for this role. As an HCA you, too, will be part of your organization's culture, but you also influence it through your actions and leadership role.

Because of its mission, your organization must deal with regulations from external agencies that place stringent requirements on its actions. The nature of the healthcare industry means that it is highly regulated. This means that regulation is part of your life as an HCA. Chapter 11 discussed on of the major regulators of the industry and administration's reaction to their efforts. The chapter also showed that compliance does not always equate to quality. For this reason, the chapter contained an overview of the definitions of quality and the efforts of payers, advocates, and patients to secure it. It also discusses how health care has adapted quality assurance ideas from other industries. The chapter ends with a presentation of the ethics theories and principles that support quality assurance in health care.

Your ethics practice as an HCA must be centered on your raison d'être: the patient. Recently, there has been a call for more patient-centered care from payers, regulators, and the patients themselves. To address this issue, you must ascertain the patients' satisfaction levels regarding their care (Chapter 12). Measuring this experience brings its own set of ethical issues and temptations. Finally, you must be able to implement a more patient-focused model of care in your facility. How will this change influence your practices as an ethics-based manager? What are the costs versus the benefits of making this paradigm shift?

After looking at some of the influences from the organization and the community, you were in a position to examine ethics on a personal level. It is ultimately your choice whether or not you use ethics as part of your daily practice. As you saw in Section IV, it is not always an obvious or easy decision to make. You will be tempted by the shadow side of leadership to use your abilities and power to improve your personal bottom line, often at the expense of the organization. In fact, there are people who would even consider you a "winner" if you took advantage of your position.

The resources mentioned in Chapters 13 and 14 should help you to resist those temptations and remain true to the tenets of your profession and personal moral foundation. Remember that with power comes responsibility. Even if you are not "caught," ultimately you are accountable for your actions. Finally, Chapters 15 and 16 offered some practical advice for practicing as an HCA in the real world of health care. This advice came from both the literature and "practice sense." Chapter 16 offered some insight into issues for your future so that you can maintain ethics vigilance.

The challenges set forth in the text are designed to assist you to practice as an ethics-based HCA, even when it is not expeditious to do so. They ask you to use what you have learned to improve your daily decision-making and practice and provide a workplace where ethics is the norm. You are the future of this industry. The patients, staff, organization, profession, and community will count on you to go beyond compliance to excellence. They will expect you to balance your business acumen with your ethics wisdom. They will expect you to maintain at least an I-YOU ethics relationship in your dealings with patients, professionals, and staff members. They also expect you to maintain currency and competency in your profession through lifelong learning. You will be expected to bring honor to the profession that you have chosen. Yes, much is expected of you, but you are up to the challenge. You are a professional ethics-based HCA.

■ THE FUTURE, OR WHO HID THE CRYSTAL BALL?

As I write this last section of the text, I am reminded of how fast the future can challenge everything. News of economic challenges all over the world seems to cast a pall over people's faith in their future. The healthcare industry is somewhat exempt from these challenges, but we must not ignore them. Recession leads to job loss in the community and loss of healthcare insurance. It also means that the supplies and materials that we use to heal may be more costly or difficult to obtain. We may also become more ethically challenged as we try to balance mission and margin. We cannot ignore the economic challenges of our time.

How do we prepare for the future? What new man-made challenges might we face? Will Mother Nature bring us more floods, hurricanes, fires, or earthquakes? The answer unfortunately is "Yes, we will face challenges of all types and severity." Given the certainty that something will happen, our duty is to be prepared to the best of our abilities. Preparedness will require foresight, a plan for action, and the courage to take that action when it is needed. Remember that your ethics can be challenged during times of great change.

As you can imagine, your challenge alerts will come from many sources. Keep your eyes, ears, and mind open. Remain active in your community and state to keep track of the pulse of change and be ready for it. In this last section, I would like to suggest four future ALERTS for your consideration.

ALERT: Disaster Preparation

The alert for disaster preparation is a logical place to start because we are aware of them. Natural disasters are well covered in the news media. Healthcare facilities must be prepared to provide service during natural disasters such as hurricanes, tornados, and earthquakes. Disasters that are not created by an act of nature must also be addressed by a specific organization. It can be the result of a human-created event such as acts of terrorism, airplane crashes, multidwelling fires, chemical spills, or multiple-victim violence.

When any disaster occurs, the community expects you to provide compassionate care, even when reimbursement is not immediate. During the crisis, you are supposed to put mission first. This cannot happen unless you are proactive and work with **"what if" plans**. There are even computer programs that can assist you to work out logistics and financials for these plans. I suggest that ethics also needs to be part of contingency planning. For example, what is your ethics responsibility to your staff members who must provide the care? Do you have to build into your budget counseling resources? Do you have any ethics responsibility to the community beyond the provision of care? Considering ethics as part of a contingency plan for any disaster can broaden the scope of the plan and assist you to address needs more compassionately, if or when a disaster occurs.

ALERT: Technology Changes

Technology is another area where you must be alert to future changes because it can challenge both your ethics and your bottom line. As you read in Chapter 8, the future holds the potential for some amazing technologic advances, some of which are already being tested. Prominent scientists were polled about the greatest breakthroughs for the next 25 years ("Thinktank," 2005). Many of these scientists cited technologies derived from the human genome project as strong contenders. Diseases and conditions that exist today can be greatly improved or even eliminated through knowledge of their root causes and gene-specific treatments. Can you imagine the business opportunities here? What ethics issues might they create?

This is just one aspect where technology can create great benefits and challenges. Endoscopic surgery, brain mapping, cell replacement therapy, stem cell research, implanted computer systems, and other potential applications are just around the corner. From a business standpoint, executive and physician decision-making computer systems are getting more and more sophisticated. In the future, it might even be considered malpractice if a computer analysis is not part of diagnosis or business decisions. Imagine the ethics discussions around these issues.

How do you prepare for such major change? The key is to stay vigilant. Keep reading both professional and popular sources of information. Attend conferences where technology is featured. Talk about the potential implementation of technology before it is imminent so that you can do an unbiased cost-benefit analysis. In other words, do not get complacent—stay ahead of the technology curve. Remember to consider the ethics ramifications of any technology before you invest your economic and human resources on it. Technology promises much, but challenges even more.

ALERT: The Boomers Are Coming! The Boomers Are Coming!

You cannot overestimate the impact the Baby Boomers will have on healthcare delivery. This generation changed every American institution that it touched, from public schools to the housing industry. As a driver of the consumer and integrated medicine movement, they have already begun to change healthcare delivery. Even more change will occur as they retire and need more services. Will you be ready? What challenges to ethics will they present?

Keep in mind that the Boomers have a different attitude toward health care than previous generations. They are likely to expect quality care (as they define it) and tolerate less inconvenience. They also want to have fair value for their economic investment and be a partner in their own care. You can see that these attitudes will challenge the paternalism of traditional health care, but they can also create new markets for service. The key will be to balance the ethics of what is truly needed with what is desired and profitable. There will also be challenges attached to health care for all of the Boomers and not just for those who are well insured or well funded.

In addition, you will face ethics challenges when the Boomer health professionals reach retirement age. It is feared that there might be a **brain drain**. Sufficient numbers of professionals from the younger generations may not be able to fill the caregiver void. Some hope comes from the Boomers who remain healthy and want to work into their seventies, but the potential shortage must be addressed. You cannot wait until you are in a shortage-based crisis to act. Keep track of the aging of your work force and their intentions for retirement. In addition, establishing policies and practices to make a positive work environment should help attract future employees and decrease your chances of being understaffed as people retire. To be proactive, perhaps you could join in career fairs and events at high schools and colleges. Some healthcare organizations have established affiliations with colleges and universities. By offering internships, guest lecturers, and seminars, the organization can help "grow their own professionals."

ALERT: A New Kind of Workforce

There are several current concerns about the healthcare workforce that promise to affect the future of the industry. The first is the shortage of nurses and other health professionals. According to the American Association of Colleges of Nursing (2008), if there is no change in current practices, there could be a shortage of one million nurses by 2020. The retirement of boomer nurses, insufficient numbers of students in nursing programs, and a lack of qualified nursing faculty will contribute to this shortage. In addition, nurses are leaving the profession because of low job satisfaction, high stress, and increased job availability in nonclinical sectors. Similar patterns emerge for other healthcare professionals. Such shortages have the potential to affect the quality of patient care, patient safety, and the overall image of health care in a negative way.

According to Briles (2009), a **toxic work environment** is one reason why healthcare professionals are leaving the profession for other career opportunities. She conducted a major study of over 3000 health professionals. Abusive behavior or bullying was common in work environments. Most of the **bully behavior** was conducted by managers and most of the manager bullies were female. Despite the significant mission of health care, the environment was filled with discontent employees who sabotaged each other, failed to communicate, and did not act as team players. This kind of environment can only enhance the nursing shortage.

As an HCA, you have to ask, "What do employees want from work?" and "How can I provide this kind of environment?" These are important questions to ask and answer for the future of the healthcare workforce. Increasingly, employees are looking for more than paychecks and bonuses. Even in times of economic distress, work is more than a paycheck. This is especially true given the nature of work in a healthcare setting. Money alone cannot motivate people to go the extra mile when patients are difficult or when the situation is traumatic. There needs to be an internal motivation that keeps the employee caring even when caring is difficult.

Pierce (2001) suggests that employees are seeking a spiritual connection to their work. This means that work has to have meaning and purpose and a connection to something higher. They are seeking a sense of community and support. They also want to balance work and family so that life is enhanced. Freeman and Morrison (2009) note that spirituality at work includes the ability to use creativity, compassion, integrity, and stewardship to make a difference in the lives of others. For some, work in health care is not a job; it is a true calling. They are seeking an environment that respects them as a whole human being and offers an opportunity to fulfill their potential.

Spirituality at work is also connected to what Pink (2006) has defined as the next age of our society. He thinks that we are entering an age where so-called right brained (innovative) people will be critical to success no matter what the business. He calls this the Conceptual Age (p. 3). In order to be a valued employee in this new workforce, you would need the ability to design new products, communicate effectively, synthesize ideas, function with logic and empathy, and play. In addition, he stresses that work must have meaning and purpose. Pink (2006) presents ways to find that meaning through expressing gratitude, clarifying why you work, and identifying your spiritual needs. Just as movies and books are dedicated to someone or something, he also asks you to dedicate your work each day to someone who is important to you.

What is the ethics connection? Think about the four principles of ethics. How do they relate to the needs of the new workforce? First, there is autonomy. Respecting the individuality of your employees means that you must respect them as whole human beings. You cannot ignore their spiritual need for meaning and purpose in their work. From a practical standpoint, if staff members do not feel connected to the larger purpose of your organization, then it would be easy for them to be disloyal or give poor patient care. After all, it would be just a job.

Nonmaleficence and beneficence are strongly connected to the workplace that will attract your future workforce. First, you have a legal and ethical obligation to provide a workplace that is safe physically and emotionally. This includes an awareness of the potential of bullying and establishing a no-tolerance policy toward it. On the positive side, you can use your words and actions to feed employees' spirits through true appreciation for the work that they do. Your ability to lead with justice also will appeal to the workforce of the future. They will expect to be treated with fairness and respect as they participate in the provision of quality patient care. Remember that the competition for well-qualified staff members will be high. An environment that is both welcoming and respectful will go a long way toward hiring and retaining those valuable employees.

Lastly, you should never ignore your own spiritual connection to your work. Sometimes, HCAs feel that they are less valued because they do not provide direct patient care. However, you need to consider yourself the foundation of that care. After all, if you do your work correctly, patient care is supported and made possible. For example, the lights will be turned on, the supplies in place, the records maintained, and the staff members paid. In addition, you will need to renew your own spirit by working toward balance between life and work, practicing self-assessment, and engaging in life-long learning. Always remember that you are the role model for the employee behavior that you seek.

Final Summary

Writing the new edition of this textbook has challenged my thinking about ethics as it applies to healthcare administration, I hope this book has also challenged your thinking and made you more aware of ethics in the practice of health administration. I also hope that you will have the courage to use what you have learned to become an ethics-based administrator and to create an environment where ethics is a normal part of practice. By making this choice, you will honor your profession, organization, community, and yourself. I wish you all the best in your career and your life as an HCA.

Web Resources

Office of the Inspector General
http://oig.hhs.gov/

Sample Disaster Plans
http://dhfs.wisconsin.gov/rl_DSL/Providers/SamplEmergPlans.htm

References

American Association of Colleges of Nursing. (2008). *Nursing short-age fact sheet.* Available at: http://www.aacn.nche.edu/Media/pdf/ NrsgShortageFS.pdf. Accessed March 19, 2009.

Briles, J. (2009). *Stabotage! How to deal with the pit bulls, skunks, snakes, scorpions & slugs in the health care workplace.* Aurora, CO: Mile High Press.

Freeman, D., & Morrison, E. E. (2009). Spirituality and ethics in healthcare organizations. In E. E. Morrison (Ed.). *Health Care Ethics: Critical Issues for the 21st Century* (2nd ed.). Sudbury, MA: Jones and Bartlett, pp. 321–336

Pierce, G. F. A. (2001). *Spirituality at work: 10 ways to balance your life on the job*. Chicago: Loyola Press.

Pink, D. H. (2006). *A whole new mind: Why right-brainers will rule the future*. New York: Penguin Group, Inc.

"Thinktank." (2005, February). *Discover*, 24(2), 66–70.

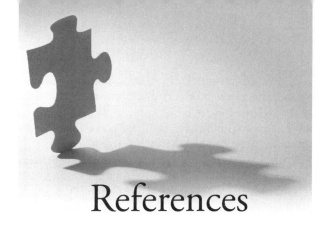

References

Adams, G. B., & Balfour, D. L. (1998). *Unmasking administrative evil.* Thousand Oaks, CA: Sage.

Adams, P. (1993). *Gesundheit!* Rochester, VT: Healing Arts Press.

Agency for Healthcare Research and Quality. (2008). *AHRQ profile: Quality research for quality healthcare.* Rockville, MD: Author.

American Association of Colleges of Nursing. (2008). *Nursing shortage fact sheet.* Available at: http://www.aacn.nche.edu/Media/pdf/NrsgShortageFS.pdf. Accessed March 19, 2009.

American College of Healthcare Executives. (2005). *Policy statement: Ethical issues related to a reduction in force.* [Electronic version]. Chicago: Author.

American College of Healthcare Executives. (2007a). *American College of Healthcare Executives code of ethics.* [Electronic version]. Chicago: Author.

American College of Healthcare Executives. (2007b). *Ethical decision making for healthcare executives.* [Electronic version]. Chicago: Author.

American College of Healthcare Executives. (2009). *ACHE healthcare executive competency assessment tool 2009.* Chicago: Author.

American Hospital Association. (2003). *The patient care partnership: Understanding expectations, rights, and responsibilities* [Brochure]. Chicago: Author.

American Medical Association. (2008). *Health information technology.* Available at: http://www.ama-assn.org/ama/pub/category/16195.html. Accessed November 28, 2008.

American Nurses Association. (2005). *Code of ethics for nurses.* Available at: http://www.nursingworld.org/. Accessed February 15, 2009.

Anderlik, M. R. (2001). *The ethics of managed care: A pragmatic approach.* Bloomington, IN: Indiana University Press.

Annison, M. H., & Wilford, D. S. (1998). *Trust matters: New directions for health care leadership.* San Francisco: Jossey-Bass.

Ashcroft, R. E., Dawson, A., Draper, H., & McMillan, J. R. (2007). *Principles of health care ethics.* West Sussex, UK: John Wiley & Sons, Ltd.

Barton, G. M., & Morrison, E. E. (2006, January/February). What happens when harassment is personal? *Journal of Medical Practice Management*, 21(4): 1–4.

Beauchamp, T. L., & Childress, J. E. (2008). *Principles of biomedical ethics* (6th ed.). New York: Oxford University Press.

Block, P. (1996). *Stewardship: Choosing service over self-interest.* San Francisco: Berrett-Koehler.

Boyle, P. J., Dubose, E. R., Ellingson, S. J., Guinn, D. E., & McCurdy, D. B. (2001). *Organizational ethics in health care: Principles, cases and practical solutions.* San Francisco: Jossey-Bass.

Briles, J. (2009). *Stabotage! How to deal with the pit bulls, skunks, snakes, scorpions & slugs in the health care workplace.* Aurora, CO: Mile High Press.

Brinkman, R., & Kirschner, R. (1994). *Dealing with people you can't stand: How to bring out the best in people at their worst.* New York: McGraw-Hill.

Brooks, R. G., & Menachemi, N. (2006). Physicians' use of email with patients: Factors influencing electronic communication and adherence to best practices. *Journal of Medical Internet Research*, 8(1), e2. Available at: http://www.jmir.org/2006/1/e2/. Accessed May 19, 2009.

Buber, M. (1996). *I and thou.* New York: Touchstone.

Budinger, T. F., & Budinger, M. D. (2006). *Ethics of emerging technologies: Scientific facts and moral challenges.* Hoboken, NJ: John Wiley & Sons, Inc.

Cahn, S. M., & Markie, P. (1998). *Ethics: History, theory, and contemporary issues.* New York: Oxford University Press.

Caplan, A. L. (Ed.). (1992). *When medicine went mad: Bioethics and the holocaust.* Totowa, NJ: Humana.

Center for the Study of Ethics in the Professions. (2008). *Codes of ethics online.* Chicago: Illinois Institute of Technology.

Cisco Systems, Inc. (2008). *Collaberation.* Available at: http://www.cisco.com/en/US/netsol/ns870/index.html. Accessed November 30, 2008.

Coddington, D. C., Fischer, E. A., Moore, K. D., & Clarke, R. L. (2000). *Beyond managed care: How consumers and technology are changing the future of health care.* San Francisco: Jossey-Bass.

Collis, J. W. (1998). *The seven fatal management sins: Understanding and avoiding managerial malpractice.* Boca Raton, FL: St. Lucia Press.

Cottone, R. R., & Travydas, V. M. (2003). *Ethical and professional issues in counseling* (2nd ed.). Upper Saddle River, NJ: Pearson Education.

Covey, S. M. R. (2006). *The speed of trust: The one thing that changes everything.* New York: Free Press.

Covey, S. R. (1989). *The 7 habits of highly effective people.* New York: Simon & Schuster.

Covey, S. R. (1992). *Principle centered leadership.* New York: Free Press.

Crichton, M. (2006). *Next.* New York: HarperCollins.

Daft, R. L. (2006). *Organizational theory and design* (9th ed.). Cincinnati, OH: South-Western.

Darr, K. (2005). *Ethics in health services management* (4th ed.). Baltimore: Health Professions Press.

Dickens, C. (1997). *A tale of two cities.* Mineola, NY: Dover Publications.

Dosick, R. W. (2000). *The business bible: Ten commandments for creating an ethical workplace.* Woodstock, VT: Jewish Light Publishing.

Dunn, R. (2006). *Haimann's healthcare management* (8th ed.). Chicago: Health Administration Press.

Dye, C. F. (2000). *Leadership in healthcare: Values at the top.* Chicago: Health Administration Press.

Eisenberg, D. M., Kessler, R. C., Foster, F. C., Norlock, F. E., Calkins, D. R., & Delbanco, T. L. (1993). Unconventional medicine in the United States. *New England Journal of Medicine, 328,* 246–252.

Eisenberg, D. M., Davis, R. B., Ettnes, S. L., Appel, S., Wilkey, S., Van Rompay, M. V., & Kessler, R. C. (1998). Trends in alternative medicine use in the United States, 1990–1997. *JAMA, 280,* 1569–1575.

Epstein, R. A. (2007). Conflicts of interest in health care: Who guards the guardians? *Perspectives in Biology and Medicine, 50*(1), 72–89.

Erikson, S., Höglund, A. T., & Helgesson, G. (2008). Do ethical guidelines give guidance? A critical examination of eight ethics regulations. *Cambridge Quarterly of Healthcare Ethics, 17*(1), 15–30.

Ethics Resource Center. (2004). *PLUS—A process for ethics decision making* [Electronic Version]. Washington, DC: Author.

Faass, N. (2001). *Integrating complementary medicine into health systems.* Gaithersburg, MD: Aspen.

Fitzpatrick, M. A. (2003, April). The JOINT is jumpin! [Electronic version]. *Nursing Management, 34*(4), 4.

Fottler, M. D., Hernandez, S. R., & Joiner, C. L. (1997). *Strategic management of human resources in health services organizations* (2nd ed.). Albany, NY: Delmar.

Frampton, S. B., & Charmel, P. A. (2009). *Putting patients first: Best practices in patient-centered care* (2nd ed.). San Francisco: Jossey-Bass.

Frankl, V. (1971). *Man's search for meaning: An introduction to logotherapy.* New York: Pocket Books.

Freeman, D., & Morrison, E. E. (2009). Spirituality and ethics in healthcare organizations. In E. E. Morrison (Ed.). *Health Care Ethics: Critical Issues for the 21st Century* (2nd ed.). Sudbury, MA: Jones and Bartlett, pp. 321–336.

Gastmans, C. (Ed.). (2002). *Between technology and humanity: The impact of technology on health care ethics.* Belgium: Leuven University Press.

Gilbert, J. A. (2007). *Strengthening ethical wisdom: Tools for transforming your health care organization*. Chicago: Health Administration Press.

Glandon, G. L., Smaltz, D. H., & Slovensky, D. J. (2008). *Austin and Boxerman's information systems for healthcare management* (7th ed.). Chicago: Health Administration Press/AUPHA.

Graber, G. C. (2009). The moral status of gametes and embryos: Storage and surrogacy. In E. E. Morrison (Ed.). *Health care ethics: Critical issues for the 21st century*. Sudbury, MA: Jones and Bartlett, pp. 61–70.

Greenspan, B. J. (2004, May/June). Certifying financials. *Healthcare Executive*, 19(3), 42.

Griffith, J. R. (1993). *The moral challenges of health care management*. Ann Arbor, MI: Health Professions Press.

Harvey, J. B. (1998). *The Abilene paradox*. San Francisco: Jossey-Bass.

Harvey, J. B. (1999). *How come every time I get stabbed in the back my fingerprints are on the knife? And other meditations on management*. San Francisco: Jossey-Bass.

Health Enhancement Systems. (2007). *Keeping healthy people healthy: A business case*. Midland, MI: Author.

Hemsath, D., & Yerkes, L. (1997). *301 ways to have fun at work*. San Francisco: Berrett-Koehler.

Hofmann, P. B. (2006). Evaluating ethical fitness. *Healthcare Executive*, 21(3), 34–35.

Hoffman, P. B., & Nelson, W. A. (Eds.). (2001). *Managing ethically: An executive's guide*. Chicago: Health Administration Press.

Holland, S. (2007). *Public health ethics*. Malden, MA: Polity Press.

Hoover, J. (2004). *How to work for an idiot: Survive and thrive without killing your boss*. Franklin Lakes, NJ: Career Press.

Institute for the Future. (2003). *Health & health care 2010: The forecast, the challenge* (2nd ed.). San Francisco: Jossey-Bass.

Institute of Medicine. (2001). *Crossing the quality chasm: A new health system for the 21st century*. Washington, DC: National Academy Press.

Institutes for Healthcare Improvement. (2009). *20/20 vision: 2009 progress report*. Cambridge, MA: Author.

Johnson, C. E. (2009). *Meeting the ethical challenges of leadership: Casting light or shadow* (3rd ed.). Thousand Oaks, CA: Sage.

Joint Commission on Accreditation of Health Care Organizations. (2008). *History tracking report: 2008 to 2009 requirements accreditation program: Hospital chapter: Ethics, right, and responsibilities*. Available at http://jointcommission.org/NR/rdonlyres/8C588. Accessed November 3, 2008.

Joint Commission on Accreditation of Healthcare Organizations. (2008a). *A journey through the history of the Joint Commission*.

Available at: http://www.jointcommission.org/AboutUs/joint_commission_history.htm. Accessed January 19, 2009.

Joint Commission on Accreditation of Healthcare Organizations. (2008b). *The Joint Commission*. Available at: http://www.jointcommission.org/. Accessed January 19, 2009.

Kalina, K., Pew, S., & Bourgeois, D. (2004). *Don't go there alone! A guide to hospitals for patients and their advocates*. Kansas City, MO: 33-44-55 Publishing.

Kohlberg, L. (1984). *The philosophy of moral development: Moral stages and the idea of justice*. New York: HarperCollins.

Kubler-Ross, E. (1997). *On death and dying*. New York: Scribner.

Leapfrog Group. (2008). *Fact sheet*. Available at: http://www.leapfroggroup.org. Accessed November 26, 2008.

Leebov, W. (2008). *Wendy Leebov's great patient experiences: No nonsense solutions with gratifying results*. Chicago: Health Forum Inc.

Lee, F. (2004). *If Disney ran your hospital: 9 1/2 things you would do differently*. Bozeman, MT: Second River Healthcare Press.

May, E. L. (2004, May/June). Managing the revenue cycle: Success factors from the field. *Healthcare Executive*, 19(3), 10–16, 18.

McChance, D. (2004). *Medusa's ear: University foundings from Kant to Chorla L.* Albany, NY: SUNY Press.

McGinn, P. (2005). *Leading others, managing yourself*. Chicago: Health Administration Press.

McKeon, R. (Ed.). (1971). *The basic works of Aristotle*. New York: Random House.

McNamara, C. (2008). *Complete guide to ethics management: An ethic toolkit for managers*. Available at the Authenticity Consulting Web site: http://www.managementhelp.org/ethics/ethxgde.htm. Accessed December 26, 2008.

Micozzi, M. S. (2005). *Fundamentals of complementary and alternative medicine* (3rd ed.). New York: Churchill Livingstone.

Monagle, J. F., & West, M. P. (2009). Hospital ethics committees: Roles, memberships, structure, and difficulties. In Morrison, E. E. (Ed.). *Health care ethics: Critical issues for the 21st Century* (2nd ed.). Sudbury, MA: Jones and Bartlett, pp. 251–266.

Moore, J. (2009). Ethically important distinctions among managed care organizations. In Morrison, E. E. (Ed.). *Health care ethics: Critical issues for the 21st century*. Sudbury, MA: Jones and Bartlett, pp. 267–282.

Morrison, I. (2000). *Health care in the new millennium: Vision, values, and leadership*. San Francisco: Jossey-Bass.

National Center for Complementary and Alternative Medicine. (2008). *Health information*. Available at: http://nccam.nih.gov/. Accessed November 16, 2008.

National Certification Commission for Acupuncture and Oriental Medicine. (2008). *Code of ethics.* Available at: http://www.nccaom.org/. Accessed February 15, 2009.

National Committee for Quality Assurance. (2008). *About NCQA.* Available at: http://www.ncqa.org/tabid/675/Default.aspx. Accessed November 3, 2008.

Nelson, W. A. (2005). An organizational ethics decision-making process. *Healthcare Executive,* 20(4), 8–14.

Nowicki, M. (2007). *The financial management of hospital and healthcare organizations* (4th ed.). Chicago: Health Administration Press.

Office of Civil Rights. (2008). *Understanding HIPPA privacy.* Available at: http://www.hhs.gov/ocr/privacy/hipaa/understanding/index.html. Accessed May 16, 2009.

Orlikoff, J. E., & Totten, M. K. (2007). Stewardship in action. *Healthcare Executive,* 22(5), 56–59.

Palmer, P. J. (2000). *Let your life speak.* San Francisco: Jossey-Bass.

Pearson, S. D., Sabin, J. E., & Emanuel, E. J. (2003). *No margin, no mission: Health-care organizations and the quest for ethical excellence.* New York: Oxford University Press.

Perry, F. (2002). *The tracks we leave: Ethics in healthcare management.* Chicago: Health Administration Press.

Pierce, G. F. A. (2001). *Spirituality at work: 10 ways to balance your life on the job.* Chicago: Loyola Press.

Pink, D. H. (2006). *A whole new mind: Why right-brainers will rule the future.* New York: Penguin Group, Inc.

Press, I. (2002). *Patient satisfaction: Defining, measuring, and improving the experience of care.* Chicago: Health Administration Press.

Purtilo, R. B., & Criss, M. L. (2005). *Ethical dimensions in the health professions* (4th ed.). Philadelphia: Elsevier Saunders.

Ransom, E. R., Joshi, M. S., Nash, D. B., & Ransom, S. B. (Eds.). (2008). *The healthcare quality book* (2nd ed.). Chicago: Health Administration Press.

Roberti, R. (2008). Frequently asked questions. *Radio Frequency Identification Journal.* Available at: http://www.rfidjournal.com/faq. Accessed November 30, 2008.

Roth, W., & Taleff, P. (2002). Health care standards: The good, bad, and ugly in our future [Electronic version]. *Journal of Quality and Participation,* 25(2), 40–45.

Shi, L., & Singh, D. A. (2008). *Delivering health care in America: A systems approach* (4th ed.). Sudbury, MA: Jones and Bartlett.

Shortell, S. M., Gillies, R. R., Anderson, D. A., Erickson, K. M., & Mitchell, J. B. (2000). *Remaking health care in America: The evolution of organized delivery systems* (2nd ed.). San Francisco: Jossey-Bass.

Squazzo, J. D. (2008). Ethics and excellence: The making of a profession's values, standards. *Healthcare Executive*, 23(2), 30–33. Available at: ABI/INFORM Global database. (Document ID: 14459954410). Accessed February 15, 2009.

Summers, J. (2009). Theory of healthcare ethics. In E. E. Morrison (Ed.). *Health care ethics: Critical issues for the 21st century*. Sudbury, MA: Jones and Bartlett, pp. 3–40.

Swayne, L. E., Duncan, J., & Ginter, P. M. (2006). *Strategic management of health care organizations* (5th ed.). Malden, MA: Blackwell.

Tapping, D. (2008). *The simply Lean pocket guide*. Chelsea, MI: MCS Media, Inc.

"Thinktank." (2005, February). *Discover*, 24(2), 66–70.

Tong, R. (2007). *New perspectives in healthcare ethics: An interdisciplinary and crosscultural approach*. Upper Saddle River, NJ: Prentice Hall.

Tulchinshky, T. H., & Varavikova, E. A. (2000). *The new public health: An introduction for the 21st century*. San Diego, CA: Academic Press.

Turnock, B. J. (2004). *Public health* (2nd ed.). Sudbury, MA: Jones and Bartlett.

Worthley, J. A. (1997). *The ethics of the ordinary in healthcare: Concepts and cases*. Chicago: Health Administration Press.

Worthley, J. A. (1999). *Organizational ethics in the compliance context*. Chicago: Health Administration Press.

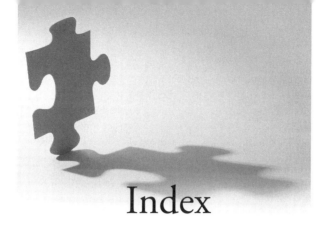

Index